Praise for *The Little Black Book of Violence* . . .

"Kane and Wilder's *Little Black Book of Violence* will save liv prison. Their insightful and informative text is an invaluable resou.... ioi anyone who follows the warrior's path and deals with violence, or who is interested in this life or death topic.

The hard-won wisdom of the two authors, combined with research, quotes, and passages from others, provide a guidebook on why and how to avoid violence, what to do when it cannot be avoided, and how to survive the physical and legal aftermath that follows most violent encounters.

Do yourself a favor. Answer all of the questions in Appendix A – "How Far Am I Willing to Go?" Then read this book in its entirety. Answer the questions again, and take the time to think seriously about your answers. Sure, there are many of them, but this mental exercise could very well make the difference in your surviving and staying free versus ending up behind bars or becoming a statistic due to a violent encounter. Violence has consequences, many of them permanent. This *Little Black Book* will help you understand them and, more importantly, avoid the worst of them.

As an attorney, a self-defense instructor, and someone who has experienced violence, I was most impressed with the practical and realistic information Kane and Wilder provide in their *Little Black Book*. This is a must read for anyone who deals with violence, anyone who thinks he may encounter violence, or anyone who wants to increase his knowledge regarding avoiding, confronting, and surviving the aftermath of violent encounters. I commend both Kane and Wilder for providing this much-needed resource. Thank you gentlemen. You have just saved lives.

> — **Alain Burrese, J.D.,** former U.S. Army 2nd Infantry Division Scout Sniper School instructor and author of *Hard-Won Wisdom From the School of Hard Knocks*, and the DVDs *Hapkido Hoshinsul, Streetfighting Essentials, Hapkido Cane,* and the *Lock On* series.

Kane and Wilder's *Little Black Book of Violence* is a well thought out and detailed book of tactical thinking. Reminiscent of Musashi's *Book of Five Rings*, *Little Black Book of Violence* gives the reader insight way beyond punching and kicking back. Elements of psychology, street smarts, and martial strategy make this book worthy of inclusion in everyone's library. Well done and comprehensive.

> — **Kancho John Roseberry**, three-time All Services Judo Champion, seven-time All Marine Judo Champion, 10th *dan* Goju Ryu karate, 7th *dan* judo, 3rd *dan* aikido, (honorary) 5th *dan* Daito Ryu Aikijujutsu.

Every parent of an adolescent should read this. We need to be reminded sometimes of how certain we were at that age, and how little we really knew. It takes a well-adjusted grownup to put things in perspective for our kids without losing it and shutting down all communication. As the mother of an adolescent son, I know what a challenge that can be.

Kane and Wilder succeed in this; they slow us down and point us in the right direction. Fitted out with insight, we can help our kids through inevitable assaults on their egos, and they can strategize without violence. The sooner a they learn to choose their battles, and use wits instead of fists, the better off they'll be. This book is like a deep breath and counting to 10; it gives parents and kids the time to tell the difference.

— **Julie Van Dielen**, Producer, Law Enforcement Training for *In the Line of Duty.*

Wow. I loved this book! Authors Wilder and Kane continue to specialize in bringing to light areas of martial arts that have little or ever been discussed.

Through *The Little Black Book of Violence: What Every Young Man Needs to Know about Fighting*, Wilder and Kane have written a very important, critically timed, and far-reaching treatise on the subject of reality-based martial violence. Writing their text as a field guide to violence and violent encounters, the authors lend their knowledge and expertise to show both the "how's" and the "why's" of violent encounters that occur including the aftermath, and probably most important, the necessary steps to take to avoid them. Recognizing that no one truly "wins" in a violent encounter incident, Wilder and Kane offer tips and solutions to the reader to ensure safe passage if the situation should arise.

Drawing from multiple sources, perspectives, and personal reflections from actual martial combatants, the true flavor of down and dirty fighting is captured and revealed to the audience at large. Dispelled are the glorious myths and glamorized dramatization of "man-to-man" combative violence. The aftermath of the fight is laid bare as it really exists. The reader is left to experience the blood, injuries, guilt, regret, and post-traumatic stress that sometimes plague the individual combatant involved.

This book was relevant to my own experiences having conducted hundreds of traffic, summary, misdemeanor, and felony arrests over the course of a fifteen-year police career. During that time I often was required to "lay hands" on those arrestees and bring them into custody. The times I recall most vividly were those where I was fighting, grappling, and attempting to subdue my subject opponent. Those real-life incidents were engaged in with pure adrenalin where I fought to protect myself and to fulfill my duty, knowing there was no margin for error. At times, after the arrest, I would find myself with cuts, scrapes, and holes ripped in my uniform or my badge and other accoutrements pulled off and missing. However, I still considered myself fortunate to have survived all of those years without serious injury. Why are these statements important to you then, the potential reader? They are a testament to the powerful truthfulness, veracity, and accuracy of the knowledge and advice contained in this book. In my opinion, this book is as relevant to any police officer, soldier, or martial artist as it is to any student of criminal justice or psychology.

In my opinion, this wonderful book fills a necessary void of knowledge in the realm of martial science. I rate it at five out of five stars. Bravo!

— **Jeffrey-Peter A.M. Hauck, J.D.**, Entrepreneur, Professional Consultant and Trainer, Former U.S. Army 82nd Airborne Infantry Pathfinder, Martial Arts Instructor, retired Municipal Police Sergeant, and co-author of *Ports and Happy Havens.*

The Little Black Book of Violence is a hip, easy-to-read manual on how to identify potentially violent situations and avoid them. Or, failing that, how to best deal effectively with violence should one be forced to do so. Everyone with a pulse should read this book, but it's a must read for teenaged boys, who aren't likely to get this kind of a tutorial at home or school.

> — **William C. Dietz**, bestselling author of more than thirty science fiction novels and thrillers including *Halo: The Flood*, and *Hitman: Enemy Within*.

Lawrence Kane and Kris Wilder have written a comprehensive book about violence, more specifically, how to recognize situations where violence might occur and how to deal with those situations should one be unable to avoid them. Sometimes it is prudent to fight, other times less so. For example, when faced with a threat to one's life, and verbal defense has proven insufficient, one might be forced to resort to physical battle. However, if the situation involves only an attempt to avoid losing face, one might be wise to remember that physical battle, with or without weapons, is seldom as glorious as one might have imagined. While you are thinking "fight," your adversary may well be thinking "combat," with the intent to permanently maim or kill. There will be blood and injuries, some severe, even in situations that do not involve a weapon.

The Little Black Book of Violence: What Every Young Man Needs to Know about Fighting raises a number of excellent questions that one should ask in order to learn about self. It teaches one how to examine a potentially violent situation with a critical eye, how to use the indicators (such as the "tell") to discern when violence is imminent, and how to ensure that one's message is heard when emotions are running hot. Having an understanding of the process that leads to a violent situation will fuel one's confidence and, at least partially, help lift the "fog" of battle.

Young men have their heroes and their dreams. Kane and Wilder, through their knowledge of fighting and their ability to use the written word supported by graphic images and real-life stories, have managed to present a very cool yet frightening perspective on violence, a book where the dreams of heroism and adventure are acted upon with proper forethought and intellect.

> — **Martina Sprague,** martial arts instructor and author of seven books on martial arts and two books on history.

Although I've been training in the fighting arts for over four decades, I found this book to be rich with innovative ways to apply techniques, insightful observations on self-defense, and a mother lode of gold nuggets on the nature of violence and how not to be its next victim. The dynamic writing team of Kane and Wilder just gets better and better with each new book. While martial arts schools show you how to kick and punch, *The Little Black Book* fills in crucial information about street survival that most instructors don't teach or even know.

> — **Loren W. Christensen,** 8th *dan* black belt, author of 38 books on the fighting arts including *Warriors, Defensive Tactics, On Combat,* and *Fighter's Fact Book.*

Today we live in a society replete with criminal, professional, and recreational violence. Beyond mere acceptance, a culture of violence is being nurtured by the portrayal of brutality, cruelty, and aggressive behavior in movies and on TV, by its simulation in video games, and by access via Internet that can provide the worst acts of inhumanity that the world has to offer 24/7.

As a result, our society has raised an entire generation of youth who are desensitized to most forms of violence. Whereas our government has dictated that our public schools are responsible for educating our teens on the subject of sexuality, there is little to be found in any educational program to address the avoidance, prevention, or protection from violence. Maybe it is in this new world order that books like *The Little Black Book of Violence* can provide some semblance of rational thought.

This book is an important work that all youth of any post-elementary school age should read or at least should have portions read to them (with the caution that the graphic nature of some of the words and illustrations could be overwhelming to some adolescents). I was hooked from the first 15 words in the Prologue all the way through Appendix E. I suggest you read it, re-read it, memorize some of the more basic "rules," and keep the book handy. Unlike most books, the appendices are interesting and valuable material; I recommend studying them first. In the appendix describing vital area targets, you will be amazed at how many descriptions of a blow to one of these areas end in the phrase "paralysis or death." I'm sure most "non-violent" types that might find themselves in some kind of violent encounter will be busy trying to protect their genitals without giving much concern to the other 39 areas, and this could be very unfortunate.

Pain is about the only thing left to the imagination today. This book tries to help the reader "visualize" pain. I like to call this book *Scared Smart* or at least *Scared Thoughtful*. As a minimum, after reading this book you will learn to be more observant and more aware of the potential for violence and certainly more knowledgeable about the possible physical and financial consequences of a violent encounter. Whatever the circumstances, this book will help you spot potentially violent situations, find your way around them, or give you the best chance at surviving them. Don't wait for the movie!

> — **Michael F. Murphy**, School Board Director, Bellevue, WA School District.

Great book! A must read for any man or woman who is interested in learning not only how to defend oneself, but how to read other people's aggressions and understand both the mental and physical aspects of violence.

> — **Staff Sgt. Bryan Hopkins**, USMC, 1999 Armed Forces Judo Champion, US Marine Corps Martial Arts Instructor.

The Little Black Book of Violence is an exceptionally modest title for a volume so comprehensive. Dividing their subject sensibly enough into before, during, and after, Kane and Wilder use quotes, anecdotes, and expert commentary to shine an unflinching light on the realities of violence, with a focus on what can be done to avoid it, or when avoidance is impractical or impossible, to prevail. Despite the complexity of the subject matter and the comprehensiveness of their approach, Kane and Wilder maintain an engaging, readable, and occasionally humorous style that makes the book not just incredibly useful, but hard to put down, as well. It was a privilege to get a sneak peek at this fine book and I have no doubt it'll do for many others what it's done for me—help me live more sensibly, more sanely, and more safely.

> — **Barry Eisler**, internationally bestselling author of the John Rain series, *shodan* in *Kodokan* judo.

The **Little Black Book** *of*

VIOLENCE

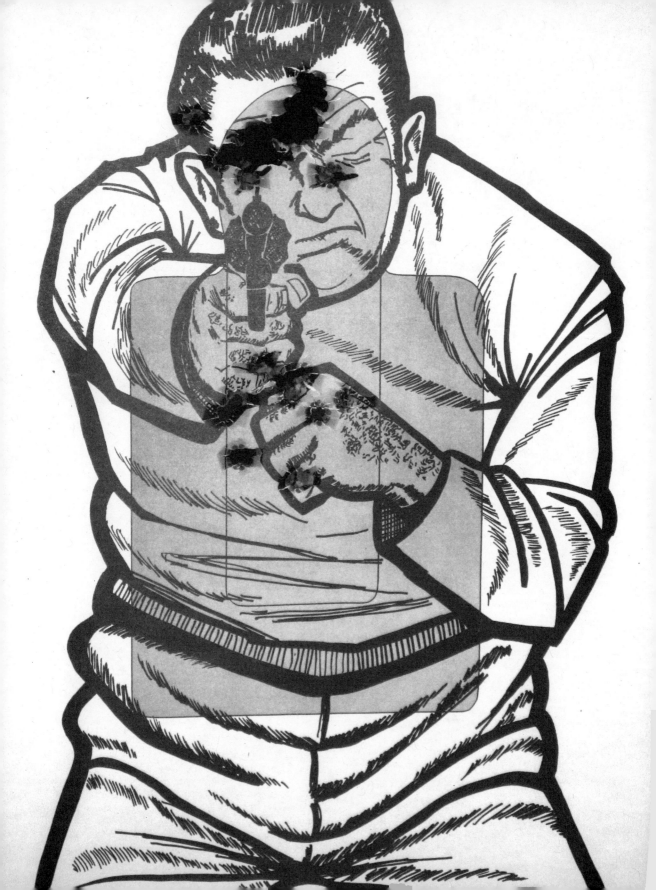

The Little Black Book *of* VIOLENCE

What *Every* Young Man Needs to Know about *Fighting*

Lawrence A. Kane and Kris Wilder

YMAA Publication Center
Wolfeboro, N.H., USA

YMAA Publication Center
Main Office: PO Box 480
Wolfeboro, NH 03894
1-800-669-8892 • www.ymaa.com • ymaa@aol.com

ISBN-13: 978-1-59439-129-3
ISBN-10: 1-59439-129-7

Cover design by Richard Rossiter
Edited by Susan Bullowa

10 9 8 7 6 5 4

Publisher's Cataloging in Publication

Kane, Lawrence A. (Lawrence Alan)

The little black book of violence : what every young man needs to
know about fighting / Lawrence A. Kane and Kris Wilder. --
Wolfeboro, N.H. : YMAA Publication Center, c2009.

    p. ; cm.

    ISBN: 978-1-59439-129-3
    Includes bibliographical references and index.

    1. Violence--Prevention--Handbooks, manuals, etc. 2. Assault
and battery--Prevention--Handbooks, manuals, etc. 3. Self-
defense--Handbooks, manuals, etc. 4. Young men--Conduct of life.
I. Wilder, Kris. II. Title.

GV1111 .K275 2009
613.6/6--dc22   0904

Warning: While self-defense is legal, fighting is illegal. If you don't know the difference you'll go to jail because you aren't defending yourself; you are fighting—or worse. Readers are encouraged to be aware of all appropriate local and national laws relating to self-defense, reasonable force, and the use of weaponry, and act in accordance with all applicable laws at all times. Understand that while legal definitions and interpretations are generally uniform, there are small—but very important—differences from state to state. To stay out of jail, you need to know these differences. Neither the authors nor the publisher assumes any responsibility for the use or misuse of information contained in this book.

    Nothing in this document constitutes a legal opinion nor should any of its contents be treated as such. While the authors believe that everything herein is accurate, any questions regarding specific self-defense situations, legal liability, and/or interpretation of federal, state, or local laws should always be addressed by an attorney at law. This text relies on public news sources to gather information on various crimes and criminals described herein. While news reports of such incidents are generally accurate, they are on occasion incomplete or incorrect. Consequently, all suspects should be considered innocent until proven guilty in a court of law.

    When it comes to martial arts, self-defense, and related topics, no text, no matter how well written, can substitute for professional, hands-on instruction. These materials should be used **for academic study only.**

Printed in Canada.

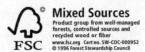

Mixed Sources
Product group from well-managed forests, controlled sources and recycled wood or fiber
www.fsc.org Cert no. SW-COC-000952
© 1996 Forest Stewardship Council
FSC

Dedication

This book is dedicated to those who understand that their life focus should be on something greater than themselves. Those with such understanding rarely find resolution in fighting.

Table of Contents

Prologue

"When I felt the knife blade grate across my teeth, I knew I was in trouble, and then my lower lip fell open like overcooked chicken dropping from the bone."

At eighteen, I found myself outside an all-ages pool hall in Redmond, Washington. If Redmond sounds familiar to you, it should; it is the home of Microsoft corporate headquarters, the home of programmers, computer geeks, and ninety-eight pound nerds. I was standing in the heart of suburbia bleeding badly from my face. The three men who jumped me outside the pool hall started hitting me hard, driving me onto the ground that was more dirt than gravel. I tried to fight but they had got the first strike in, a slash with a knife that was designed to shock, disfigure, and terrify me. It worked.

What brought me some thirty miles from my home to fight in the parking lot of a pool hall? My buddy's name was on the line. He was losing face so I decided that I needed to defend him. It was a matter of friendship, of honor. So, in my senior year of high school, five close friends and I cut the deal for a fight—five on five at the appointed pool hall—and just to add drama, we were going to do it at midnight.

I got there early to hang out with my buddies and amp ourselves up for the confrontation. It was maybe a quarter to midnight when I stepped outside for a smoke. One of the three guys hanging around near the door gave me a hard look and then spat out, "Wadda you looking at?" "Nothing," I replied and turned to go back inside. I heard one of them move and looked back to see what was going on when I was met by a knife slash across my face, striking my teeth and making my mouth an "X" instead of the nice, straight line my momma gave me. When I felt that blade grate across my teeth, I knew I was in trouble, and then my lower lip fell open like overcooked chicken dropping from the bone.

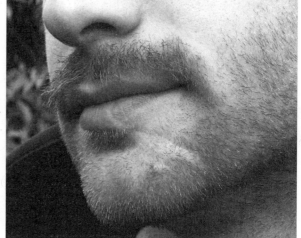

This wasn't the glorious battle I'd imagined. It was pain and blood and terror. What would the victor get from this fight? Absolutely nothing! No turf, no money, nothing, save perhaps a little pride. And the loser? I wound up with eighty stitches and a missing tooth. It cost me a day in the hospital, a big medical bill, and this scar you are looking at right now.

"Andy"
Seattle, WA

Foreword

Sergeant Rory Miller

Kris and Lawrence are nice guys.

They're tough guys, and they have the skill to put a hurtin' on you. They've both spilled blood and smelled it. But they're nice and intelligent and a little naïve—because they think they can convince you that violence is something you want to avoid just using facts.

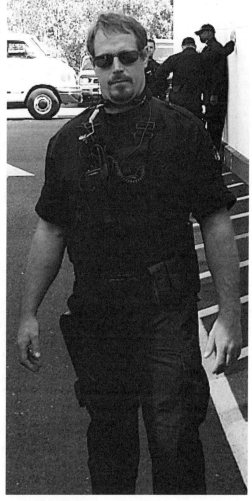

There are tons of facts in here. Facts and stories, and really good advice. Whatever you paid in money for the book, someone else paid in blood for the lessons. All that advice came at a price. All of Lawrence's statistics were originally written in some poor bastard's blood on some sidewalk.

Lawrence and Kris think that they can get this through your head with facts and words. I don't think you're that smart.

When they write how hard it will be looking in the mirror every morning knowing that you have killed someone, they know this is true—because every non-sociopath they have talked to tells them how hard it is. Just words. In your adolescent fantasy (and even in your fifties, many of your fantasies are purely adolescent) being a 'killer' seems pretty cool.

Let me lay it out as these two fine men tried to lay it out in this *Little Black Book*; there are tons of things that are cool to think about that suck to do. Some suck so badly that the memory becomes a pain separate from the thing you are remembering.

You will read about heroes in here. Your little eyes will get all shiny and you will think, "I could do that!" And it's a good feeling because in your little Hollywood-influenced world, the hero gets the acclaim of people and the love of a beautiful stranger. In the world of this book, the same hero gets months of physical therapy, torturous surgeries and "it" (the arm, the knee, the hand, the eye, the back) never, ever works the same way again. Never.

Or maybe it goes another way. Maybe the relatives of the guy who attacked you, though they have been afraid of him for years, come out of the woodwork and get a small army of attorneys and start remembering how he was "a good boy, very caring" or he "was turning his life around." That small army of attorneys will have a mission—to take money from you to give to the family of the person you injured or to the person himself. If a home invasion robber can sue, and win for "loss of earnings," there's very little hope that good intentions will protect you. What seems worse, to me, is that you wind up giving your earnings, your money, and your assets to someone you don't even like, possibly someone with a long history of crime, certainly to someone who doesn't deserve it.

That's the good option because the boys in blue may show up. You may find some special stainless steel bling ratcheted over your wrists and get a nice ride to the big building with the laminated Lexan windows and sometimes real bars for doors. When you hear and feel that cold electronic lock slam shut behind you, you will know that your life has changed forever. Then you might meet me or someone very like me. If you decided to sip twice at the well of violence, it will be my job to stop you, and I will stop you cold. It will hurt quite a lot.

> When you hear and feel that cold electronic lock slam shut behind you, you will know that your life has changed forever. Then you might meet me or someone very like me. If you decided to sip twice at the well of violence, it will be my job to stop you, and I will stop you cold. It will hurt quite a lot.

Lawrence and Kris tell good stories about fights and killings that don't happen. A strategist takes the lesson and they hope, in their naïve and sincere way, that the reader (that's you) wants to be a strategist. I know better. You'll skim those stories and get to the bloody ones, imagining what a knife can do in vivid Technicolor, just like at the movies. But the movies never get the screams quite right and sometimes the real memories that stay with you are the smells: rotten sh*t and fresh blood and decomposition and the soapy, meaty smell of fresh brains.

Kris and Lawrence are so careful to go over the complexity of the subject. Violence isn't just violence. It happens in a social context, a legal context, and a medical context, and they all play off of each other. They put it in your face that you may lose your home, your career, your family, your sight… to save a wallet with fourteen dollars or so that some strangers won't think bad thoughts about you. Is it enough for them to put it in your face? Will you read it?

I don't think you're that smart. I don't think you can see past your own ego. I think that you will risk your own life and piss away good information to protect your daydreams.

Maybe not. Prove me wrong. Read the book; read it carefully. Follow the advice, avoid the risks, and become a *strategist*. Prove to me that you are smarter than I think you are.

I won't hold my breath.

Sgt. **Rory Miller**
www.chirontraining.com
www.chirontraining.blogspot.com

Sergeant Rory Miller is the author of Meditations on Violence: A Comparison of Martial Arts Training and Real World Violence. *He has studied martial arts since 1981. He has received college varsities in judo and fencing, and holds mokuroku (teaching certificate) in Sosuishitsu-ryu jujutsu. He is a corrections officer and tactical team leader who teaches and designs courses in defensive tactics, close quarters combat, and Use of Force policy and application for law enforcement and corrections officers. A veteran of hundreds of violent confrontations, he lectures on realism and training for martial artists and writers.*

Foreword

Marc "Animal" MacYoung

One of the harder things for a young man to hear is that many of the things that he is willing to fight for aren't worth fighting for. In fact, often all you seem to hear from older people is "don't fight."

Unfortunately, that is kind of hard to do. As a young man, you have many opportunities to get involved in violence. And in the heat of the moment, it really does seem like the only way to handle the problem. Older people who tell you 'not to fight' just

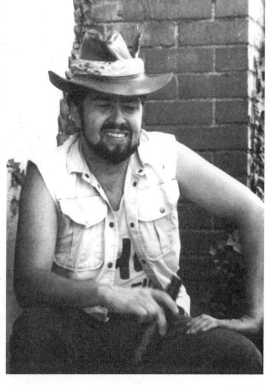

never seem to realize that, often, the repercussions of not fighting look to be a bigger problem than all those bad things that 'might' happen if you do fight. While 'don't fight' because of what might happen seems to make sense to older people, that advice doesn't do you much good about dealing with the problems that WILL happen if you don't fight.

I mean sure, you may get a bloody nose if you fight the guy, but how much grief and suffering are you going to have to endure when word gets out that you're a wimp for not fighting him? How does not fighting help you deal with the feelings of being less than a man for not standing up for yourself? Will your girlfriend think you're a wuss for not defending her honor? And, will she still be willing to sleep with a wuss? These are the kinds of problems that "don't fight" doesn't answer.

You hold in your hands a rather unique book, a book that will help you understand something that will be, at first, confusing. But the more you know about the subject of violence, the more you realize that both sides are right.

How can that be? How can two totally opposite points of view be right?

Well, let's start with the idea that it isn't black or white. There are all kinds of shades of gray. Both groups are right to a degree. It's just that often these different points of view can't see what the other group sees because of the years in between them.

Now to really muck things up, let's throw in something else that complicates things. How much of what you are feeling right now is based on biological patterns? Patterns that ALL human beings have—even though most of the time they are neither consciously aware of the patterns or know how to talk about them.

Oh and guess what? These patterns are seriously influenced by age. As a young man, you are very concerned with establishing social status, finding a mate, and making your own territory. This is primate behavior and it often includes violence. It's when you remember that humans are primates that should make you go, "Oh…" Now for the big shocker, the people who are telling you 'not to fight' are the ones who have already dealt with these primate drives. That means they're secure with their social status, have established territories, and live with long-term mates. Good for them, but it doesn't help you now does it?

When you are in the middle of an emotional storm, being pushed along by the need to establish yourself, violence can look like a perfectly logical thing to do. On the other hand, to those who've established themselves, it looks pretty stupid. They've forgotten what it was like not having these issues squared away. And this is why their answer of 'don't fight' looks as stupid to someone trying to establish himself as fighting looks to them.

Lawrence and Kris have written a book that will help young men understand how violence happens, how it can be avoided (without losing face), how situations can escalate into violence because of a reaction to something that you thought would solve the problem and the life-long consequences that violence can have. Sometimes resorting to violence is necessary, but more often than not it is better—for all kinds of reasons—to find a peaceful way to resolve the problem.

The trick is to know when each of these times are. And this book will help with that too.

Marc "Animal" MacYoung
www.nononsenseselfdefense.com

Growing up on gang-infested streets not only gave Marc MacYoung his street name "Animal," but also extensive firsthand experience about what does and does not work for self-defense. Over the years, he has held a number of dangerous occupations including director of a correctional institute, bodyguard, and bouncer. He was first shot at when he was 15 years old and has since survived multiple attempts on his life, including professional contracts. He has studied a variety of martial arts since childhood, teaching experience-based self-defense to police, military, civilians, and martial artists around the world. His has written dozens of books and produced numerous DVDs covering all aspects of this field.

Lawrence and Kris have written a book that will help young men understand how violence happens, how it can be avoided (without losing face), how situations can escalate into violence because of a reaction to something that you thought would solve the problem, and the life-long consequences that violence can have. Sometimes resorting to violence is necessary, but more often than not it is better—for all kinds of reasons—to find a peaceful way to resolve the problem.

Preface

Both the victor
and the vanquished are
but drops of dew,
but bolts of lightning-
thus should we view the world.
– Ouchi Yoshitaka (1507–1551)[1]

This book is about violence. It is about running into something that you have probably never encountered in your life, but that will change your whole world if you do. We're not talking about a schoolyard brawl or a fistfight between buddies here, but rather the deeper, darker kind of altercations, the ones where oftentimes someone doesn't walk away, and win or lose you may very well be scarred for life.

If you picked up this book because you are interested in self-defense and want to give yourself the best chance of surviving a violent encounter, you've come to the right place. If, instead, you've just had a run-in with the dark side, are trying to make sense of what occurred, and are looking for strategies to ensure that it will not happen again, well, you've come to the right place for that too.

We will introduce you to a world of hatred, anger, fear, and lies where you will come to understand sociopaths, career criminals, thieves, cheats, bullies, misogynists, and various other twisted personalities that you might one day run across in real life. We hope that you will never experience the violence wrought by such people. Yet, if you do, and most will at one point or another in their lives, we will prepare you to better understand and more likely survive the experience.

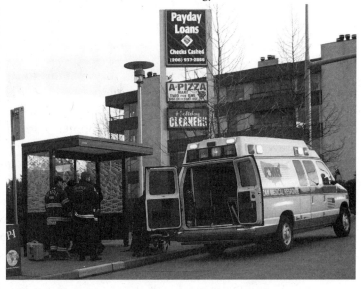

We have taken a no-nonsense approach in reflecting the world of violence. Consequently, you may well be offended by some of what you read. You might even disagree with certain things we have written in this book. If you find the contents provocative, or even shocking, then we have succeeded in making you think. That's what this book is about, opening your mind. And, of course, filling it with practical, sensible knowledge and tools to protect yourself from violence.

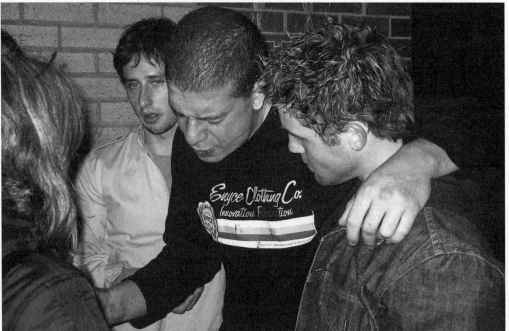

Photo courtesy of Al Arsenault

According to the Bureau of Justice Statistics, men commit about 80 percent of all violent crimes in the United States, serious stuff like homicides, rapes, robberies, and assaults. Men are twice as likely as women to become victims of those same violent crimes, except for rape.* Furthermore, males are more likely to be victimized by a stranger, whereas females are more likely to be victimized by a friend, acquaintance, or intimate. (Although when women engage in violence, they are more likely to assault someone physically they know than a stranger—which still leaves you in the crosshairs.) Consequently, while bad things can happen to anyone, males are the ones who really need to understand aggression and be prepared for sudden encounters with violence. That is why this book was written especially for you. Let us make it clear; although we may present situations or vignettes from one gender's perspective, violence is an equal opportunity employer that knows no gender.

When it comes to violence, all the statistics confirm that younger people are far more inclined toward aggressive behavior than older people are. For example, many bars and most nightclubs are populated by younger people. Take an emotionally charged atmosphere, stir in a generous dose of alcohol and/or drugs, and you've got a good recipe for conflict and violence.

Young males tend to have a long list of things to prove, whether they are conscious of them or not. Often their motives are unconscious because they are based

---

* Almost 90 percent of reported rapes are perpetrated against female victims, though the rate of reporting by males who were sexually assaulted is thought to be very low, so that number might be a bit skewed.

on biological patterns of the human species. You probably don't realize how much of what you think and feel is based on these patterns—and this especially applies to territoriality and status.

Young men typically do not truly understand or fully appreciate the physical, psychological, and legal costs of violence. They often feel immortal, never considering the possibility of becoming maimed, crippled, or even killed in a confrontation. Consequently, young men will fight for any number of reasons—affiliations, self esteem, social status, not to be considered a wimp, the clothes they wear, revenge for some perceived slight, to impress a cute girlfriend, or just to blow off a little steam, to name a few.

So, what do the participants of violence look like? Well, they look like you, the reader. You might simply find yourself in the wrong place at the right time. Perhaps some seemingly harmless behavior on your part will be the spark that sets things off, or you may be minding your own business and fail to notice impending danger until you walk into it unaware. Either way, it's a precarious place to be.

The goal of this book is to help you understand and avoid behavior that will get you involved in violence by giving you a roadmap to a conscious decision-making process that takes the non-thinking response out of your behavior. We will enable you to reach up into your head and flick the switch on the violence control panel from "react" to "respond." You need to ask yourself, "Is this really worth fighting over?" While in some instances, the response could legitimately be "Yes," more often than not, it ought to be "No."

Simply put, some yahoo spewing insults about your favorite sports team is worlds apart from a drug-crazed lunatic coming at you with a knife in a parking lot. There is a large gray area between those two extremes where hard and fast rules don't always apply. This is where wisdom, oftentimes hard-earned wisdom, is the difference between a good decision and a bad one. It's not always a life or death decision, yet a bad choice could have serious consequences, the kind of stuff that can change a life completely, for the worse.

> The goal of this book is to help you understand and avoid behavior that will get you involved in violence by giving you a roadmap to a conscious decision-making process that takes the non-thinking response out of your behavior. You need to ask yourself, "Is this really worth fighting over?" While in some instances, the response could legitimately be "Yes," more often than not, it ought to be "No."

Recognize that every time you engage in violence, no matter how small and trivial, it has the potential of escalating into something that has life-long consequences. What *is* really worth fighting for when you might end up spending the rest of your life behind bars with a sociopathic roommate, dreading the moment you might accidentally drop the soap in the shower, confined to a wheelchair peeing through a catheter and sh*tting into a colostomy bag, or declaring bankruptcy under the crushing weight of a massive civil lawsuit?

Is it really worth fighting over a comment that hurts your feelings or makes you feel less than a man? Is it really worth fighting with the mugger over your wallet? Is it really worth fighting the other driver who flipped you the bird in traffic? Is it worth fighting over a threat to your child? Is it worth fighting someone who bumped into you at a party and refused to apologize for spilling your drink? Is it worth fighting someone trying to break into your car? Is it worth fighting a drunk who copped a feel on your girlfriend?

What if it's not just one guy who's messing with you but rather a gang of thugs? What about fighting to protect a pregnant woman or disabled friend who cannot get away from a hostile individual? What if he's got a knife or a gun? What if it's your intoxicated brother or your drugged-up best friend pointing the weapon at you with malevolence in his eyes?

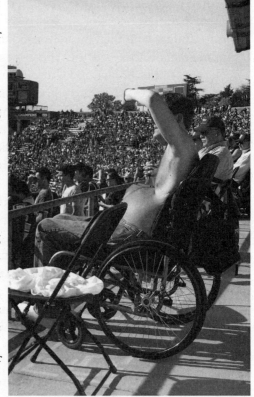

These are all situational; they are decisions that without forethought could, and most likely will, be poorly made.

We hope to give you a strategic view of what is happening, a view that is more practical than emotional. It is then up to you to establish a goal and to adhere to tactics that serve that goal. An example of establishing these goals comes from a police officer friend of ours. Long before encountering violence, he had already built an internal list of things he simply will not allow in his world. An example is, "I will not allow myself to be tied up." He knows from experience and training that being tied up is a precursor to being moved to a secondary crime scene or killed outright. For him, physical restraint by a criminal means certain death. In his mind, it is far better to fight now and have some chance of survival than to comply and face near certain slaughter later on.

How would you respond to that type of scenario? It is not only useful, but also critical, to determine what you are willing to do, or have done to you, during a violent encounter, in advance of such incidents occurring. That way, during the heat of the moment, you can act without hesitation.

Here's your chance to really think about it. At the end of the book in Appendix A is a checklist titled "How Far Am I Willing to Go?" To use this checklist properly, **stop reading this book now, flip to the back, and fill in your answers. Once you have finished reading the book, go back and do it again.** There is no answer key. There is no right or wrong when it comes to responding to these questions. The answers that you put will be whatever is right for you at the time. Once filled out, this list will be composed of your limits and thresholds, the ones you will use as a guide. This exercise will help you understand how you will operate in the world and especially in the world of violence.

Once you have read this book you will recognize behaviors from people around you and, more importantly, you will recognize your own. If you can recognize such behaviors, especially those within yourself, then you are halfway toward winning any conflict. As you begin to understand these behaviors and situations, it will help you make the right choices for success in terms of conflict resolution. Ultimately, what you have learned will help you live a longer and more peaceful life as a result. Be smart, be informed, and be safe.

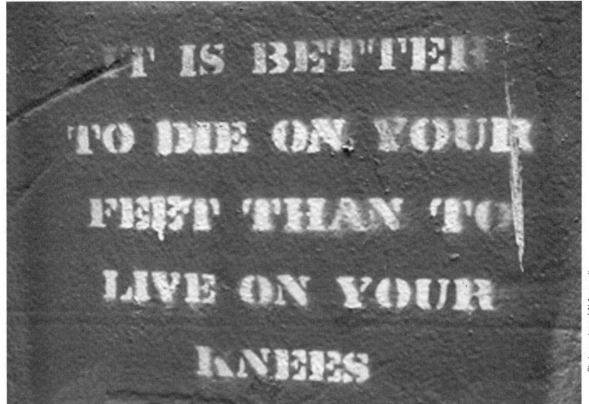

Acknowledgements

Laura Vanderpool has helped with all of our books over the years. Once again, she reviewed the draft manuscript, gave us insightful feedback, and helped shore up our sometimes overt grammatical shortcomings. Her keen insight and ongoing assistance is, quite simply, invaluable. Without her, we would be grunting cavemen not knowing if we should eat the paper or write on it.

We are also enormously grateful to Loren Christensen who has always been very supportive of our work. For this book, he graciously shared his first-hand experience and in-depth research on gang culture and crowd violence. Great stuff man, thanks! We sincerely appreciate Marc MacYoung's insight into the brutal realities of violence; he has probably forgotten more than most people will ever know about the subject. Not only was his hard-won wisdom invaluable on this project, but he also donated some great photographs as well. Sergeant Rory Miller helped us benefit from the vast experience at the sharp end of conflict. His discerning feedback has been tremendously helpful and very much appreciated. Lt. Colonel John R. Finch (ret.) graciously shared his unique insight and personal experience with the "cost" and aftermath of violence. Tracy Getty and Jeffrey-Peter Hauck contributed some outstanding photographs. Finally, a big thank you goes to David Organ for sharing his amusing drunk wrangling experience. Thanks guys, you rock!

Posed photos in this book feature Frank Getty, Tracy Getty, Lawrence Kane, Joey Kane, Sophal Keo, Lance Kilgore, Lou Kings, Andy Orose, Joyce Walters, and Kris Wilder. These pictures were taken by Joey Kane, Lawrence Kane, and Kris Wilder. This book also contains several gruesome visuals that graphically illustrate the effects of real-life violence. While some of these pictures were taken by Lawrence Kane, who carried a camera around with him for several months while keeping an eye out for trouble, many were provided by Al Arsenault.

Al is the Executive Director of the famed Odd Squad, a cadre of Vancouver police officers who worked, fought, and filmed in the seedy underbelly of Canada's infamous Skid Road. This blighted area is infested with drugs, crime, mental illness, and every possible social problem imaginable. These pictures capture but a bit of the human degradation and suffering Al has witnessed in his 27 years as a street cop with the Vancouver Police Department.

A more poignant rendition of the essence of drug Hell can be found in *Tears for April: Beyond the Blue Lens* (2007), a gut-wrenching feature-length documentary film about the lives, deaths, and the horrible suffering in between, of a handful of addicts who live in what Al calls the "Chemical Gulag" (www.oddsquad.com).

Al is currently in Thailand on a sabbatical from the Vancouver Police Judo Club and Odd Squad to write a book about his experiences with Odd Squad, drug abuse, and policing. He is also starting on two more practical martial arts books for civilians and police. For a sample of his work, see his book *Chin Na in Ground Fighting* published in 2003.

Introduction

Spitting blood
clears up reality
and dream alike.
—Sunao (1887– 1926)[2]

Violence is everywhere—on the street, in the workplace, on campus, and in the community. It can be instigated by everyone from drunken fools who hit like Jell-O to drug-crazed lunatics who cannot only throw a good punch but will slash your throat for good measure, and everything else in between. The danger can come from fists, feet, or flying objects. You might encounter or deploy impromptu weapons such as bricks, bottles, or bludgeons, or more conventional ones such as blades, buckshot, or bullets.

You might be the instigator, the victim, a witness, any or all of the above. You might see violence coming or it might catch you totally by surprise. Aggression can come from friends, relatives, acquaintances, or total strangers. It can be logical or illogical, easily predictable or totally unexpected. It might be some crackhead trying to score a few bucks for his next rock, an irate driver in the grip of road rage, or a neighborhood bully intimidating you to make his point. Or it might be from your drunken brother at your cousin's wedding, or it might be your best friend having a drug reaction at a party.

Aggression doesn't have to make sense at the time, and often won't. Whenever the face of violence is glaring at you with that cold, hard stare, however, you must deal with it effectively in order to survive. For example, a friend of ours was putting some dishes away one afternoon when his sister tried to kill him with a steak knife. One moment he was leaning over the dishwasher and the next there was a wedge of razor-sharp steel whistling toward his lower back. Why? She simply wanted to know what it would be like to murder someone, though he did not know that, nor frankly care about that, at the time. All he was concerned with was not dying. Fortunately, he caught a reflection in his peripheral vision, reacted appropriately, disarmed her, and survived unscathed without even a minor scratch.

That's where situational awareness comes into play. If you see violence coming early enough, you can easily walk, or more often, run away. With sufficient warning to prepare yourself mentally and physically, you can choose to fight or not to fight. When you are caught by surprise, however, you frequently have no choice but to fight… and on his terms rather than yours. Not exactly an ideal situation when it comes to survival. This is, of course, why predators like to jump their victims, catching them by surprise rather than facing up to them on even terms. The other guy doesn't want to fight. He wants to *win*.

Though street predators, bullies, and thugs are not typically all that intelligent, they are generally very crafty. It doesn't take a genius to know that if he attacks you out in a highly traveled, public place, he will have less control over the encounter and will more than likely

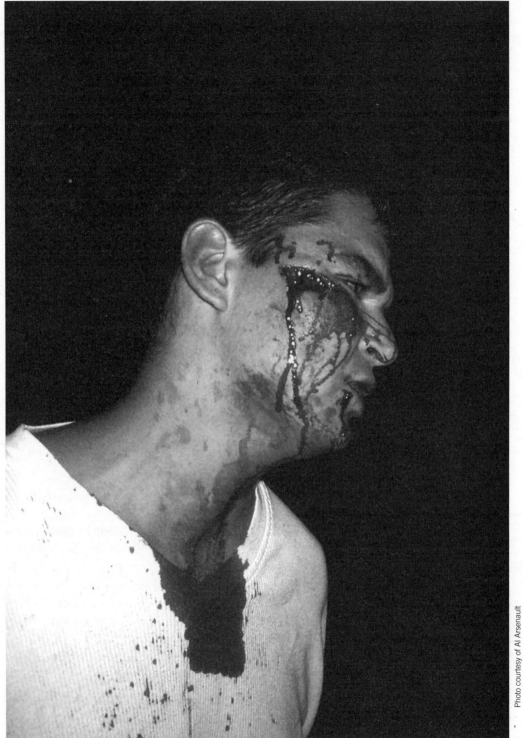

Photo courtesy of Al Arsenault

Aggression doesn't have to make sense at the time, and often won't, yet you must lean to deal with it effectively in order to survive.

be seen. And if not get caught, then at least he should have his plans interfered with. While he might want to take you to an isolated place in order to have the privacy he needs to assault, rape, murder, or rob you, he is not likely to find too many victims wandering around in remote, secluded locations. Consequently, fringe areas adjacent to heavily traveled public places are where the majority of violent crimes occur. That is where you need to pay the most attention to your surroundings. This includes areas such as parking lots, public parks, bike paths, alleyways, bathrooms, stairwells, ATM kiosks, bus terminals, train platforms and the like, particularly at night when few bystanders are hanging around.

Sometimes you're confronted by a violent person who has not yet attacked you, but is in the process of working himself up to a fight. You may have the chance to talk him down if you know how to de-escalate a situation, as opposed to trying to show him you aren't afraid of him, and that he needs to back off (that usually escalates a conflict rather than preventing it). But before you can de-escalate a situation, you need to know what kinds of things will escalate it from a verbal confrontation into violence.

Even if you cannot verbally de-escalate a bad situation, your words can be a powerful weapon for defending yourself on the street. For example, if you are in a public place you may have the opportunity to solicit help from bystanders or create friendly witnesses by using words that point out your danger and clearly articulate who's the aggressor and who's the victim. Anyone who stumbles across a fight that's already in progress has no way of knowing who the bad guy is if you don't make it clear for him. Furthermore, clever words can distract your adversary and facilitate your escape.

Escape is an admirable goal. Self-defense really isn't about fighting like most people think. Self-defense is primarily about not being there when the other guy wants to fight. Fighting is a participatory event. It means you were part of the problem. Even if you think you were only 'defending' yourself, if your actions contributed to the creation, escalation, and execution of violence then you were fighting. And remember, fighting is illegal.

Not fighting is good because whenever you do get into an altercation there will be repercussions. Perhaps you win, beating the other guy down with your fists only to find that he's come back afterward with the police, his lawyer, or a gun. Perhaps you lose and take the beat down yourself. If you're lucky you may end up with nothing more than a few bruises or minor bleeding, yet it's not unusual to suffer injuries that are far more serious. Go visit an emergency room in an urban area on a Friday or Saturday night and you'll see what we mean. Such visits can be quite enlightening.

The brutal reality of a violent encounter is that if you are knocked out, severely busted up, or otherwise placed in a position where you can no longer defend yourself during a fight, you are completely at the other guy's mercy. And often in the heat of the moment, mercy is in short supply. There is only a thin veneer of civilization, laws written on paper and enforced by folks who are much too far away to intervene right here, right now, standing between you and his wrath. He may very well break off the fight when you

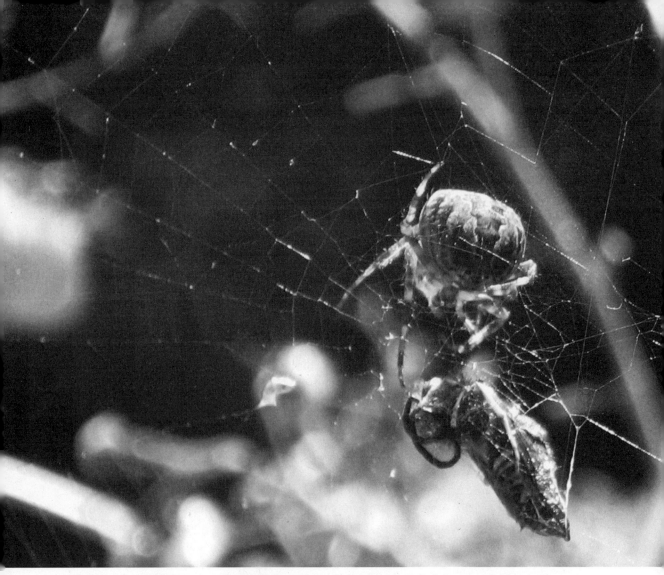

The hornet's deadly stinger was no match for the spider's nefarious trap. Similarly, it doesn't matter how tough you are if you never see the other guy coming. Good situational awareness, on the other hand, can keep you safe.

are curled up into a little ball of agony at his feet. Unfortunately, he may, in his drunken fury, decide to put the boots to you.

Since not fighting is so important, that's what the first section of this book is all about—becoming aware of and learning how to avoid violent confrontations. It explains some of the brutal realities of violence so that, perhaps, you won't want to fight either. You will learn about important concepts such as escalato (the "game" whereby events escalate into violence), victim interviews, predatory positioning, cutting from the herd, verbal self-defense, understanding your adversary, knowing when he's eager to attack, understanding gang culture, and identifying weapons before they can be deployed against you, among other things.

Unfortunately, there are instances when you have no choice but to fight and others where it is prudent to do so. If so, you need to know how to do it effectively. The second section of this book is about what actually happens during a violent encounter, helping you understand smart things you might want to try and dumb things you should attempt to avoid during a fight. It teaches important principles that help you know when you can legally get away with going physical and identifies appropriate levels of force that you might be able to employ while keeping yourself out of jail whenever you have to get hands on.

The last section covers the aftermath of violence, showing that it's almost never over when it's over. Surviving the fight is just the beginning. There is a host of other consequences to address, including first aid, legal issues, managing witnesses, finding a good attorney, dealing with the press, interacting with law enforcement, and dealing with psychological trauma.

The book is laid out as a series of vignettes within each section, each describing a different aspect of what happens before, during, or after violence. You will find quotes from legendary warriors Sun Tzu (*The Art of War*) and Miyamoto Musashi (*The Book of Five Rings*) at the beginning of each vignette, demonstrating that these concepts have been around for a very long time.

Sun Tzu (544–496 B.C.) is an honorific that means "Master Sun." According to historians, his given name was Wu. His mastery of military strategy was so exceptional that he supposedly transformed 180 courtesans into trained soldiers in a single session in order to secure a generalship with King Ho-Lu. Whether that particular episode is true or not, it is well known King Ho-Lu, with Sun Tzu at his side, defeated the powerful Chinese Ch'u state in 506 B.C., capturing their capital city of Ying. He then headed north and subdued the states of Ch'i and Chin to forge his empire. Sun Tzu recorded his winning strategies in a book titled *The Art of War*. It was the first and most revered volume of its type, one that is still referenced by military and business leaders throughout the world today.

Miyamoto Musashi (1584–1645) was born Shinmen Takezō. He grew up in the Harima Province of Japan. Arguably, the greatest swordsman who ever lived, Musashi slew his first opponent, Arima Kihei, at the age of 13. Considered *Kensei*, the sword saint of Japan, Musashi killed more than sixty trained *samurai* warriors in fights or duals during the feudal period where even a minor battle injury could lead to infection and death. He was the founder of the *Hyōhō Niten Ichi-Ryu* style of swordsmanship, which translates as "two heavens as one" or "two sword style." Like most *samurai*, he was skilled in the

> Aggression doesn't have to make sense at the time, and often won't. Whenever the face of violence is glaring at you with that cold, hard stare, however, you must deal with it effectively in order to survive. The brutal reality of a violent encounter is that if you are knocked out, severely busted up, or otherwise placed in a position where you can no longer defend yourself during a fight, you are completely at the other guy's mercy. There is only a thin veneer of civilization, laws written on paper and enforced by folks who are much too far away to intervene right here, right now, standing between you and his wrath.

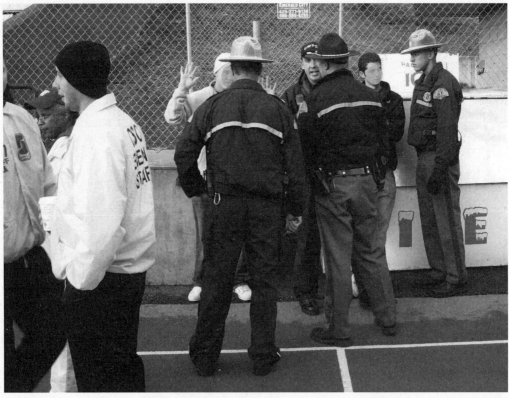

Violence is almost never over when it's 'over.' There are a host of consequences to deal with including recovering from physical and/or psychological trauma as well as navigating the legal system, among others.

peaceful arts as well, an exceptional poet, calligrapher, and artist. Two years before he died, Musashi retired to a life of seclusion in a cave where he codified his winning strategy in the famous *Go Rin No Sho* which, in English, means *The Book of Five Rings*.

Each chapter in this book begins with a poem penned by a *samurai* warrior or *haiku* poet on the verge of death. These perspectives are fascinating and, we think, worth your consideration. In the interest of making this book as useful for the reader as possible, however, we have attempted to limit our philosophical commentary in favor of real-life examples and practical advice, using actual people and situations from which you can learn.

A key aspect of this book is the checklist in Appendix A. If you have not already done so as directed in the preface, stop reading the book now, flip to the back, and fill in your answers. This exercise is designed to make you think, putting the information you are about to read into a context that will be meaningful and real for you when you must make decisions under pressure or threat out in the real world. Once you have finished reading the book, go back and do the exercise again. See what you have learned, evaluate

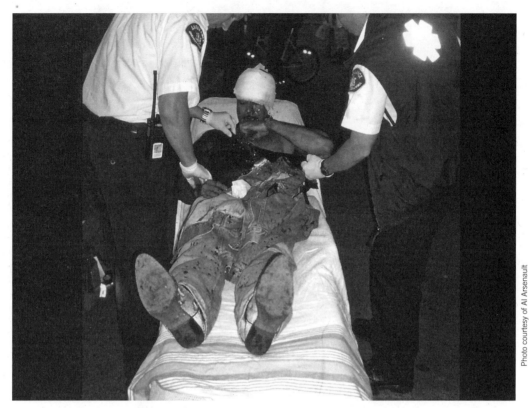

Photo courtesy of Al Arsenault

Self-defense really isn't about fighting; it's primarily about not being there when the other guy wants to fight. Knowledge and good sense are your main weapons for self-defense.

if and how your attitude has changed, and reflect on what you might do next time you run across aggressive or violent behavior on the street.

Our goal is to help you put things into perspective and give you the tools necessary to navigate the world of violence without running into any insurmountable rocks, pitfalls, or traps along your way. It's a serious topic, yet we have tried to make it interesting, meaningful and, most of all, thought provoking. After all, knowledge and good sense are your main weapons of self-defense.

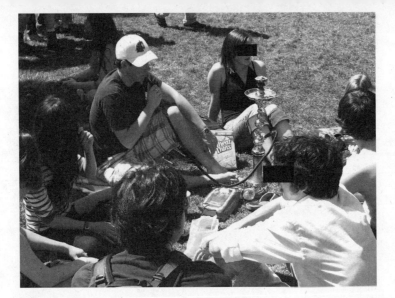

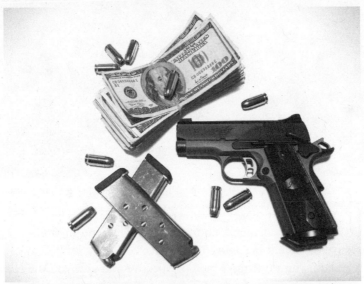

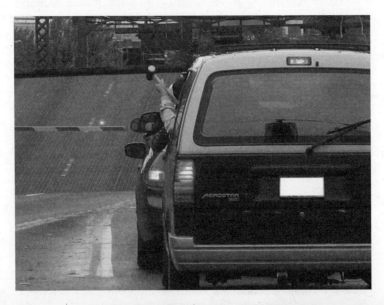

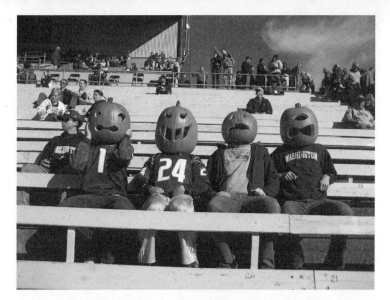

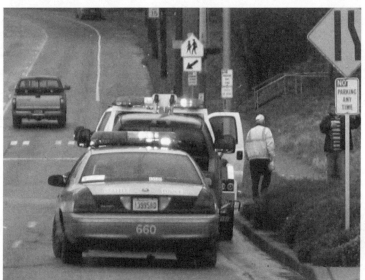

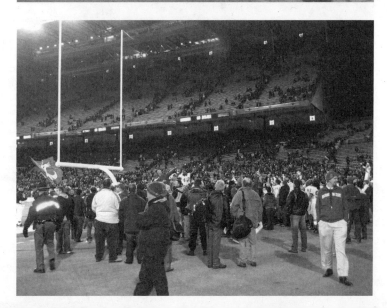

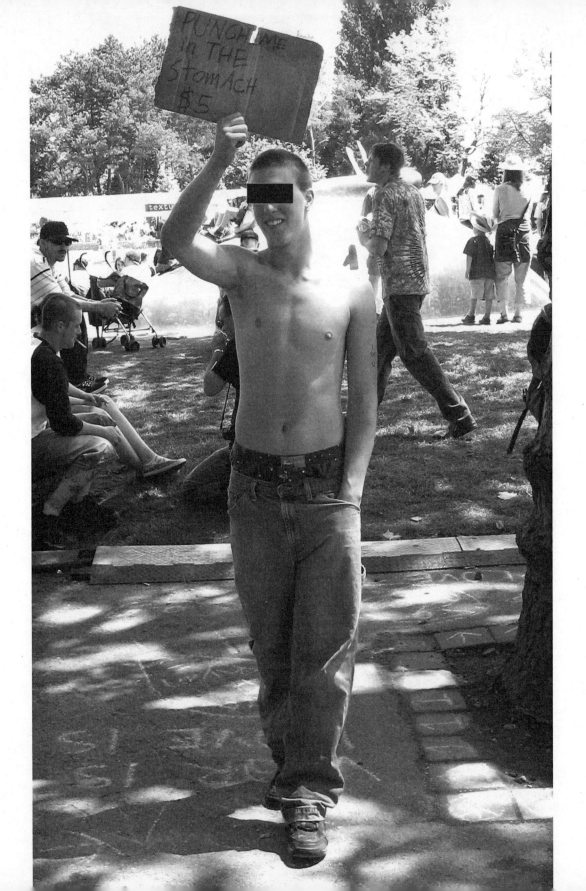

SECTION ONE

Before Violence Occurs

When autumn winds blow
not one leaf remains
the way it was.

— *Togyu (1705–1749)*[3]

Rule number one of self-defense is, "Don't get hit." Sounds simple at first blush but it's really more complicated than that. At best, it's about avoiding situations or locations where violence is most likely to occur. Sadly, we often don't think about such things or we blow them off as irrelevant, stuff that happens to other guys. Juanita Watkins, a friend of Marc MacYoung's, summed it up best when she sagely wrote, "Just because something is dangerous doesn't automatically mean that you are going to get hurt if you do it. I have noticed that the young, inexperienced—or simply imagination impaired—take this to mean there is no danger at all."

Let's face it; we all do dumb stuff from time to time. Oftentimes nothing bad happens. When there are no adverse consequences for our behavior, it's easy to keep on taking risks. Heck, risks can be fun. That doesn't mean, however, that it's a good idea to keep pushing the envelope. Traveling through the wrong neighborhoods, hanging out with the wrong people, or frequenting the wrong night spots will have consequences sooner or later, especially if you act out inappropriately while you are there.

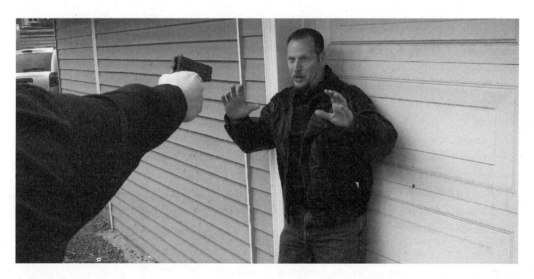

Most people who find themselves involved in violence think that they were just minding their own business and when they look up, suddenly this problem comes out of nowhere. It just seems like this at the time, though. There is virtually always some type of build up, something they didn't see or didn't recognize the significance of until it became a problem. That's why it appears to have come out of nowhere. Oftentimes what you think is an innocent comment, gesture, or look is what gets you clobbered.

Self-defense is about keeping your cool, not being the instigator, even inadvertently. It's about paying attention, being aware of and evading threats before it's too late. Less ideally, if the violence is right in front of you, it's about doing all you can to avoid a fight. After all, the only fight you know you'll win, the one you are guaranteed to walk away from with all your parts and pieces fully intact, is the fight you never get into. This is what Sun Tzu meant when he wrote, "To subdue an enemy without fighting is the highest skill," more than 2,500 years ago.

This section covers everything you need to know and do to avoid getting into an actual fight. In addition to helping you identify potential threats and how to evade them, it also helps you develop the emotional fortitude you need in order to walk away from a confrontation when the other guy gets in your face and you really, really want to thump him.

Awareness is Your Best Defense

To see the sun and moon is no sign of sharp sight; to hear the noise of thunder is no sign of a quick ear.

— *Sun Tzu*

If you know the Way broadly you will see it in everything. Men must polish their particular Way.

— *Miyamoto Musashi*

Again, the best self-defense is being aware of and avoiding dangerous people and hazardous situations. When that is not possible, when you've failed to identify and act upon signs of impending threat, self-defense can still be about verbally de-escalating a tense encounter before it turns violent. Fighting is your last resort to keep yourself safe after you've blown your self-defense, when awareness, avoidance, and de-escalation have all failed.

Since it is fundamental to personal safety, we'll begin by discussing awareness. Situational awareness means a solid understanding of time and place and how they relate to you, your family, friends, and others around you at any given moment. In some ways, it's more of an attitude than a skill. Any time you are near others, especially strangers, it pays to be vigilant, striking a good balance between obliviousness and paranoia. If you can sense danger before stumbling across it, you have a much better chance of escaping unscathed.

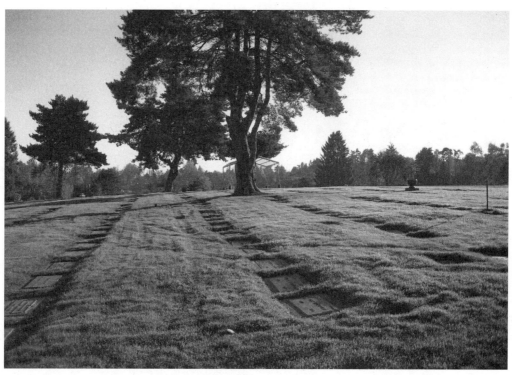

Whenever someone throws a punch, launches a kick, pulls out a knife, or draws a gun something bad is going to happen. The question is not one of 'if' but rather of "how much."

Whenever someone throws a punch, launches a kick, pulls out a knife, or draws a gun—something bad is going to happen. That's "bad" in a *Ghostbusters* "don't cross the streams Egon" kind of way.[4] If you are on the receiving end, you are the one who is going to get hurt, maimed, crippled, or killed. Fortunately, with a little training the majority of all that bad stuff is easily recognizable and avoidable before it gets to the physical part.

Most self-defense experts agree that nine out of ten dangers can be identified and avoided simply by learning how to look out for them. Since it is still possible to talk your way out of more than half of the potentially violent situations that you do get yourself into, this means that you should only need to fight your way out of three, four, or at worst, five of every hundred hazardous encounters. With good situational awareness, you may never have anywhere near a hundred such confrontations in your lifetime so those odds really aren't all that bad, huh?

Knowing when it is time to leave a party is a common example of good situational awareness. Fights at parties tend to happen after a certain time of night. It's not the hour on the clock that's important, but rather the mood of the crowd. Most people have a good time and leave long before the sh*t starts. Just about everyone who's going to hook up has already done so; they've found a date, left together, and are off having fun. As the

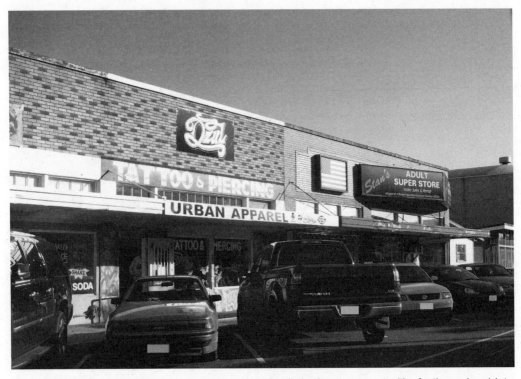

Good situational awareness helps make you a hard target by eliminating easy opportunities for those who wish to do you harm. Constant vigilance is emotionally and physically draining, however, so you need a process for knowing when to ratchet your level of alertness up or down.

crowd starts to thin, those who have nothing better to do than cause trouble are the ones who are left. Buzzing with frustration and raging hormones, those who insist on hanging on well into the night are the ones who get caught up in it when the fecal matter is most likely to fly. If you pay attention to the behaviors of those around you, however, it's fairly easy to know when it's time to leave. If you're not there when things start to get rough, bad things can't happen to you.

The same thing happens on the street. Criminals may be strong, fast, crafty, and mean, but in general, they are neither exceptionally bright nor hardworking. We are stereotyping here, but seriously, how many rocket scientists or Mensa members are there on death row? Further, many crimes are quick fix substitutes for earning a living the old fashioned way via hard work. Why then would a street thug go out of his way to tangle with a tough, prepared target when easier prey is readily available?

By constantly surveying and evaluating your environment, you achieve more control over what ultimately happens to you. Good situational awareness helps you make yourself a hard target by eliminating easy opportunities for those who wish to do you harm. It's not a guarantee of perfect safety since there truly are no absolutes when it comes to

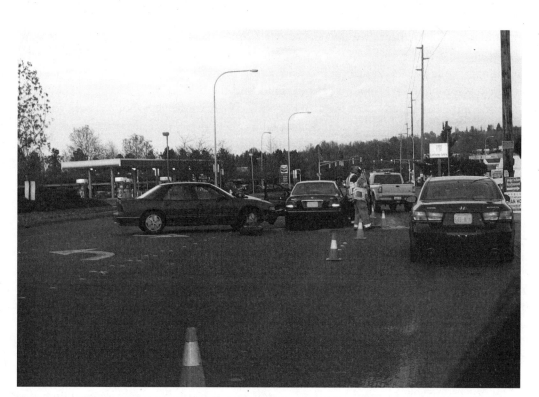

Remember a time when you were driving along minding your own business when you suddenly "knew" the car beside you was going to swerve into your lane and took evasive action to avoid an accident? This ability to predict what other drivers are going to do is an excellent example of good situational awareness.

self-defense, yet good situational awareness can let you predict and avoid most difficult situations.

Situational awareness is something that everyone instinctively has, yet few individuals truly pay attention to. In most cases, you should be able to spot a developing situation, turn around, and walk (or drive) away before anything bad happens. Once you understand the basic concepts and begin to pay attention to your built-in survival mechanisms, situational awareness can also be refined and improved through practice. Sometimes, however, try as you might to avoid it, trouble finds you and you will have to react accordingly. Good awareness helps you be prepared for that as well.

Can you remember a time when you were driving along the highway, suddenly "knew" the car beside you was going to swerve into your lane, and took evasive action to avoid an accident? Almost everyone who drives has done that on numerous occasions. It is so common that most people forget about such incidents shortly after they happen. This ability to predict what other drivers are going to do is an excellent example of good situational awareness.

However, vigilance in this area is emotionally and physically draining. No one can maintain an elevated level of awareness at all times in all places. There is a difference between being aware and becoming paranoid. Consequently, many self-defense experts use a color code system to help define and communicate appropriate levels of situational awareness for whatever situation people could find themselves in.

The most commonly used approach, codified by Colonel Jeff Cooper, was based in large part on the color alert system developed by the United States Marine Corps during World War II and later modified for civilian use. These color code conditions include White (oblivious), Yellow (aware), Orange (alert), Red (concerned), and Black (under attack). This code should not be confused with the similar U.S. Department of Homeland Security threat level alerts that use similar colors.

> Any time you are near others, especially strangers, it pays to be vigilant. Bad guys don't want to fight. They want to win. Consequently, tough, prepared targets are usually left alone in favor of easier prey. You cannot, however, walk around in a constant state of hyper-vigilance or paranoia. Self-defense experts often use a color code system to define appropriate levels of situational awareness that help you strike the right balance, paying attention to what's important, and keeping yourself safe. The colors themselves are far less important than the overall concept—different levels of awareness are appropriate for different situations.

The mindset and attitude of each condition are described below. While it is possible to move up and down the entire scale, clearly hitting each condition in turn, it is also possible to skip from one level to another very quickly. Consequently, while it is valuable to think of each condition as a distinct state along a continuum like rungs of a ladder, don't get too hung up on each level. The important concept is that the diverse tactical situations you face will warrant various levels of vigilance. It is prudent to consciously choose the appropriate level of situational awareness.

Condition White (Oblivious). In Condition White, you are pretty much oblivious to your surroundings, completely unprepared for trouble if it arrives. You are a lemming, distracted or unaware, thus unable to perceive any existing danger in your immediate area or be alert for any that may be presented to you. Drivers carrying on conversations with passengers, people talking on cell phones, joggers wearing headphones and jamming to their music, and other generally preoccupied individuals fall into this category.

You may remember a time when you were driving along with the stereo cranked up and grooving to the music when suddenly the police officer you didn't know was behind you lit off his siren and lights. Nearly jumping out of your skin, you checked your speedometer only to find you'd been speeding and knowing you'd been busted. That's an example of being in Condition White. While almost everyone has done it, it's not too cool, huh?

An interesting exercise is to do a little people watching, trying to identify those around you in this mode. Their heads will commonly be tilted downward toward the ground in front of them or fixed on a spot in the distance such as one might do when looking at a tourist map, reading a book, or searching for a distant address or landmark. These folks are easy marks for just about any pickpocket, mugger, rapist, or other deviant they stumble across.

Try watching a crowd at a mall, nightclub, or other public area with a predator mindset sometime; it can be an illuminating experience. Try to read people's body language as they pass by you. Who looks like a victim and who does not? Oblivious people in Condition White stand out from the crowd once you know how to look for them.

If you are attacked in Condition White, you are likely going to be hurt. If armed, you can easily become a danger to yourself or others. Even police officers, who have access to much better training than the average civilian, have been killed by their own weapons when they relaxed their vigilance at the wrong times or places.

Condition Yellow (Aware). Although you are not looking for or expecting trouble in Condition Yellow, if it comes up you will have a good chance to identify it in time to react. People in this condition are at ease, not immediately perceiving any danger,

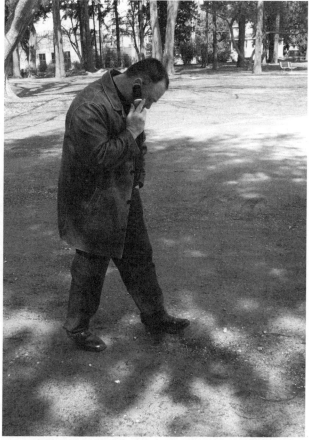

In Condition White, you are pretty much oblivious to your surroundings, completely unprepared for trouble if it arrives.

but pretty much aware of their surroundings. You can identify, without looking twice, generally who and what is around you—vehicles, people, building entrances, street corners, and areas that might provide concealment and/or cover should something untoward happen. To clarify the difference between these two concepts, concealment (for example, a bush) keeps bad guys from seeing you but does not provide much physical protection, while cover (for example, a stone wall) can keep the bad guy and/or his weapon from getting to you should he wish to attack.

Body language is important. People in Condition Yellow should be self-assured and appear confident in everything they do, yet not present an overt challenge or threat to others. Predators typically stalk those they consider weaker prey, rarely victimizing the strong. We're not just talking about hardcore criminals here, but also bullies and petty thugs as well. People in this state look confident, walking with their

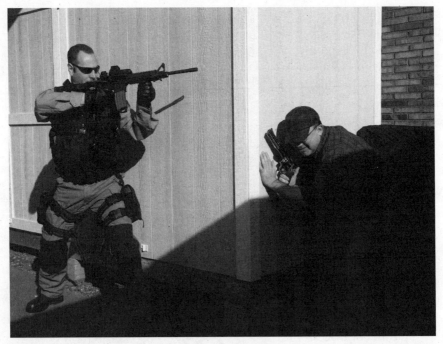

Cover, such as this sturdy, equipment-filled shed, creates a physical barrier between you and the adversary. He can neither see nor reach you without moving.

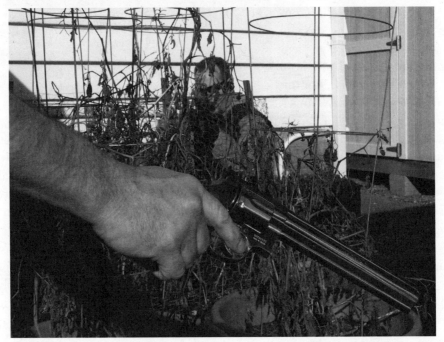

Concealment such as this bush can keep the other guy from spotting you but offers little, if any, physical protection.

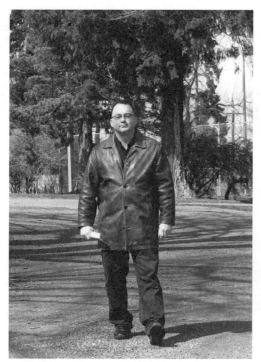

Although you are not looking for or expecting trouble in Condition Yellow, if it comes up you will have a good chance to identify it in time to react.

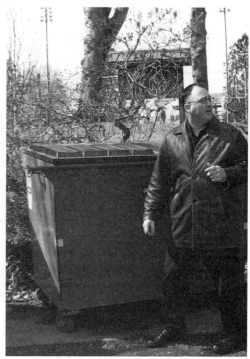

In Condition Orange, you have become aware of some non-specific danger and need to ascertain whether there is a legitimate threat to your safety.

heads up and casually scanning their immediate area as well as what is just beyond. They see who and what is ahead of them, are aware of their environment to each side, and occasionally turn to scan behind them.

Condition Yellow is appropriate any time a person is in public. If you are armed in any way, it is essential. You should notice anything out of place, anyone looking or acting in an unusual manner, or anything that is simply out of context and further evaluate for potential threat. Examples might include a crowd gathered for no apparent reason, someone wearing heavy clothing on a summer day, a person studiously avoiding eye contact, anyone whose hands are hidden from view, a person moving awkwardly or with an unusual gait, or someone who simply stares at you for no apparent reason. Anything that stimulates your intuitive survival sense, suspicion, or curiosity should be studied more closely.

Condition Orange (Alert). People in Condition Orange have become aware of some non-specific danger (typically via Condition Yellow) and need to ascertain whether there is a legitimate threat to their safety. The difference between conditions Yellow and Orange is the identification of a specific target for further attention. You may have heard a nearby shout, the sound of glass breaking, or an unidentified sudden noise where you

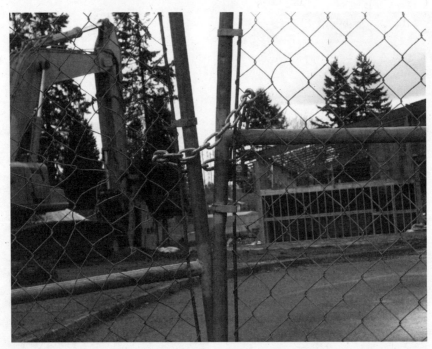

Be aware of potential escape routes before you need to use them. It does no good to attempt to flee danger only to find yourself trapped because you didn't know that your path was blocked.

would not have expected one. You might also have seen another person or a group of people acting abnormally, someone whose demeanor makes you feel uncomfortable, or somebody whose appearance or behavior stands out as unusual.

In this state, you should focus on the nebulous danger, but not to the exclusion of a broader awareness of your surroundings. Trouble may be starting in other places in addition to the one that has drawn your attention (for example, an ambush situation). It is wise to look for escape routes and nearby areas of cover or concealment. If unarmed, you should also try to spot objects that can be used as makeshift weapons or distractions. It may be prudent to reposition yourself to take advantage of cover, escape routes, or impromptu weapons should it become necessary to use them. It is usually premature to make any aggressive moves at this point.

If armed, it is a good idea to be sure that your weapon is accessible, though it is probably not prudent to call attention to it at this point. If in a lonely area like a parking garage, bathroom, or alley, it is usually wise to move into a better-lit or populated area like a restaurant or store. Denying privacy for criminal acts to occur or escalate once started is one of the most fundamental principles of self-defense.

This is also a good time to prepare a plan of action, contemplating what you might have to do should the danger become an imminent threat. If the trouble is immediate, but not directed at you it may be prudent to move to safety and then call for help to alert authorities to the incident. If the combatants overhear your call you may inadvertently make yourself a target of their wrath.

If, on the other hand, it turns out that trouble is not brewing, you simply return to Condition Yellow, abandoning the plan. Consider your effort good practice, be thankful that nothing untoward happened, and go on with your day. There is a pretty good chance that if the other guy was thinking of jumping you that he sensed your preparation and changed his mind. If, on the other hand, you become convinced that trouble truly is likely forthcoming, you will need to escalate to Condition Red.

Condition Red (Concerned). People in this condition have been confronted by a potential adversary or are in close proximity to someone who is becoming aggressive and is near enough to confront them quickly. Condition Red means that you have every reason to believe that the other guy(s) poses a clear and present danger to you or someone with you.

You must be prepared to fight, hopefully taking advantage of the plan you visualized in Condition Orange (assuming you had sufficient warning). At this point it is prudent to begin moving away toward escape routes, locations with strategic cover, or areas of concealment if you can do so. If the confrontation is immediate, it is often a good idea to try to move away from any weapons being brandished or distractions being made, while at the same time keeping well aware of them.

If you are armed and the situation warrants a lethal response, this may be the point where you draw and ready your weapon or at least make its presence known (see "Use Only as Much Force as the Situation Warrants" in Section Two to understand when lethal force may be appropriate). If you are carrying a gun, for example, this might include reaching under your jacket to grab a hold of your pistol and thumbing your holster's safety release. A verbal challenge at this point may prove useful if time permits. De-escalation may still be an option but it can also backfire so you must be prepared in case it does not work. Every reasonable attempt should still be made to avoid a fight yet you must resign yourself to the very real possibility that it will be unsuccessful.

While a show of ability and readiness to resist with countervailing force may stop the confrontation in its tracks, it could also elevate it to the next level, open conflict. Either way, your intent should be to stop the potential assault that is forthcoming, escape to safety, or stay safe until help arrives, and doing so without harming anyone including those threatening you. You must not want to kill or hurt anyone nor teach him a lesson. Such attitudes can make you the aggressor in the eyes of the law. In addition, even if you are never charged with a crime, you will still have to live with yourself afterward.

Condition Black (Under Attack). People in Condition Black are actively being attacked. Although it is possible to skip nearly instantly from Condition Yellow all the way up to Condition Black, encounters generally escalate at a pace where you can adjust your level of

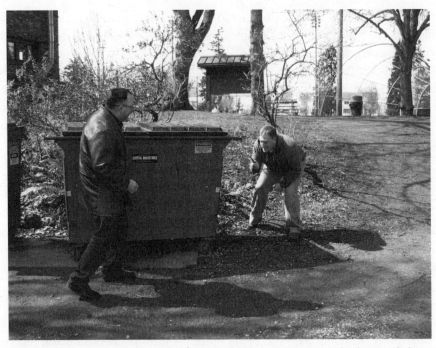

In Condition Red you have been confronted by a potential adversary or are in close proximity to someone who acting aggressively.

awareness incrementally so long as you did not start off in Condition White. This gives observant individuals a leg up in dealing with dangerous adversaries.

Once you have been assaulted, verbal challenges and de-escalation attempts are no longer useful. You must flee or fight back, using any appropriate distractions and/or weapons at your disposal. If armed and confronted by an armed attacker or multiple unarmed assailants, you may decide to use your weapon in self-defense. Shooting to "wound" and firing "warning" shots are Hollywood falderal; anytime you pull the trigger, it's very serious business. The same thing goes for knives, blunt instruments, and other impromptu weapons as well. Be sure that you are legally, ethically, and morally entitled to do so before employing potentially lethal countervailing force. Your intent must be to stop the assault that is in progress so that you can escape to safety or otherwise remain safe until help arrives. Your goal is to be safe, not to kill your attacker or teach him a lesson.

Each encounter is different; its unique characteristics will determine an appropriate response. It is important to use sufficient force to effectively control the situation and keep yourself safe without overreacting. You will, no doubt, want to treat a drunken relative at a family reunion quite differently than a homicidal street punk coming at you in a drug-induced rage. We'll talk more about this in Section Two.

Any time you are near others, especially strangers, it pays to be vigilant so as not to be

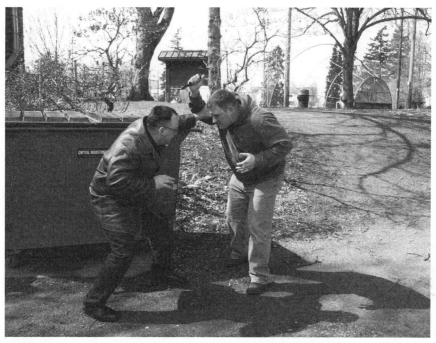

In Condition Black, you are actively being attacked. Verbal challenges and de-escalation attempts are no longer useful; you must flee or fight back.

caught unawares by sudden violence. If you appear to be a tough, prepared target, most predators, bullies, and thugs will look for their victims elsewhere. You cannot walk around in a constant state of hyper-vigilance, however. It's emotionally and physically untenable. A color code system, therefore, gives you a mental model that defines appropriate levels of situational awareness to help you strike the appropriate balance between obliviousness and paranoia. Using it can help keep you safe.

Don't Get Caught Up in the Escalato Follies

To begin by bluster, but afterwards to take fright at the enemy's numbers, shows a supreme lack of intelligence.

— Sun Tzu

Speed is not part of the true Way of strategy. Speed implies that things seem fast or slow, according to whether or not they are in rhythm. Whatever the Way, the master of strategy does not appear fast.

— Miyamoto Musashi

The "escalato follies" refer to the one-upmanship cycle that almost inevitably leads to physical violence unless one party backs down and breaks off the game. The term escalato was originally coined by musician, comedian, and political satirist Tom Lehrer to describe the process of irrational commitment where people continue to increase their investment in a decision despite evidence suggesting that it was the wrong thing to do. The current term in business and political circles is "escalation of commitment." It is also very closely tied in with threat displays. Actions that you do hoping the other guy will back off, so you don't need to use violence—sometimes they work, sometimes they make it worse.

You know the drill—you think I just ogled your girlfriend's ass so you glare at me. I was actually minding my own business, nursing a beer and spacing out, so I don't know what the heck you're pissed off about and flip you the bird in response to your getting in my face for no apparent reason. Now you're really mad 'cuz I'm a serious dickhead so you get in my face and start spewing insults. I'm not about to let you get away with that so I toss my beer in your face. You haul back to hit me but I beat you to the draw and kick you in the 'nads. You stumble backward, grab a pool cue, and bust it over my head.

> Escalato is a cycle of one-upmanship that inevitably leads to physical violence unless one party backs down and breaks off the game. The tougher you truly are, the less you should feel a need to prove it. Even if the other guy is a complete ass, it is far better to lose a little face than it is to fight to show that you are right, particularly when violence often leads to jail time, lawsuits, hospitalization, or in extreme cases, death. Do you want to be responsible for an accidental death because you lost your temper? Even if you are not charged with a crime could you live with yourself afterward knowing that you've taken a life and destroyed a family? While it may be pretty easy to rationalize what you did, justifying your actions in your own mind for the first few years, it's really tough to wake up every day for the rest of your life to the knowledge that you are a killer.

Things go downhill from there. By the time the dust settles, one of us is carried out on a gurney while the other gets to wear a stainless steel bracelet, earns a trip to the local police department, takes out a second mortgage to cover legal expenses, and quickly discovers that he's seriously screwed up his life.

While this example makes light of a truly significant incident, this kind of scenario plays itself out all the time in real life. Seriously, these escalato follies are a supremely dangerous game—one you really, really do not want to play. Win or lose, there's always a cost to it, usually a big one.

One way to avoid getting caught up in the escalato game is by knowing how to respond rather than react. Responding is a planned course of action, one that leaves you in control of your emotions and actions. Reacting, on the other hand, cedes control to the opponent. If you become angry, defensive, or otherwise emotionally involved, it is easy to get caught up in the cycle.

It is supremely important that you respond to an aggressor's actions rather than react to them. Even if the other guy is a complete ass, it is far better to lose face while remaining alive and free than fighting to prove you're right. While violence often results only in bruises to the body and/or ego, it can easily end with someone's disfigurement, death, or imprisonment. It is never worth such extreme consequences just to prove your point.

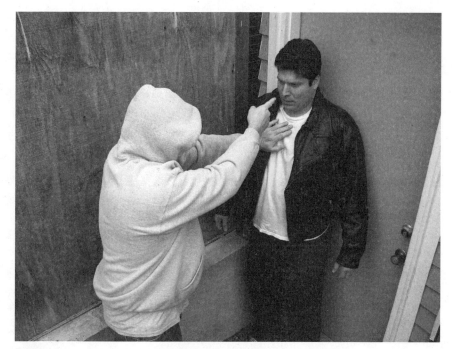

Responding is a planned course of action, one that leaves you in control of your emotions and actions. Reacting, on the other hand, cedes control to the opponent.

So, you may be asking yourself, "Does that sort of thing really happen in real life? Come on, man, dying from a fistfight? That's outrageous." Unfortunately, it is not only possible, but also even probable. It happens all the time.

For example, Mark Leidheisl, 39, a regional senior vice president for Wells Fargo Bank, died on April 20, 2005, from a blunt force trauma injury to the head. Sacramento police reported that the incident that led to Leidheisl's death might have been fueled by road rage and that he appeared to have been the aggressor. An unmarked medicine bottle in Leidheisl's car contained Paxil (an antidepressant), morphine (a powerful painkiller), and an unidentified third pill type. Tests later found that he had a blood alcohol level of at least 0.13 (more than the legal driving limit of 0.08) and opiates in his system. Drugs, alcohol, and violence frequently go together, with very bad results.

Here's what happened: Reports state that Leidheisl allegedly cut off another vehicle while driving out of Arco Arena's parking lot after the Wednesday night game. Leidheisl, a friend and the two men in the other vehicle reportedly exchanged heated words, stopped and got out of their vehicles on a nearby street. During the subsequent fight, Leidheisl fell and hit his head on the pavement, causing the fatal injury. The suspects from the other vehicle, ages 43 and 44, reportedly left but contacted police after seeing news reports about how seriously Leidheisl was hurt.

District Attorney Jan Scully told reporters, "After a thorough review of the police investigation, it is clear that Mark Leidheisl died as a result of mutual combat between him and Jeffrey Berndt. One punch thrown in self-defense by Jeffrey Berndt struck Mark Leidheisl in the face, causing him to fall backwards striking his head on the asphalt pavement. This fall fractured Leidheisl's skull, causing his death."

A few moments of road rage, or perhaps more accurately parking lot rage, and a guy was dead. Not just any guy, mind you, but someone with a great career, a ton of friends, a wonderful family, and a whole lot to live for. Now, Leidheisl's wife Holly and his 12-year-old son Taylor will never see him again. It was not intentional, of course, but accidents can and do happen. Do you want to be responsible for an accidental death because you lost your temper? Even if you are not charged with a crime, could you live with yourself afterward knowing that you've taken a life and destroyed a family? While it may be pretty easy to rationalize what you did, justifying your actions in your own mind for the first few years, it's really tough to wake up every day for the rest of your life to the knowledge that you are a killer.

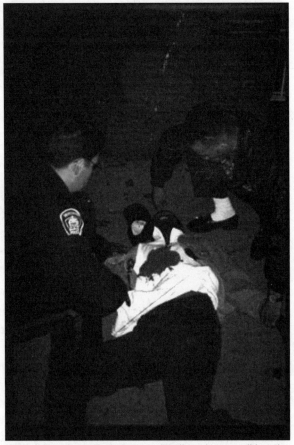

While it may be pretty easy to rationalize what you did at the time, particularly if it was truly was self-defense, it's really tough to wake up every day for the rest of your life to the knowledge that you are a killer.

Anger should be used strategically as a tool, never as an unchecked emotion. If you really are upset about something, you generally cannot afford to show it. On the job, you can be perceived as a "loose cannon" by your manager and/or co-workers, facing disciplinary action or possible termination. At home or among friends, you can irreparably harm your interpersonal relationships. Walking away until you can control your anger is best.

If you need to prove a point and you are not actually furious, on the other hand, feigned anger can sometimes be an effective tool. Consider disciplining children—if you yell at them too often they become desensitized. If you do it judiciously, they may learn important life lessons and grow up to become better people. The same thing applies to venting feigned rage. You can get away with it only rarely, however, since the vast majority of people remember negative emotions longer than positive ones, hence a long memory of your actions. That means that you really need to save this tactic for the time at which you need it the most.

In his best-selling book, *The 7 Habits of Highly Effective People*, business guru Steven Covey described a concept called idiosyncratic credit. You can think of it as an emotional bank account. Whenever you do good things for the people you are close to and treat them with dignity and respect, you build up credit in your account. Whenever you become abrasive or insensitive, you make withdrawals. So long as the balance remains positive, you remain on their "good" side. Blowing up at someone uses up a huge amount of idiosyncratic credit so make your withdrawals wisely.

Avoid the escalato follies at all costs. Keep your ego in check. In addition, do your best to verbally de-escalate a confrontation before it becomes violent. Apologizing for some perceived slight, even when you did nothing wrong, often beats the alternative.

The Victim Interview

Thus, what enables the wise sovereign and the good general to strike and conquer, and achieve things beyond the reach of ordinary men, is foreknowledge.
— *Sun Tzu*

It is important in strategy to know the enemy's sword and not to be distracted by insignificant movements of his sword. You must study this. The gaze is the same for single combat and for large-scale strategy.
— *Miyamoto Musashi*

Muggers, thugs, robbers, bullies, gang bangers, and rapists all have one thing in common: They are happy to dish out pain, but are quite reluctant to be on the receiving end of it. Consequently, before a bad guy tees off on you, he will evaluate his odds of success. This evaluation is often called an "interview." Unlike a job search, however, this is one interview that you really do not want to pass. Passing means that you appear to be an easy target. To the other guy, you've got a giant "V" for victim stamped on your forehead. This interview may be conducted by a single individual or a group of thugs. Either way, knowing the common tactics people who mean you harm might employ can help you respond appropriately.

During these interviews, your goal is to be both calm and resolute. This is Condition Red stuff, a specific threat aimed squarely toward you, so be prepared to act accordingly. If you are approached by a single individual, be wary of bystanders who may join him. Don't forget to glance behind you when prudent because his partner(s) may

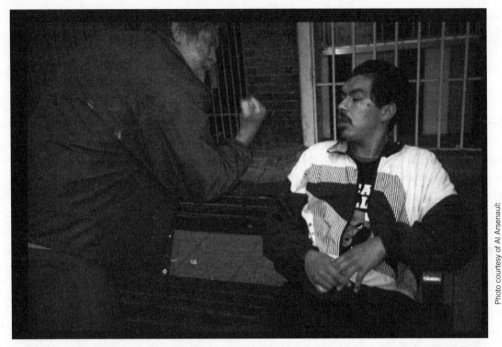

Photo courtesy of Al Arsenault

Before a bad guy attacks he will evaluate his odds of success. In general, the less you look and act like a victim during this "interview" process, the safer you will be.

be approaching from that direction. Use reflections and shadows to sense what's going on. Furthermore, pay attention to escape routes should you need to fight your way free. Be wary of the bad guy's hands, particularly if you cannot see both of them, as he may very well be armed and preparing to use his weapon against you.

The less you look and act like a victim during the interview process, the safer you will be. It helps to know what you might face and visualize how best to respond ahead of time. There are five different types of interviews, which you may encounter: (1) hot (spur of the moment), (2) escalating, (3) regular, (4) silent, and (5) prolonged.

If you are in a martial arts program or sign up for a weekend self-defense course, you may have the opportunity to practice responding to "woofers" who play the bad guy's role in the interview process. Instructors can help you learn the right ways to deal with tense situations by play-acting, leading you through various scenarios and then debriefing your performance afterward. If you do not have access or are not interested in this sort of training, it is still prudent to at least visualize such encounters and think about what your response options might be.

The following types of interviews were first codified by Marc "Animal" MacYoung in his book *Safe in the City: A Streetwise Guide to Avoid Being Robbed, Raped, Ripped Off, Or Run Over* (co-written with Chris Pfouts).

1. Hot Interviews. Hot interviews are sudden, unexpected, and frequently powerfully emotional. Maybe you are minding your own business nursing a beer when suddenly a guy gets in your face and begins shouting obscenities. Or, perhaps, you get the classic, "What are you looking at?" line. This is not a physical attack yet, but rather an emotional one. If you are not accustomed to dealing with this type of extreme outburst and react in a dazed or confused manner, you will almost certainly be perceived as an easy victim. Physical violence will surely follow while you are too disoriented to respond coherently.

You must immediately shift to Condition Red, demonstrating resolute commitment to defend yourself with countervailing force in order to fail this type of interview. This means you look and act as if you're ready to tee off on the guy without actually taking any action (yet). If you are a trained martial artist, straighten your spine, control your breathing, and set yourself for attack while verbally fending off the adversary. Keep your hands in front of you and make a fence that allows you sufficient space in which to work. A calm, prepared demeanor can be quite intimidating to folks who know how to read it. Most thugs are very astute at reading body language; after all, they don't survive too long on the street without that skill.

If you are not a trained fighter, you can do a good job of faking it by centering yourself, keeping your hands up with your arms bent and elbows down to keep some space between you and the bad guy, and balancing your weight evenly on both feet. Rather than getting ready to fight, be prepared to bolt to safety. Ask a police officer sometime, it's very hard to contain someone who really wants to get away from you. Use this to your advantage.

Regardless of your level of training or preparedness, remember that he has not attacked yet. You legally cannot thump him first in most cases. Demonstrating that you are ready to do so, however, may very well end the encounter without the need for violence.

> Criminals, bullies, and thugs choose their victims carefully, preying on oblivious, feeble, or otherwise ill-prepared individuals who make easy targets. Before they strike, they look you over to evaluate their odds of success, using hot, escalating, regular, silent, or prolonged interviews. After all, it's best when pain only goes one way—from them to you. Consequently, the less you look and act like a victim during this examination process, the safer you will be. It helps to know what you might face and visualize how best to respond ahead of time. The set up typically involves four elements, dialogue, deception, distraction, and destruction. If you can see through his ruse, you can force the other guy to abort short of the fourth step, the actual attack.

2. Escalating Interviews. Unlike a hot interview, which begins with immediate hostility, an escalating interview starts out fairly benign yet rapidly turns hostile. The bad guy will test your boundaries by making increasingly outrageous demands or exhibiting more and more contemptible behavior. This type of thing is much easier to shut off early than late. Each concession in each encounter establishes a pattern or habit of conceding. For example, he might begin with a statement like, "You're in my chair!" and then proceed to demand payment for rent. Every time he succeeds in pushing your boundaries, his confidence will grow. He will go from abrasive, to abusive, to outright physically violent.

The key to stopping an escalating interview is the same as it is for a hot one, demonstrating that you are prepared to respond violently if necessary. The good news, however, is that you get a bit more time to wrap your mind around what is happening and formulate a proper response. Pay attention to escape routes, impromptu weapons, bystanders, and other factors that might come into play if things get rough.

3. Regular Interviews. Regular interviews generally begin with some type of distraction such as asking for directions, the time, or a cigarette. While he is talking to you, the adversary will be evaluating your awareness, calculating his odds of success, and stealthily positioning himself to attack. This is a common tactic of muggers and criminals who want to steal your stuff but can also be used by bullies looking for a fight as well.

Be wary of the dialogue; it is a set-up. The appropriate response to whatever the other guy asks for is "no." Furthermore, insist that he keeps his distance. A five-foot rule is useful. Shout something along the lines of "back off... give me five feet." There are few legitimate reasons for a person you don't know to be closer than five feet from you in a public place. Five feet gives you enough space to spot threat indicators, weapons, and offensive movements and get a moment of time in which to take defensive action.

Sneak attackers may use just about any dirty trick to disguise their intent, get close enough to launch their assault, and keep you from responding until it is too late to defend yourself. This process, sometimes called the "four Ds" by self-defense experts, includes dialogue, deception, distraction, and destruction.

Dialogue creates a distraction while letting your adversary control the distance between you. It is the set up to get him close enough to his intended victim where he can use the element of surprise to strike with impunity. That means that he must be within three to five feet away in order to hit you with anything other than a projectile weapon. The closer he is the less warning you get and the harder it is to defend yourself.

Deception disguises the predatory nature of the adversary, letting him blend into the crowd and making him appear as harmless as possible until it is too late. Much of deception is based on body language and behavior, though it can include things like wearing clothing designed to blend in and disguise the presence of weapons too.

Distraction sets up the attack, typically by asking a question or otherwise using verbal techniques. It can also include gestures or body movements such as when he suddenly widens his eyes and looks over your shoulder to get you to look behind you and expose your back.

Destruction is the physical assault, robbery, rape, or murder. It could be something more innocuous such as a pick pocketing too. When violence is in the cards, if he can successfully distract you he can get in at least one or two good blows before you realize what is going on and attempt to respond. It's very tough to fight back once you are surprised, behind the count, injured, and reeling from the pain.

Despite these four Ds, it is exceedingly rare for the victim to be caught totally unaware. For example, even if he was sucker punched, most assault victims report that they saw the blow coming but did not have time to react. Even when long-range weapons are involved (such as firearms), fights typically begin close up. Unarmed confrontations always take place at close range. If you can see your attacker, you should not be surprised by an attack. Your level of awareness and preparedness should ratchet up a bit whenever a stranger is close enough to strike, at least until you have given him a thorough once-over and dismissed any threat.

4. **Silent Interviews.** A silent interview is when a bad guy puts himself in a position to observe and evaluate you. If you look wary and confident, he will very likely select someone else to pick on; whereas, if you are oblivious and unprepared, he will mark you as a target. Unlike a hot, escalating, or regular interview, he may never utter a word. The whole thing takes place in his head.

For example, he might position himself near an ATM, waiting for potential victims who withdraw large amounts of cash. Or, perhaps, he might be sitting in a box van in a parking lot waiting for victims to wander by so that he can pull them into the vehicle and drive off. Once he makes his presence known, you may have only seconds to react. If you can shift from Condition Yellow to Condition Red fast enough, he may sense your preparedness and break off his attack, turning into a "just messing with you, ha, ha, ha" kind of scenario. Because you were not aware that you were being interviewed, you may very well have to fight your way out of such encounters.

The key to fending off silent interviews is good situational awareness. If you look like a tough, prepared target, or can spot the other guy fast enough, he may balk, break off his attack, and go off in search for an easier victim. Put yourself in the bad guy's place. Any time you are near a potential ambush position, kick your awareness up another notch. Pay attention not only to the place, but also to the time as well. Using an ATM kiosk during broad daylight in a crowded mall during the holiday shopping season is safer than using an identical one in the parking lot of that same mall late on a summer night. You get the idea.

5. **Prolonged Interviews.** Prolonged interviews take place over long periods and may be combined with other types of interviews. Stalkers, con artists, and serial rapists often watch their victims for days if not weeks before they act. Consequently, maintaining an adequate level of awareness whenever you are in a public place is a good idea. Even within your own home, it is smart to retain a level of vigilance. Take precautions such as keeping your doors and windows locked, trimming back concealing foliage, installing motion sensor lights that turn on when intruders enter your yard, using a monitored alarm system, and paying attention to passers-by.

Regardless of how you are interviewed by a potential aggressor to evaluate their odds of success, the less you look and act like a victim during the interview process the safer you will be. Knowing what you might expect and practicing (and/or visualizing) how you might respond ahead of time places you in a position of strength when you encounter these behaviors on the street.

Know When He's Eager to Hit You

Therefore, the good fighter will be terrible in his onset, and prompt in his decision.

– Sun Tzu

In single combat, also, you must use the advantage of taking the enemy unawares by frightening him with your body, long sword, or voice, to defeat him. You should research this well.

– Miyamoto Musashi

Violence rarely happens in a vacuum. There is always some escalation process—even a really short one—that precedes it. Hot, escalating, regular, silent, or prolonged interviews take place while the other guy sizes you up and determines whether or not you will be an easy mark. Glaring, staring, shoving, arguing, threatening, yelling, or other clear signs of escalation precede the majority of violent encounters.

Insults and other forms of verbal abuse are common precursors to a fight. Oftentimes, the other guy is trying to intimidate you. He might also be trying to goad you into throwing the first blow so that he has a legitimate excuse to stomp a mud hole in you. Swallow your pride and walk away if you can. The more dangerous you are, the less you should feel a need to prove it.

There are typically two types of aggressors who might confront you on the street, dominance attackers and predators. Dominance attackers want to feel superior to their victim. If you walk away from one of these individuals, he will generally be happy to let you go in peace. He feels that he has won by making you back down. Predatory attackers, on the other hand, want a victim who will not put up a fight. If you walk away from one of these individuals, you may trigger the very attack you were trying to avoid.

Nevertheless, trying to leave puts you on better legal ground if you ultimately have to fight back, particularly if witnesses observe what happened or the incident ends up being captured on film or video. With the prevalence of closed-circuit security monitors, cell phone cameras, traffic cams, and other forms of electronic surveillance out there, that's not an unrealistic situation.

While the escalation process varies from encounter to encounter, there are certain common behaviors that may lead to violence. Possible trouble indicators include

- Glaring, staring, or otherwise "sizing you up."
- Attempts by an individual or group to follow, herd (control your direction), flank, or mirror your movements.
- Making unprovoked accusations, threats, aggressive requests, demands, or using foul language for no apparent reason.
- Baiting or attempting to provoke an aggressive response from you (for example, "What's your problem?" or "What are you looking at?").
- Closing, moving into a range that enables the other guy to attack, particularly when the movements are covert or sudden.
- Unusual or out-of-place body movements, aggressive gestures, agitated pacing, clenched fists, forward weight shift, straightening the spine, or adopting a fighting stance.

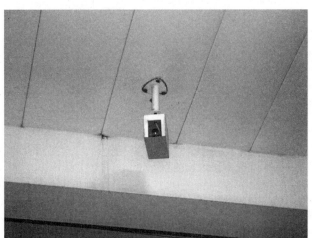

With ubiquitous closed-circuit security monitors, cell phone cameras, traffic cams, and other forms of electronic surveillance out there it is reasonable to assume that everything you do during a violent encounter will be captured on film. Act accordingly.

- Clearing space to move or draw a weapon.
- Hands and/or teeth clenched, neck taut, or other stiff or shaking body movements.
- Shouting to startle or paralyze you as an attack begins.

While it is common to experience this type of obvious escalation, ambushes also occur. In such situations, the escalation has already occurred, yet the victim is unaware of it because it took place solely within the mind of the attacker. He has already looked you over, conducted a mental interview to ascertain that you are an easy target, and decided upon a course of action against you. This summing up can cause a situation where you have no choice but to fight.

Regrettably, most people are simply not mentally prepared to react to sudden violence, needlessly being hurt or killed despite the fact that they saw it coming. It does not matter why you were attacked, simply that you were attacked. Do not deny what is happening at the time, but rather respond appropriately to defend yourself. Worry about making sense of the encounter afterward.

The good news, however, is that there are physiological, behavioral, and verbal indicators that you can spot to warn you of imminent conflict. Some are subtle and may indicate nothing of an alarming nature. Other indicators are overtly hostile and should cause immediate action. Most fall in between and require judgment to be applied before taking action.

As a general rule, you should err on the side of caution, trying to avoid or evade problem situations before they spin out of control. It is important to trust your instincts in such situations. Whether you see it or not, there will often be some indicator that can warn you of a person's intent just before he attacks.

This indicator is often called the "tell." Poker players coined this term, which refers to some movement or gesture that lets them figure out when an opponent is bluffing. In the self-defense and martial arts communities, the tell has been called many things, such as the adrenal dump or the twitch. If you do not see the tell you are bound to lose. Even if you are really, really fast, action is always faster than reaction. In other words, missing the tell is what gets you sucker punched. Recovery after the first strike is challenging, though not impossible.

Looking for the tell involves noticing the really small physical movements a person might make to signal intent to attack as well as subtle changes in the person's energy. Physical signs are essentially manifestations of an adrenal response that implies a person is about to attack. These indicators could include a slight drop of the shoulder, a tensing of the neck, or a puckering of the lips. You will also want to trust your intuition here to discern a change in the person's energy, virtually undetectable from a physical standpoint but easy to spot once you know what you are looking for.

Some examples of where changes of energy may constitute a tell include:

> Violence doesn't happen in a vacuum. There is always some type of escalation process beforehand, even if it is really short or takes place solely in the mind of the aggressor. By understanding the indicators of a forthcoming attack you will have a better opportunity to avoid confrontations altogether, or where necessary, defend yourself effectively. If you miss these vital clues, you will have a tough time responding to sudden violence. It is even worse if you are thinking "fist," failing to notice the knife in his grip. Armed or unarmed, if you don't see an attack until the last moment you will be at a severe disadvantage. It takes a certain amount of time to realize what is happening, shift your mental gears, form a plan of action, adopt a defensive posture, and ward off the attack. Unless you're highly skilled and very well trained, you won't have enough time to respond to a surprise attack without getting hurt.

- A person who was standing still moves slightly. A weight shift is far subtler than a step, but the change is possibly preparation for attack.
- A sudden pallor or sudden flushing of the person's face (that is, an adrenaline-induced vasoconstriction).
- A person who was looking at you suddenly looks away or, conversely, a person who was looking away suddenly makes eye contact.
- A change in the rate, tone, pitch, or volume of a person's voice. An overt example is when someone who is shouting becomes suddenly quiet or, conversely, one who has been quiet begins raising his or her voice.

• A sudden change in the person's breathing (i.e., shallow and fast for untrained adversaries; slow and deep for trained opponents)

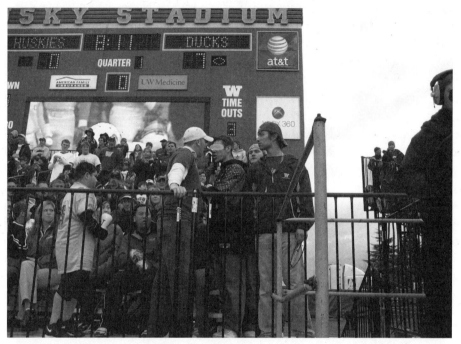

Whether you see it or not, there is almost always some indicator that warns you of a person's intent just before he attacks. Missing this "tell." is what gets you sucker punched.

By understanding the indicators of a potential attack, you will have a better opportunity to avoid confrontations altogether, or where necessary, defend yourself effectively. Action being faster than reaction, the earlier you identify these indicators, the better prepared and safer you will be. Know when he is eager to hit you; it gives you a leg up when it becomes necessary to counterattack.

Don't Let Them Get Into Position for Attack

You can be sure of succeeding in your attacks if you only attack places that are undefended.

— Sun Tzu

What is big is easy to perceive; what is small is difficult to perceive.
— Miyamoto Musashi

It's common knowledge that bad guys cheat to win. These people aren't going to pick a fair fight with someone when they stand a good chance of getting hurt in the process. Your adversary, therefore, will want to surprise and overwhelm you whenever possible. He may very well deploy a weapon as well. Furthermore, thugs often work together in small groups to stack the odds even higher in their direction.

The good news is that the bad guys cannot hurt you if they cannot reach you. In order to pull off a successful attack, the other guy needs to close distance and move into a position from which he can strike. Fists, feet, knives, blunt instruments, and other hand-held weapons require close range to be effective. Even gunfights typically take place at close range. According to Federal Bureau of Investigation statistics, about half of all gun murder victims are killed from a range of five feet or less. Consequently, the aforementioned five-foot rule is good to remember.

Unless a lot of alcohol or drugs are involved, however, you will rarely be attacked in the middle of a crowd. Here the adversary has less control over the encounter and is more likely to get caught. Further, while a bad guy may attempt to take you to an isolated place to commit the violence he intends, he is not likely to find too many victims in remote, secluded locations. Consequently, fringe areas adjacent to heavily traveled public places are where the majority of violent crimes occur. This includes areas such as parking lots, bathrooms, stairwells, laundry rooms, phone booths, ATM kiosks, and the like.

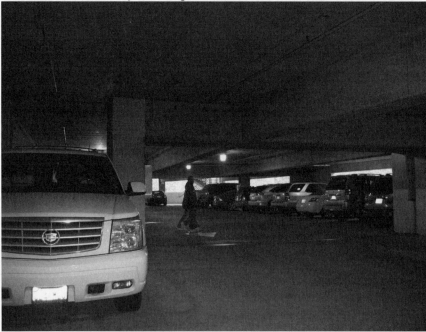

Fringe areas adjacent to heavily traveled public places are where the majority of violent crimes occur.

Your level of awareness should be kicked up a notch whenever you travel through these fringe areas. Pay attention to other individuals and behaviors that may constitute a threat. There are a variety of tactics that bad guys might use to get themselves into position to attack you. These include closing, cornering, surprising, pincering, herding, or surrounding.

Closing

Fights, even most gunfights in civilian settings, begin up close. Consequently, the most common method of getting close enough to attack is simply by walking up to the victim. This is often combined with some type of distraction, typically verbal, to help the bad guy seem less threatening while he maneuvers himself into position to strike. Remember the four Ds (dialogue, deception, distraction, and destruction)? The goal is to move in close so that he can surprise and overwhelm you with the attack.

There is no legitimate reason for a person you do not know to get closer than five feet from you on the street unless you are in the middle of a large crowd or sitting on public transportation (for example, busses, subways, trains). Trust your intuition. If he makes you uncomfortable and tries to close distance, warn him away. Don't worry about being rude or breaking some social norm. It is better to be a little embarrassed and safe than beaten to a pulp and sorry. After all, this is someone you've never met before and will likely never meet again. Anyone who insists on closing after you have warned him away has clearly announced that his intentions are less than honorable. Demand space and be prepared to fight if it is not given.

> Fringe areas adjacent to heavily traveled public places are where the majority of violent crimes occur. This includes areas such as parking lots, bathrooms, stairwells, laundry rooms, phone booths, ATM kiosks, and the like. In order to initiate an attack, the bad guy(s) must close distance and/or control your movement in order to get into range. They can do this by closing, cornering, surprising, pincering, herding, or surrounding you. Spotting these behaviors ahead of time gives you a fighting chance.

Cornering

Cornering or trapping is another common approach, one that is a bit more strategic than simple closing. The bad guy angles his approach in a manner that traps you between him and a solid object such as the wall of a building or a parked vehicle if you are outside on the street. A variation you might find indoors is to block the only doorway into a room so that you need to go through him in order to escape.

A common cornering method is to approach a person when he's getting into his car, particularly in store parking lots where you are also carrying encumbering purchases and valuables such as cash and credit cards. Think about how long it takes to pull your keys out of your pocket, insert them into the lock, turn the lock, open the door, slip inside, close and lock the door, start up the vehicle, and drive away. You are vulnerable during most of those steps, trapped between the bad guy and your vehicle or stuck in the vehicle with the door open before you can get it closed and drive away. It takes even longer if you need to drop a bunch of packages into the trunk or back seat first.

Cornering behavior should always be a concern, particularly in fringe areas where attacks are more likely to occur. When traveling in these areas pay close attention to alternate routes you might take in order to effect an escape. If your awareness is sufficient, you should be able to spot this behavior and move in an alternate direction before you can become effectively trapped.

Surprising

Surprising requires a source of concealment from which the bad guy might spring when he chooses to attack. This can include trees, bushes, doorways, parked vehicles, garbage bins, or any other barriers behind which he can hide yet track your movements and step out to attack. Even pools of darkness between streetlights can be used for surprise if you are inattentive.

Pay careful attention to your environment, particularly in areas you frequent such as the sidewalk near your home, office, school, and so on. Look at these areas through the lens of a mugger. What are the sources of cover or concealment? If you were the bad guy, where would you hide? Once you know these locations, you can give them a quick once-over before you pass by, thwarting most surprise attacks.

Don't forget that he needs free access to be able to move out and attack you quickly, so he won't be in something like a garbage bin but rather hiding alongside it. Doors, on the other hand, facilitate rapid egress so he could be sitting in a vehicle or standing behind the entrance to a building.

Pincering

Bad guys often work together. If you wind up running across two adversaries working in tandem, they have additional tricks to get you into position for attack. The most common of these is a pincer movement where one guy distracts you so that the other can sneak up on you from behind. The bad guys might split up as they approach you or spread out so that you pass one before being accosted by the other. That way one is already behind you since you have walked past him on your own accord.

Be wary of individuals who ping your radar as you approach. Don't worry about embarrassing yourself by overreacting; just turn around and walk away. Similarly, if one or more individuals who were together split up as they approach you, angle off in another direction. If they start to follow, their intent will be clear. More often than not, your awareness marks you as a difficult target and they will find someone else to pick on.

Herding

Groups of bad guys working together have a bigger bag of tricks with which to maneuver you into position for attack. Another method that can be performed by two or more thugs working together is called herding. This is similar to what carnivores do in the wild. An individual makes his presence known in a manner that causes you enough concern to want to move to a safer location. As you attempt to flee, the bad guys control available routes along which you can travel in order to herd you toward a choke point where one or more members are waiting and planning to act. If you fail to take the hint and move, the assault takes place where you first made contact with the individual or group.

It is important to pay attention to your environment at all times. Your best defense, particularly in areas that you are familiar with, is to know a variety of available escape routes for wherever you plan to travel. Of course, travel during daylight when you can and avoid choke points to the extent practicable, particularly in fringe areas at night. If you begin to feel uncomfortable with a developing situation, move toward highly populated, well-lit areas. This denies the bad guys the privacy necessary to attack you without being observed and increases their chances of getting caught, hence encourages them to target someone else.

If you think you have thwarted this type of trap, it's a good idea to dial 9-1-1 or your local emergency number to report the suspicious activities. Just because you were able to avoid the ambush doesn't mean that the next guy who happens along will too. As a good citizen, you can help others avoid becoming victims by drawing police attention to the area.

Surrounding

It gets even tougher when three or more bad guys work in concert. Again, one will often try to distract you while the others move to surround you and cut off all avenues for escape. Typically, they will casually drift apart as you approach. Like the pincer movement, the group might also spread out so that you pass alongside them before being accosted. When you reach the midpoint of the group, the wings fold in to trap you.

Once again, be wary of individuals who ping your radar as you approach. If it is a large group, turn around and walk away. Listen for signs of pursuit and calmly check back over your shoulder after fifteen feet or so to see if they are starting to follow you. Do your best to show no fear but rather resolute preparedness. Similarly, if one or more individuals who were together split up as they approach you, angle off in another direction. If they start to follow, their intent will be clear. Fighting a large group is a losing proposition. Your best defense is good situational awareness. Never get close enough to the bad guys to be in danger.

Don't forget that fringe areas adjacent to heavily traveled public places are where the majority of violent crimes occur. Do your best to avoid such areas late at night. Maintain a higher level of awareness whenever you must travel through or visit areas like parking lots, bathrooms, bus terminals, subways, train stations, stairwells, laundry rooms, or phone booths. Assaults can occur at any time of the day or night.

Be extra vigilant if you ran afoul of someone in a sporting venue, party, or drinking establishment, even if it never came to blows. He may be lurking, hoping to cut you off as you travel through a fringe area to get to your vehicle, catch a cab or a bus, or walk home. Similarly, be cautious around banks, pawnshops, check cashing establishments, casinos, and ATM kiosks where predators may be looking to separate you from your money.

In all of these situations, the bad guy must close distance or control your movement in order to get into range to attack you. Don't let him do it.

Avoid Being Cut from the Herd

By discovering the enemy's dispositions and remaining invisible ourselves, we can keep our forces concentrated, while the enemy's must be divided.
— *Sun Tzu*

In large-scale strategy, we deploy our troops for battle bearing in mind our strength, observing the enemy's numbers, and noting the details of the battlefield. This is at the start of the battle.
— *Miyamoto Musashi*

If you ever get the chance to ask a rancher or somebody who has raised farm animals about the phrase, "cut from the herd," you will hear them talk about picking one animal as a target and then using a dog and horse to separate it from the group. There aren't all that many ranchers around to interview so you are more likely to have experienced this type of behavior on television. Predators hunting in the wild do not want to tangle with tough targets that might cause them injury, so they try to cut a weak, infirm, or young animal from the herd, isolating it from the protection of the group prior to moving in for the kill. This is done to gain advantage, to make the kill as easy and efficient as possible.

This same type of behavior occurs within the human realm as well. Predators stack the deck in order to increase their odds of winning. Cutting from the herd means that the bad guy gains the advantage in numbers, determines the time, chooses the place, has the element of surprise, and is not observed by others. These points are elaborated as follows:

- **Gains the advantage in numbers.** No intelligent animal will pick a fight unless it believes it will win (or has far more to lose by not fighting). Changing the numbers to create an advantage is, therefore, fundamental. This means either separating the victim from a larger group to battle one-on-one without interference or working with other predators to outnumber the chosen victim before the fight. Similarly, choosing a weak opponent or making him weaker is just as fundamental.

A numbers advantage makes even a strong adversary weaker.

• **Determines the time.** Odds are that you will not be attacked when you're ready and raring to go. If the time of attack is determined by the aggressor, then it is by definition not chosen by the victim. In choosing the time of the attack, the aggressor is prepared while the victim is not. The predator can wait until his prey is distracted, encumbered, preoccupied, or otherwise ill prepared to fight.

• **Chooses the place.** When the attacker determines the place, he can take the high ground, spring from ambush, attack when the glare of the sun reduces the victim's ability to see, or otherwise take tactical advantage of the terrain. Scouting the best site for attack means that the predator knows the environment, anticipates escape routes, identifies sources of impromptu weapons, precludes intervention from bystanders, and otherwise takes best advantage of the optimal place to fight.

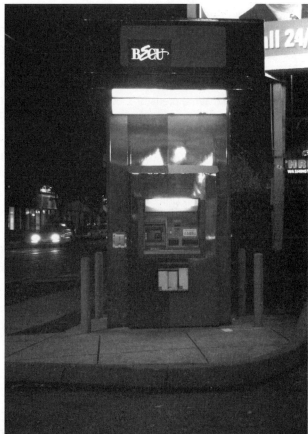

Be extra cautious around banks, pawnshops, check cashing establishments, casinos, and ATM kiosks where predators may be looking to separate you from your money.

• **Has the element of surprise.** When time and place are chosen by the aggressor, the element of surprise completes the preparation triad for the perfect attack. There is no guarantee, of course, but action being faster than reaction, surprise is a powerful advantage indeed. By the time the victim realizes what has occurred, it is already too late to escape without a fight.

• **Is not observed by others.** As a general rule, the more public the situation the safer you will be insomuch as violent crime is concerned. Certainly, riots run counter to this principle and certain crimes such as pick pocketing are facilitated by the anonymity that crowds provide. Terrorist bombers also target populated areas at peak traffic times. People who are showboating to gain social status also crave attention, as exemplified by all the fight videos you can find posted on

Animals in the wild cut from the herd to single out weaker prey. Violent individuals use the same tactic in the human jungle to waylay their victims. Cutting from the herd means that the predator gains the advantage in numbers, determines the time, chooses the place, has the element of surprise, and is not observed by others. That's a seriously unfair fight, one you are bound to lose. Don't let yourself be cut from the herd.

YouTube.com. Nevertheless, the majority of violent acts are perpetrated by one attacker against one victim or among small groups. Relatively few violent acts occur in front of large numbers of witnesses unless the perpetrator is mentally deficient and/or under the influence of drugs that limit his or her inhibitions. If the predator is unobserved by witnesses or surveillance cameras, no one can testify about his actions. Similarly, there is no one hanging around who might choose to intervene. Consequently, he has a better chance of getting away with his crime.

Let's review an everyday example of how "cutting from the herd" actually works. You have been drinking at the local tavern, and eventually visit the restroom. You are standing at the urinal minding your own business when suddenly a guy comes up behind you, and growls, "That's my girl, you SOB. You need to stay away from her!"

Let's evaluate your predicament against the predator checklist:

✓**Gains advantage in numbers: Check.** By waiting for you to go to the men 's room, he is able to isolate you from your friends or anyone who may come to your aid, physically or verbally. This includes the referee of the tavern, the bouncer. If you're really unlucky, he might have brought his friends in with him.

✓**Determines the time: Check.** He waited for you to go to the men's room, but it also took him three or four beers and twenty minutes of internal dialogue to screw up the courage to wait for you there. By the time he confronts you, he has worked himself into a frenzy, injected plenty of liquid courage, and is raring to go. You, on the other hand, are literally caught with your pants down, well unzipped anyway. Not exactly your best time to fight.

✓**Chooses the place: Check.** He could have jumped you at your table, waited for you in the parking lot by your car, hung out in the hallway for you to use the phone, or selected any other location, yet the men's room is the optimal choice. You are less likely to be prepared to fight. Furthermore, it is more confined, has better privacy, and is easier to control. He's picked the ideal place to do you in.

✓**Has the element of surprise: Check.** You are busy. In order to use the urinal, you must have your back to anybody who decides to approach you. Furthermore, you are unlikely to pay much attention to other people around you. It's socially unacceptable to look at other guys in the men's room, right? Similarly,

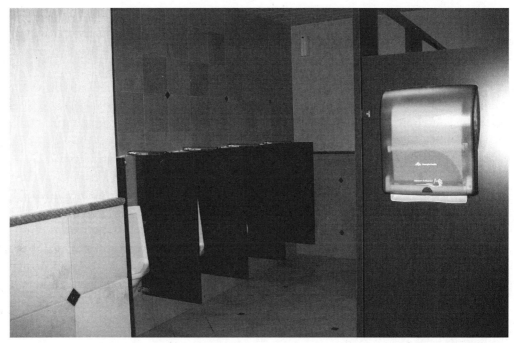

While it is socially unacceptable to look too closely at those around you in a public restroom, it is an isolated area that can give a bad guy the privacy he needs to attack. If ambushed you may be caught with your pants down, ill prepared to fight.

you are equally unlikely to turn around quickly when you hear him come in. He intuitively knows that you expect to be left alone when going to the bathroom so this will catch you off guard.

✓ **Is not observed by others: Check.** The restroom has only one way to enter or leave. It is small, constrained by stall walls, and provides little room to maneuver. It is relatively easy to lock the door, block or jam it with something, and assure a moment of complete privacy for the attack.

In this scenario, if a fight ensues you are almost certain to lose. You may still have some tricks up your sleeve like peeing on his foot to distract him, but it's still awful tough to fight when you've been taken by surprise and need to make sense of what's happening before you can respond effectively. And it's psychologically tough to fight with your dick hanging out...

Cutting from the herd is an age-old technique. It is instinctual, and it works. Be aware of where and when it might be used on you. Do your best to avoid isolated areas like parks, trails, alleys, elevators, and empty buildings, especially at night, unless you have someone else you trust with you. Even if you are in a group, don't take any unnecessary chances.

If you are attacked in this type of situation, it makes sense to call attention to your predicament. Even in an isolated location, there may still be people around who can hear what's going on and might choose to investigate. In order to attract attention, however, you need to yell something that stands apart from a generic cry of "help."

Many self-defense experts recommend screaming "fire" under the assumption that it will make people pay attention since a fire can affect everyone around you. We're not sure that's the best choice, particularly if your assailant has a gun. "Oh my god, don't kill me with that knife," on the other hand, is a pretty cogent statement. Not only may this tactic have a better chance of attracting attention of a prospective rescuer than a generic shout for help, but it also demonstrates to potential witnesses that you are in legitimate fear for your life should you have to kill your attacker in self-defense. Further, the mere presence of other attentive individuals may make a bad guy stop trying to hurt you and become more concerned about how to escape successfully before authorities arrive to arrest him.

Don't let yourself be cut from the herd. In such situations, your adversary gains the advantage in numbers, determines the time, chooses the place, has the element of surprise, and is not observed by others. You may be able to attract attention by shouting for help if you do so creatively, but there is no guarantee that it will arrive in time to do you much good. It is far better, therefore, to be aware of this tactic and avoid locations where it might be used against you.

Don't Be Afraid to Call in Support

In war, the general receives his commands from the sovereign, collects his army and concentrates his forces.

> – *Sun Tzu*

It is said the warrior's is the twofold Way of pen and sword, and he should have a taste for both Ways.

> – *Miyamoto Musashi*

Bullies often look for victims who are eager to preserve their social status or are afraid to lose face, the kinds of guys who are willing to play the escalato game. They are reluctant, however, to take on a challenge that they cannot win. A large group of people changes the equation in your potential opponent's eyes very quickly. If you are willing to call in support rather than going it alone, you are no longer a helpless victim, but rather a well-protected target.

If you have friends that are willing to help you, call them in immediately before a bad situation comes to blows. This can often end a fight before it begins. If you are dealing with an antagonistic group of guys or, God forbid, a criminal gang, they are already assembled so you are on the short end numbers-wise, or in other words outnumbered, if you cannot gather additional support.

Before he founded his own *dojo*, Wilder taught karate at a local YMCA. Walking through the hallway in his karate uniform before class one night he discovered a crowd of about half a dozen people looking intently through the gymnasium window. He discovered that the basketball game in the gym had deteriorated into a shouting match and believed that it was rapidly going to escalate to violence. A number of young men, strong and angry, were not only ready to throw down, but very likely to seriously injure each other.

"Somebody should do something." A woman said, and all heads turned expectantly toward Wilder, the karate black belt. "Like what?" he thought, then, deciding he should take responsibility to act, he turned down the hall, rounded the corner and opened the door to the gym. He then let out the best karate *kiai* (spirit shout or loud yell) he could muster. Startled by the shout, the youths in the gym paused their argument for a moment and looked over at him in all his "karate glory."

"Hey," he said, signaling with his thumb over his shoulder. "The front desk just called the cops; thought you should know."

With that, he backed the two steps out the door, turned, and left without saying another word. He had advantage of a martial arts outfit that conveyed some level of authority. Using that influence, he yelled at them, made his statement, and left. The threat of repercussions was enough to end the fight before it began, as the players quickly dispersed and exited the building.

Despite what he had told the youths, however, the front desk was located at the other end of the building. Since they were so far away from the action, the desk staff had no idea that anything untoward had occurred, and in fact, had not called the police. Regardless, the police were very real in the minds of the basketball players. Wilder solved the problem by appearing to call in support, and that was all that counted at that moment.

You cannot always bluff though. Simply saying that your friends who are all karate experts are outside, or, "You're gonna get it when..." is not effective, so don't bother taking that route. It doesn't play well in court either. A plausible and instantly believable threat, on the other hand, can be very effective.

Wilder's intervention not only solved the problem, but kept him safe as well. Standing in the doorway and shouting, he was never close enough to the youths to be at risk. Furthermore, they were only wearing shorts and shoes, so the chances of a hidden long-distance weapon such as a gun were practically non-existent. Upon launching the "cop bomb" he left immediately, knowing that interfering in somebody else's fight could mean trouble.

> Calling in support is often a useful way of cutting short a fight before it begins. A large group of people changes the equation in your adversary's eyes very quickly. You are no longer a helpless victim, but rather a well-protected target. A plausible threat of authority, such as contacting 9-1-1 might work too. Don't be afraid to call in support when you need help.

Calling in support is often a useful way of precluding the imperative to fight. Use it when you can to make yourself a harder target.

Your Words are a Weapon, Use Them Wisely

Humble words and increased preparations are signs that the enemy is about to advance. Violent language and driving forward as if to the attack are signs that he will retreat.

— *Sun Tzu*

There is a time and place for use of weapons.

— *Miyamoto Musashi*

What you say during a tense encounter can make a crucial difference between your ability to walk away from a potential adversary versus a requirement to fight your way clear. On the one hand, you might be able to verbally de-escalate a tense situation, while on the other you can just as easily set the other guy off if you are not careful. Consequently, while sticks and stones may break your bones, your words can actually kill you. Doesn't quite match the nursery rhyme, yet this insight is nothing new. The following parable from biblical times (Midrash Psalms 39 from Rapaport's book) describes the power of the tongue, the life or death impact your words can make:

How flexible is the tongue, and how great is its power! A Persian king's physicians ordered him to drink the milk of a lioness to maintain his health. Seeking favor from the king, one of his servants offered to procure this rare medicine.

Taking with him some sheep with which to lure the beast, the servant actually succeeded in obtaining milk from a lioness. Fatigued from his trials, he took a break on his journey homeward and fell into a deep sleep. During his slumber, the various members of his body began to argue about which of them had contributed most towards the success of their owner in obtaining so rare a thing as lioness milk.

The feet began the argument saying, "There can be no doubt that we are the only factors in this successful undertaking. Without us there could have been no setting out on this dangerous venture." "Not so," retorted the hands. "The facility you offered would have been of no avail had our power not been called into requisition. It is the service we rendered that enabled our owner to procure milk from the lioness." "Neither of you could have rendered any service," exclaimed the eyes, "without the sight which we supplied." "And yet," interrupted the heart, "had not I inspired the idea, no steps would have been taken to bring any of your powers into exercise."

At last the tongue put in his claim, and was utterly ridiculed by the unanimous opinions of all the other contending members of the body. "You," they scornfully replied, "You who have not the free power of action which is possessed by all and each of us. You who are imprisoned in the narrow space of the human mouth, you dare to put in a claim to have contributed to this success!" In the midst of this contention the man awoke and proceeded on his journey home.

When he was brought before the king with the much desired milk, the man, by a slip of the tongue said, "Here I have brought your Majesty the dog's milk you asked for." The king was incensed by this insulting remark. In a rage he ordered that the man to be put to death for his insolence.

On the man's way to execution, all the members of his body, heart, eyes, feet, and hands trembled and were terribly afraid. "Did I not tell you," said the tongue, "that my power is above all the united strengths you possess? And you ridiculed me for my trouble. What think you of my power now? Are you now prepared to acknowledge my supremacy?"

When all the members of the body consented to the tongue's proposition, the tongue requested and obtained a short reprieve, so that it could make a last appeal for the king's clemency.

When the man was brought to the king his tongue began speaking with great eloquence. "Is this the reward great and just king, to be meted out to the only one of your majesty's servants who was glad of the opportunity to offer his life to fulfill his king's desire, who gladly carried his life in his hand to obtain for his august master what scarcely ever was obtained by mortal man?"

"That may be true," replied the king, "yet your own statement was that you brought me dog's milk instead of the lioness' milk which you undertook to procure."

"Not so, O gracious king," replied the tongue, "I brought the identical milk that your majesty required. It was merely by an unfortunate mistake in my speech that I changed the name. In fact there is a similarity, as the word כליא in Hebrew may mean either lioness or dog. My words will be verified if your majesty will condescend to make use of the milk I procured, for it will effect the cure your majesty desires."

The milk was submitted to the test, and was found to be that of a lioness; and so the body of the man was saved and the tongue triumphantly demonstrated its great power for good or for evil.

While that fanciful tale serves to make a point, it actually has quite a lot to do with real life. Consider this incident reported in the news.

On January 27, 2005, actress Nicole duFresne was robbed at gunpoint by 19-year-old Rudy Fleming who stole her friend's purse and pistol-whipped her fiancé. What was supposed to be a simple property crime turned deadly, however, when the 28-year-old actress confronted the teenaged robber. She became furious, shoved Fleming, and snapped, "What are you going to do, shoot us?" A fatal mistake—she died shortly thereafter in her fiancé's arms.

This tragedy is an excellent case study in what not to do when confronted by an armed aggressor. Experts often state that robbery is more often about power than anything else.

Discussing the duFresne shooting, Alfonso Lenhardt of the National Crime Prevention Council said, "It's a tragedy, but in this case it sounds like the suspect felt he wasn't getting the respect he was due. When a gun is in the hands of a desperate person with low self-esteem, they're going to react that way."

Respect is paramount for gang members too, even wannabes. Mouthing off to any street punk is downright dangerous. If you are similarly confronted by an adversary, save your righteous indignation for a safer environment after the immediate danger has passed. It does you no good to be right yet dead like duFresne. Having to be right despite the cost, reacting indignantly in the face of a threat, or insulting an adversary frequently guarantees that a conflict will escalate out of control.

If you are in error about something, admit it. Honesty is a much better way to de-escalate a bad situation than lying or stubbornly refusing to acknowledge a wrong. It is tough on the ego, but it sure beats an unnecessary hospital stay, jail time, or a premature trip to the morgue.

Try not to insult or embarrass the other person in any way, particularly in public. We do not like being treated that way, we are pretty sure you do not either, and we strongly suspect that neither will an aggressive person. Giving someone a face-saving way out affords him the opportunity to back down gracefully. Put his back up against the metaphorical wall, on the other hand, and he will ultimately feel forced to lash out at you, striking back (from his perspective) to save his dignity and honor.

> While sticks and stones may break your bones, your words can actually kill you. They can also save your life. Having to be right despite the cost, reacting indignantly in the face of a threat, or insulting an adversary often guarantees that a conflict will escalate to violence. Clever words, on the other hand, can de-escalate a tense situation, stave off bloodshed until help arrives, or momentarily distract an opponent to facilitate your counterattack and escape.

Even if you are in the right, it is sometimes prudent to pretend otherwise. Do not let your ego overrule your common sense. Giving your vehicle to a carjacker, your wallet to a robber, or your apology to someone who tries to start a fight hurts a lot less than eating a blade or a bullet because you refused to back down.

Even if you cannot de-escalate a situation simply by talking, clever words may enable you to stall until help arrives or the attacker changes his/her mind and leaves. You can also use conversation as a psychological weapon to increase your chances of surviving as well as to create openings for your physical defenses. Deception, for example, is but one of the tactics you might choose to employ. Any convincing distraction you can create will be to your advantage, such as shouting for nonexistent friends. There is strength in numbers and in making an aggressor believe you are not alone.

If you realize that de-escalation is not working and that you will have no other choice but to fight, it may also be possible to cause your opponent to make a mental twitch, providing a moment of opportunity to counterattack while they mentally shift gears. This twitch is brought about by dissonance between what the person expects and what you actually say or do.

A common example is asking a question, as we saw with the four Ds. While the bad guy is focusing on your words or thinking about an answer, you have a moment in which to run or strike. This may be particularly useful when confronted with multiple assailants. Ask something completely unexpected like, "What time is it?" or something really odd like, "What was Gandhi's batting average?" Cognitive dissonance is powerful. During the opponent's momentary confusion, you will have an opportunity to act. Similarly, if you can hit an aggressor while he is talking it takes about half a second for him to switch gears mentally from communicating to fighting.

Kane saw a great example of this when he watched a police officer confront an assault suspect. The guy was shirtless in unseasonably cold weather and appeared to be drunk and/or on drugs. The suspect wasn't particularly argumentative, but he was not cooperative either. Despite the officer's questions about what he was doing and repeated orders to show his hands, he refused to respond and continued to keep his right hand in his pocket. Assuming a weapon, the officer suddenly shot one hand up to grab the guy's throat, lifted him upward a few inches to break his balance, and then stepped forward to use his entire bodyweight to slam the suspect onto the ground. Continuing in one smooth motion, he rolled the guy over,

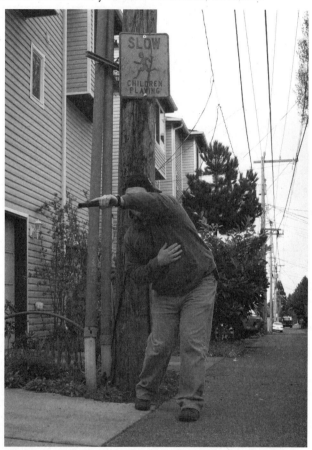

Mouthing off to any street punk is dangerous. Having to be right despite the cost can cause a conflict to escalate out of control. Giving the other guy a face-saving way out, on the other hand, affords him the opportunity to back down gracefully.

and calmly said, "Don't resist, don't resist," while simultaneously placing him in handcuffs.

This trick worked flawlessly because the officer made his move without any obvious pause or preparation, striking in mid-sentence while the suspect was focused on his words rather than his actions. It was a great example of disguising the "tell." Once the guy was on the ground, the officer's orders not to resist not only kept the guy from struggling but also helped witnesses understand that he was not using excessive force, which could prove crucial should witnesses be called to testify in court.

For better or worse, your words truly are a weapon. The challenge is that they can hurt you just as easily as they can harm your adversary. Use them wisely.

Don't Get Hung Up on Name Calling

The Book of Army Management says: On the field of battle, the spoken word does not carry far enough.

— *Sun Tzu*

Or, as the enemy attacks, attack more strongly, taking advantage of the resulting disorder in his timing to win.

— *Miyamoto Musashi*

Name-calling means absolutely nothing unless you give it value. It should be meaningless when it comes to fighting, save perhaps, as a distraction to use against the other guy. We have all heard the same old expletives and insults so many times that they no longer have significance.

Unfortunately, it is not always easy to keep this perspective. Calling one's masculinity into question, for example, is designed to attack the deepest part of your psyche. It is meant to go to the root of who you think you are, to kick your metaphorical feet right out from underneath you. And it can work if you let it.

While standing in the living room of his home, Bill's wife (now ex-wife) decided that he needed to find a windshield repair business for her to get her car windshield fixed that Monday morning. Bill, however, had a business meeting he had to get to and told her that he did not have time that morning, but would take care of it in the afternoon. Impatient, she went to the heart as quickly as she could. "Be a man," she spat out.

Bill was instantly mad. He didn't do anything about it but he was seriously upset. That is how quick three little words can take you from walking out the door thinking about a meeting to becoming instantly ticked off. Name-calling is designed to knock you off your mental equilibrium. When you are mad, you are not in total control. When you are not in control of yourself, you become vulnerable.

Think of the classic movie scene where the hero hits the villain in the face. The villain just smiles, and maybe spits out some blood, and continues the fight. Name-calling is like the first punch in a fight; it is meant to put you off balance. If you respond to the name-calling, you have reeled from the first punch. Worse yet, if the other guy can goad you into throwing the first blow, you become the bad guy in the eyes of the law (or of any witnesses). Now he has free reign to tee off on you with impunity. After all, he's defending himself from your aggression. That's another important reason to be cautious when insults start to fly.

Do your best not to respond to insults. By understanding that they're not truth but merely a way to get at you, they can become a punch you will choose not to receive.

It is important to note that often the intense emotional response that words cause may be harder to ignore than those caused by weapons. For example, you can be wounded in combat with an adversary and never know it until after the dust settles, suddenly discovering that you've been stabbed, shot, or badly mangled once the adrenaline wears off and the pain kicks in. There are hundreds of cases where soldiers on the battlefield suddenly discovered that their legs had been blown off when they tried to stand back up after a firefight.

Calm, reasoned responses will help you win in a fight, yet if you lose your cool because of what someone has said, your technique gets thrown out of whack. Fighting when enraged makes you a bit stronger and faster but far less skilled. Against a competent opponent, your rage will get you busted up pretty quickly.

> Words are meaningless unless you give them power. Name-calling is designed to knock you off your mental equilibrium. If you let them make you mad, you are no longer in control, hence vulnerable. That's when words really can hurt you.

Words are meaningless unless you give them power. Then they can hurt you.

If You Have Made a Mistake, Apologize

Success in warfare is gained by carefully accommodating ourselves to the enemy's purpose.

– Sun Tzu

An individual can easily change his mind, so his movements are difficult to predict. You must appreciate this.

– Miyamoto Musashi

Imagine this scenario: You walk out of the restroom at your neighborhood bar and accidentally smack into another guy, spilling his beer. He is clearly upset, calls you a derogatory name, and takes a swing at you. If your goal is not to get hurt, you can walk away, he can walk away, he can be dragged away on a stretcher, or he can be carried away in a box. All these options accomplish your goal of not being hurt, but some are clearly better than others are.

What might happen if you can evade his punch and say something along the lines of, "Whoa! I'm sorry, I didn't see you there. Let me buy you a new one." Conversely, what will certainly happen if you immediately begin to fight back?

You can often tell when someone is in the wrong by how he or she reacts. Anyone who is unwilling to admit that he made a mistake is almost always going to take the argument to a personal level. Rather than continuing to debate the merits of the disagreement, he suddenly changes tactics and insults start to fly. At that point, the conflict is no longer about the mistake; it is about dominance, control, and saving face. Sadly, violence will often follow.

If you are in error about something, it is usually best to admit it. Honesty is a much better way to de-escalate a bad situation than lying or stubbornly refusing to acknowledge a wrong. It is tough on the ego, but it sure beats an unnecessary hospital stay, jail time, or trip to the morgue.

Your life and physical well-being are worth fighting for while your possessions and self-esteem are not. Unfortunately, however, when you apologize to an aggressive person, it will often be seen as weakness. You may very well be verbally attacked for saying that you are sorry, hence feel compelled to fight. Don't fall into that trap.

The apology rarely goes like this: You say, *"I'm sorry! That was my mistake. I was wrong. It won't happen again."* The other guy replies, *"Thank you! It is rare that someone is willing to admit when they are wrong. You're a real stand-up guy. I hope you have a good evening."*

It is more likely to work this way: You say, *"Sorry man, my fault."* He replies, *"Damn right it is!"* You respond, *"Yes it was, sorry."* And then you walk away. Before you get too far you hear him retort, *"F%&ing pussy!"*

Your goal is not to fight. If you walk away, your goal will be achieved. There can be no fight unless he follows you. Expect to get a couple more verbal jabs as you leave though, maybe something challenging your manhood or your sexuality. Either way, leave it alone. Move on. Go somewhere else and enjoy your evening.

> Anyone who is unwilling to admit that he made a mistake is almost always going to take the argument to a personal level. At that point, the conflict is no longer about the mistake. If you are in error about something, admit it. Honesty is a much better way to de-escalate a bad situation than lying or stubbornly refusing to acknowledge a wrong. It is tough on the ego, but it sure beats the alternative. Giving someone a face-saving way out affords him the opportunity to back down gracefully. Put his back up against the metaphorical wall, on the other hand, and he will feel forced to lash out at you physically.

Name-calling is never worth fighting over. If the other person challenges you in this way, it is because he wants to fight. He thinks he can win. If he follows you and subsequently attacks, you will be on the side of the angels when things go to court. More often than not, however, he's just trying to provoke you into making the first move, or establishing dominance and will let you walk away.

The reason for this type of aggression should not be important to you. You don't care if the guy who challenged you had a bad childhood, was molested, or is just out with his posse for the evening and looking to make a good impression. You don't need a fight. You don't want a fight. Chances are, if he's spoiling for a fight, you are already outnumbered, overpowered, or something else is stacked in the other guy's favor, not yours. Maybe he's even got a weapon palmed, and is ready and able to use it.

Don't find out how he has stacked the deck unless he forces you to. Be the bigger man and walk away. After all, the tougher you truly are, the less you should feel a need to prove it. If you have made a mistake, apologize and be done with it.

Make Sure Your Intentions are Clear and Understandable

When the general is weak and without authority; when his orders are not clear and distinct; when there are no fixed duties assigned to officers and men and the ranks are formed in a slovenly haphazard manner, the result is utter disorganization.

– Sun Tzu

Really skilful people never get out of time, and are always deliberate, and never appear busy.

– Miyamoto Musashi

If you are in a face off with someone, you have already passed the interview stage and your adversary has made the decision you are an easy mark. Before he hits you, however, you might still be able to make him rethink that decision. It is still a negotiation until someone gets hit. Consequently, words are critical before fists start to fly. They can still de-escalate the confrontation or even stop it dead in its tracks.

"Don't f%&k with me!" is an old, tired expression that means nothing. The bad guy has certainly heard that before and most likely beat down the last guy who said it. Snarling something along the lines of, "I am going to rape you when I am done with you," on the other hand, changes the picture.*

While it may not play too well in court if someone hears you saying this sort of thing, and you need to have the physicality and demeanor to make it a convincing threat, your adversary will certainly get the message. Your intention, making him realize that he's picking on the wrong guy, is clear and understandable. You are scary. By breaking the conventions of what is expected, you seize the high ground militarily speaking.

Wilder remembers an incident from his college days that illuminates this point. Several friends of his were returning from a party on campus when they needed to cross the street. The combination of inebriation and young male cockiness led them to decide to cross where they wanted rather than at the designated crosswalk, which at night would have been the sensible choice. As they jaywalked across the middle of the block, a fellow student in a sports car came down the road. Seeing Wilder's pack of drunken friends, he slammed on his brakes and laid on the horn.

Of course, Wilder's friends should have been at the crosswalk waiting for the light, but the guy in the sports car should not have been going over the speed limit. And really, was the horn necessary? Add to it the driver had his girlfriend in the car, so he undoubtedly felt that he needed to yell an obscenity or two at the drunken horde to look good in her eyes. Everybody was in the wrong and alcohol was involved, a dangerous combination.

---

* If you are going to make a threat this extreme, you'd damn well better not lose the fight though. A threat of male rape after a fight could very easily sway a jury that killing you afterwards was an act of blind and justified fear. Sometimes a solution for one part of the conflict complicates all the others. Choose your words wisely.

Here's the real mistake. Because the guy was in his car he felt he was safe. We all have directed some kind of remark to another driver while in our cars that we would never say in line at the bank. However, this was a sports car with the top down so the driver and his girlfriend could enjoy the early summer night. Even if the top had not been open, windows are easy to break. At this point, the driver had made his intention clear—a verbal and public admonishment of the drunken goofballs who stepped into his path. Wilder's friend Chris, on the other hand, had another intention. He turned, placed his foot on the front bumper of the sports car, hopped up onto the hood and with two quick, and very heavy, hood-denting steps prepared to kick in the windshield. He stated, loudly and clearly, "What the f%&k is wrong with you, a*&hole!"

> A clear intent to defend yourself, along with a demonstration of ability to physically do so, can often stop a fight before it begins. Your words and demeanor must convince your adversary that he's picked on the wrong guy.

Now this vignette is not about right and wrong, or even about justification; it is about making your intentions clear. The driver's intent had been to shame these guys in front of his girlfriend for crossing incorrectly. He thought he was doing it from the "safety" of his car. The bottom line in his mind most likely was, "These guys are stupid and I am going to call them on it. They can't touch me because I'm in my car."

Wilder's friend Chris's intention was clear as well—to do violence to the driver. He demonstrated his capacity for violence for all to see, metaphorically going from 0 to 60 in the blink of an eye. Not exactly a response that the driver expected. If he were willing to do what he just did, what else would he be capable of? He literally demonstrated his intention to do so by damaging the car and asked the driver if he would like to be next.

Sure, everybody was in the wrong at several levels. What if the driver had pulled a gun? Would Wilder's friend have been able to stop it? Would you? Would you be willing to risk it? Hopefully not. Regardless, the point here is that Chris was willing to take that risk. He was willing to show just how far he was able to go. The message he conveyed by crushing a car hood was clear—"You're next!"

If you wish to preclude violence verbally or through some act, make sure that you are communicating what you intend and that you understand the risks in acting on that intention as well.

Saying Something Once Does Not Mean That It Was Understood

The Book of Army Management *says: On the field of battle, the spoken word does not carry far enough: hence the institution of gongs and drums. Nor can ordinary objects be seen clearly enough: hence the institution of banners and flags.*
— Sun Tzu

In large-scale strategy, at the start of battle we shout as loudly as possible.
— Miyamoto Musashi

When a group of nurses and/or orderlies in a mental hospital have to physically restrain a patient who has gotten out of control, they often use physical cues as well as words to communicate with each other. Not only do they get commands like, "Move over, I can help," but also they often get a tap or even a push as well.

The reason for this multi-layered communication is an attempt to circumvent the adverse impacts of adrenaline. Stress-induced accelerated heart rates can cause a loss of fine motor skills such as finger dexterity, complex motor skills such as hand-eye coordination, and depth perception. Under extreme conditions, people experience hyper-vigilance, loss of rational thought, memory loss, and inability to consciously move or react.

The same thing happens when you are facing down an adversary on the street; he can't hear you very well. He may know that you're talking, but his brain is not always processing what you say. Consequently, saying the same thing over and over is not very likely to get results. Saying the same thing in different ways is a far better option.

For example, saying, "I don't want to fight" over and over might not work because it's simply received as noise. On the other hand, saying, "I don't want to fight," followed by, "That guy just called the cops," and, "I am out of here" just might. Similarly, "This will violate my parole," combined with "We don't want to do this" has a better chance of reaching the other guy's brain and making some impact.

For example, Kane once had a frantic call at the Pac-10 football stadium where he works as a security supervisor. One of his captains had confronted a group of drunken fans who had slipped into the student section during halftime. They may have been students, but they were clearly wearing hats and jerseys for the other team, a fierce cross-state rival. Since the home team was losing badly at the time, emotions were running rather hot, making the group a target of taunts, catcalls, and an occasional thrown object from the other students.

Jim, the captain, had tried to check their tickets in order to prove that they were in the wrong section, but they claimed to have lost them. He subsequently ordered them to leave, but they weren't willing to go peacefully. By the time Kane arrived, a full-fledged shouting match was underway. It was a pretty tense situation, where a couple of the students looked ready to start swinging at the security guards and anyone else standing nearby. To make matters worse, a large group of local students was focused on the confrontation rather than on the game, heckling and shouting insults in an effort to provoke the other school's fans into a fight.

Quickly grasping what had happened, Kane managed to separate the "leader" from his little pack of rowdies, taking him aside to have a talk with him. Kane started off by pointing toward the hometown fans and saying, "Look man, you're going to get yourself hurt by sitting here. There are a lot more of them than there are of you. We can't keep all those guys off you if you're going to act like that. Why don't you go back to your own section across the way and enjoy the rest of the game."

He thought that appealing to the guy's sense of self-preservation would prove successful but he wasn't buying it so Kane changed tactics. "Look, your team's winning right? Don't you want to watch the end of the game? If you get thrown out now you'll miss it."

Once again, fear of repercussions wasn't getting the hoped-for response. The guy was drunk, full of himself, and hoping for something to prove, so Kane changed tactics once again.

> It is critical that you take steps to ensure that your message is heard, particularly when emotions are running hot. Just because you have said something once does not necessarily mean that it was understood. Repeating the same thing over and over again is far less effective than restating your message in a variety of different ways.

"How old are you?" Kane asked. "Nineteen," the student replied with a smirk. He started to say something more, but Kane cut him off. "You know that's underage, right? When the cops get here, they're not only going to throw you out for causing a disturbance, but they're also going to arrest you for drinking. That's going to look real great on your resume."

This time the message got through. The kid wasn't afraid of a fight with the hometown fans or even the security personnel, but he finally began to comprehend the downside of the situation he'd gotten himself into. While he thought he was tough enough to win any fight, he wasn't too keen on going to jail or paying a hefty fine. Once he made up his mind to leave before the police arrived, it was pretty easy to convince his buddies to go along with him. By co-opting the leader, Kane got the rest of the group to follow.

It is critical that you take steps to ensure that your message is heard, particularly when emotions are running hot. Just because you have said something once does not necessarily mean that it was heard or understood. If it does not work, change tactics and try again.

Changing the Context Can De-Escalate a Bad Situation

Those who were called skillful leaders of old knew how to drive a wedge between the enemy's front and rear; to prevent co-operation between his large and small divisions; to hinder the good troops from rescuing the bad the officers from rallying their men.

– Sun Tzu

Always chase the enemy into bad footholds, obstacles at the side, and so on, using the virtues of the place to establish predominant positions from which to fight. You must research and train diligently in this.

– Miyamoto Musashi

An angry or aggressive person may simply want to vent his outrage. In many instances, you can do much good by calmly listening to him as he rants, all the while preparing yourself to act if attacked, of course. Interjecting a few choice words as necessary to help him see the situation in a new light can be very beneficial. Changing the context in this fashion can often de-escalate a bad situation by giving the other guy an out, some face-saving way of handling things that he was unable to see before.

Here's an example: Kane stopped at an Arco station to get gas on his way home from work. Their price was roughly ten cents per gallon cheaper than anyone else in the area was so they were very crowded. Because the automated kiosks by the pumps were not working, he had to go into the store, wait in line to pre-pay, and then go back out to fill his tank. After doing so, he had to go back into the store to retrieve a couple of dollars in change.

As he approached the door, he could hear shouting coming from inside. Two women were arguing with the clerk. As he stood in line, he could not help but hear their dispute over the next several minutes. They claimed to have given the clerk twenty-two dollars to pre-pay and asserted that he put the money on the wrong pump. They said that they had received no gas and wanted him to either restart the pump or give them their money back. He first countered that they had not paid him. The argument continued with the women restating their claim and the clerk changing his response several times with such statements as they had told him the wrong pump number and that it was not his fault if someone else pumped gas on their dime. As the argument escalated, one of the women in line behind Kane went outside to call the police. Several others simply left without buying anything. Everyone was very uncomfortable.

The distraught women were dressed in quality but dirty coveralls, had some sort of ID badges that Kane could not read clipped to their waists, and were very buff. He imagined that they worked as mechanics, maintenance workers, or something similar and had just gotten off work. Neither was a small person. Kane is 5' 10" tall and they were both around his height. The clerk was shorter and skinnier than either woman was. He had a heavy accent and was a little hard to understand, especially when he raised his voice. Eventually as one of the women called the clerk a liar for the umpteenth time, he retorted that she was a "fat, uppity bitch." This, as you would probably expect, did not go over too well.

The insulted woman went stiff, then spun on her heel and headed toward the door while her friend continued to argue with the clerk. As she turned past Kane, he got a good look at her face that had jumped several notches up the threat index scale. The last time he had seen that "thousand-yard stare" was when a guy left a building, then returned a short time later with a gun.* Fearing something similar, he decided that he had better do something about it.

As she left, Kane noticed that she used her right hand to open the door and that she wore a watch on her left wrist so he assumed that she was right-handed. He followed her

---

* Kane wisely bailed before that guy returned, reading about the aftermath the next day in the local paper.

out as she stalked toward her car. She was not moving very fast so he easily caught up a dozen feet past the door. He figured that she was not armed (yet), so he took a position behind her left shoulder a couple feet back assuming that he would have the most reaction time that way if she did anything untoward.

Having positioned himself where he wanted to be, he calmly said, "You know they have half a dozen video cameras in there. Your transaction must be on tape."

She froze in place but clearly was not really processing what he said so he repeated it again adding, "All you need to do is have the manager review the tape to prove your story. There are cameras out here too so they'll know that you didn't pump any gas." What he did not add was, "… and they'll record anything stupid you're about to do too," but he suspected that she figured that out on her own. That was his intention anyway.

She slowly said, "You're right, they do have cameras in there." She paused to think for a moment and then repeated more confidently, "Yeah, they do have cameras in there." As she did so, he could virtually see the rage draining from her. She turned to face him and said eagerly, "They have cameras in there" once again, adding, "Thank you."

He replied, "No problem. You probably ought to explain that to your friend." She corrected, "She's my cousin," then said, "Yeah, I'll talk to her."

While she pulled her cousin aside and began to calm her down, he got his change from the clerk. As the clerk handed Kane the money, Kane pointed out the cameras to him too. The clerk got a goofy look on his face as the realization that everything was being recorded dawned on him too.

Kane honestly does not know who was telling the truth in this dispute, but the look the clerk gave him seemed to validate the women's claim. The guy looked very uncomfortable and real "guilty," something that Kane strongly suspected from his changing story, frustration, and personalization* during the interchange. Anyone who is unwilling to admit that he or she made a mistake is almost always going to take the argument to a personal level, sooner or later. At that point, the conflict is no longer about the mistake.

> It is possible to de-escalate a tense situation by changing the context. When an argument becomes personal, everyone gets so focused on their anger that they forgot all about their environment, the facts, and right/wrong. When the angry party is able to see the situation in a different light, however, it can give him a face-saving way out, eliminating the emotional need to fight.

The interesting thing is that while the presence of a half dozen highly visible cameras was obvious, no one in the dispute seemed to notice them. Pointing them out changed everyone's context, kicking things down several notches. Kane will never know for sure if the angry woman was going for a weapon, but he strongly suspects that he prevented something bad, probably something really bad, from happening when he intervened. He did not stick around to find out how it was all resolved because he had to pick his up son from daycare, though he did see a police car coming toward the place as he was driving away.

* Personalization is taking an argument to a personal level such as the "fat, uppity bitch" comment from the sales clerk. He was no longer focused on what happened with the $22.00 but rather on the character of his accuser.

It is possible to de-escalate a tense situation by changing the context. Kane did not choose sides or make himself a target, but rather pointed out an essential fact that everyone had overlooked. This calmed things down long enough for rational thought to overrule emotion.

Hollywood Fantasy vs. Brutal Reality

When there is much running about and the soldiers fall into rank, it means that the critical moment has come.

— *Sun Tzu*

In large-scale strategy you can frighten the enemy not by what you present to their eyes, but by shouting, making a small force seem large, or by threatening them from the flank without warning. These things all frighten. You can win by making best use of the enemy's frightened rhythm. In single combat, also, you must use the advantage of taking the enemy unawares by frightening him with your body, long sword, or voice, to defeat him. You should research this well.

— *Miyamoto Musashi*

Getting smacked in the head so hard that it stuns your brain like a blast of lightning is a sobering experience. It is virtually indescribable, though, to anyone who hasn't had the experience. There is a vast difference between living through violence and reading about it or watching it on TV. Perhaps this description can help put things into perspective: The monkey dance, metaphorically beating one's chest and throwing grass in the air, is a ritual between human opponents too. It is done to get your way or avoid a fight by intimidating the other guy. You can see it when someone puffs his chest up, gets in your face, and yells promises of the ass kicking that's going to follow. You can see it in animalistic threat displays from the schoolyard bully to the soccer hooligan to the loudmouthed drunk to other patrons in the local bar. You can hear it when the other guy spouts off about the years of *ninjutsu* training he got while working for the CIA. Until a blow is thrown, however, it simply isn't real.

When the quiet person in the corner suddenly stands up and, with focused eyes, deliberately walks your way, that's real. His thousand-yard stare means serious trouble is coming your way. There is only a thin veneer of civilization, laws written on paper and enforced by people who are much too far away to intervene right here, right now, standing between you and a guy who wants to tear your throat out and piss down your neck.

You can usually walk away from the monkey dance. At worst, you're likely to resolve things with a bit of fisticuffs and a bloody nose, yet when it turns real, you are not likely to get off that lucky. If you're smart, you won't just walk away. You'll run.

When it comes to self-defense, most people only know what they've read in books, watched on TV, or seen in the movies. That's all well and

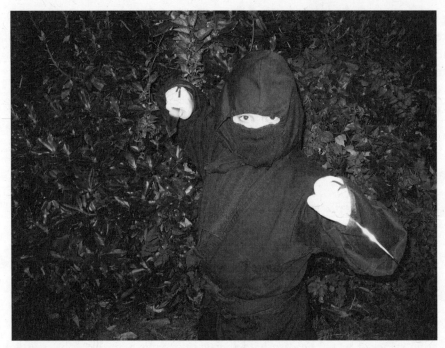

In most instances, your "deadly" ninja skills simply aren't real. Sparring in the *dojo* pales in comparison with the brutal realities of a street fight. Don't confuse sports with combat or misconstrue entertainment with reality.

good, as long as you never need to defend yourself on the street. Sadly, much of the information out there is misleading or inaccurate, sometimes dangerously so.

For example, at a 2007 shooting incident in Los Angeles, the police found a local drug dealer lying on the ground with a gun in his hand. On the sidewalk near his dead body was one live round. Imitating what he had seen in the movies, the dealer had racked the slide of his pistol, even though there was a bullet in the chamber and he could have begun firing at will. This extra movement took extra time and cost him his life.

While we may not grieve for a dead drug dealer, it is important to understand that much of what looks good in the movies has no bearing in real life. Holding a gun sideways as gangsters are frequently shown to do in movies, for example, increases the chances of a stovepipe, jam, or feeding failure. A stovepipe failure occurs when the shell casing gets pinched in the slide instead of fully ejecting from the gun. When it happens, you cannot fire a second shot without clearing the jam. Even when the gun feeds properly and ejects shells correctly, holding it sideways increases the chances of getting hot brass in your eye. Not exactly what you want to have happen during a life-or-death fight.

Another gun misconceptions from Hollywood is that people who have been shot are almost never knocked off their feet. In fact, it is rare that a shooting victim falls down instantly or is otherwise stopped dead in his tracks by a single shot, even one to the head, though it certainly does happen on occasion. They had a saying in the Old West, "dead man's ten (seconds)." It was a common experience for a gun- or knife-fighter to continue the battle for another ten seconds after suffering a fatal wound.

A defensive handgun instructor whose class Kane took reinforced this point, stating that it takes a fatally wounded person between 10 and 120 seconds to drop, so you must expect a determined attacker to continue his assault even after he has been shot. Kane was taught to fire and move rather than standing in place as you might do on a gun range. Don't relax your vigilance until the other person is clearly disabled and unable to continue the fight so that you can escape successfully to safety.

Another common misnomer is the half-hour-long fistfight. Fictional heroes are bashed, mangled, and beaten yet battle on against multiple assailants for an unbelievable amount of time. Most real fights are over rather quickly, taking minutes if not seconds before someone is knocked out, gives up, or runs off.

The intensity of a real fight is many, many times beyond what is experienced in the boxing ring or martial arts tournament. If you can imagine the other guy jumping on you, bearing down with his weight to slam you onto the pavement, and then pummeling you about the head and face until you lose consciousness, you've got some idea of what a real fight is all about. There is no jockeying for position, no sizing him up, and no trading punches then falling back to your corner at the end of the round; it's full on knock him on his ass and stomp a mud hole through him kind of stuff.

> It's all well and good to dream about how tough you are, how big, strong, or skilled in martial arts you might be, yet the realities of street violence are very different from what most people think. The boxing match or mixed martial arts tournament pales in comparison to the brutality of a street fight. Slickly choreographed Hollywood films only exacerbate the fantasy of what true violence entails. Beware of these misconceptions. Don't confuse sports with combat or misconstrue entertainment with reality.

Even if you are in great shape and an expert martial artist, you cannot expect to duke it out with another guy for half an hour and walk away unscathed. When it comes to multiple assailants, the odds are stacked against you even further. Frankly, any fight that lasts more than a few seconds is bound to result in injury. If you cannot escape a battle through awareness, avoidance, or de-escalation, then ending violence quickly should be your goal.

Adrenaline is a huge factor too. If you have ever fired a 12-gauge shotgun at a gun range, such as when shooting at targets or clay pigeons, you have no doubt noticed that those things kick like a mule, jarring your shoulder and rattling your teeth with each shot. It's even worse if you fire heavyweight 00 buckshot or slug loads as opposed to lightweight birdshot. If you are out in the wild, hunting geese, ducks, or deer with that same shotgun, however, you don't notice any adverse impact when you take a shot. There is no perceived kick at all. What's the difference between these two scenarios? Why, adrenaline of course. When you are hyped up, you simply don't feel pain, or at least don't feel it to the same degree.

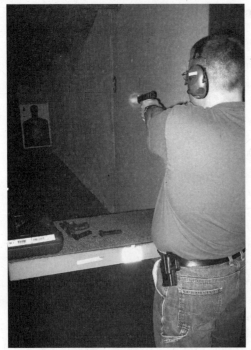

Beware of Hollywood misconceptions. For example, it is rare for a shooting victim to fall down instantly or otherwise be stopped dead in his tracks by a single shot, even one to the head.

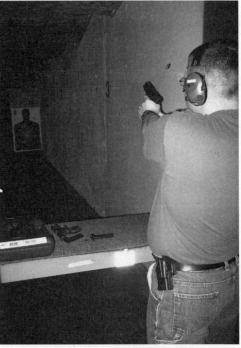

Holding a gun sideways as gangsters are frequently shown to do in movies increases the chances of a stovepipe, jam, or feeding failure that will render the weapon temporarily inoperable. If you carry a weapon, learn to use it properly.

The same kind of thing happens in a street fight. Kane vividly remembers an incident at the stadium where one guy accidentally broke his own hand punching a metal stair rail when he missed a shot at his opponent during a fight. He then proceeded to pummel the other guy without regard to his injury. In fact, he didn't even notice that he was bleeding until after the police had tackled him, dragged him off his victim, and handcuffs were snapped into place. His hand was mangled so badly that two of his knuckles were displaced and there was bone showing through at the injury site yet it had not even slowed his attack. Imagine what a dedicated attacker could do to you if you are unable to stop him.

The realities of street violence are very different from what most people think. The boxing match or mixed martial arts tournament pales in comparison to the brutality of a street fight. Sure, competitors do get seriously hurt from time to time when people beat the tar out of each other in the ring, but these competitions are first and foremost sporting events nevertheless. If they weren't, many competitors would not survive the "fighting" and the promoters would either wind up in jail or get sued out of business in short order. To help assure the safety of everyone involved, competitors use various types of gear such as padded gloves, mouth-guards, and groin protection.

Unlike actual street-fighting, sporting competitions have weight classes. Take the UFC, for instance. Under their rules competitors are grouped into lightweight (over 145 pounds to 155 pounds), welterweight (over 155 to 170 pounds), middleweight (over 170 to 185 pounds), light heavyweight (over 185 to 205 pounds), and heavyweight (over 205 to 265 pounds) divisions. On the street, you may find yourself tangling with someone much larger or smaller than yourself or potentially more than one adversary at the same time.

Sporting competitions have set time periods. Sticking with the UFC example, non-championship bouts run three rounds, while championship matches last five, with each round lasting five minutes in duration. There is a one-minute rest period between rounds. On the street, fights rarely last more than a few seconds, but when they do, there is no stopping until it's done, someone intercedes, or the authorities arrive to break things up. In the ring, you can win by submission (tap or verbal), knockout, technical knockout, decision, disqualification, or forfeiture. On the street, you win by surviving. The goal of self-defense is not to defeat an opponent but rather to escape to safety.

Unlike brawling on the street, so-called "no holds barred" events have a whole lot of rules. Of course, if you take that literally they truly do bar no holds, yet they do ban lots of other stuff that can be very effective on the street, particularly if you are a smaller and/or weaker combatant. The UFC, for example, outlaws the following:

- Head butts
- Eye gouges
- Throat strikes
- Grabbing the trachea
- Biting
- Hair pulling
- Groin striking
- Fish hooking
- Putting your finger into any orifice or into any cut or laceration on an opponent
- Small joint manipulation
- Striking to the spine
- Striking the back of the head
- Striking downward with the point of your elbow
- Clawing, pinching, or twisting the opponent's flesh
- Grabbing the clavicle
- Kicking the head of a grounded opponent
- Kneeing the head of a grounded opponent

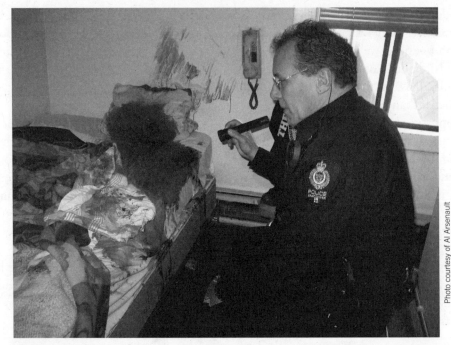

Photo courtesy of Al Arsenault

While so-called "no-holds-barred" competitions have dozens of rules designed to protect the safety of everyone involved, real-life violence has none. For example, MMA fighters don't generally get murdered in their sleep by their competitors.

- Stomping a grounded opponent
- Kicking the other guy's kidney with your heel
- Spiking an opponent to the canvas so that he lands on his head or neck
- Throwing an opponent out of the ring
- Holding the shorts or gloves of an opponent
- Spitting at an opponent
- Engaging in an "unsportsmanlike" conduct that causes an injury to an opponent
- Holding the ropes or the fence
- Using abusive language in the ring or fenced area
- Attacking an opponent during a break period
- Attacking an opponent who is under the care of the referee
- Attacking an opponent after the bell has sounded the end of a period
- Disregarding the referee's instructions
- Interference by someone in the competitor's corner.

This plethora of rules is designed to prevent serious injuries and give competitors a sporting chance to succeed. In order to keep things moving (and more interesting for the audience), they also take points away from a competitor for "timidity," including avoiding contact with an opponent, intentionally or consistently dropping the mouthpiece, or faking an injury.

There is a huge difference between sparring, fighting, and combat. Think of it this way. If you are going to face former Heavyweight Boxing Champion Mike Tyson in a match next Tuesday, you can approach it three ways—sporting competition, street fight, or combat.

- If you are thinking sports competition, you show up on time, weigh in, strap on the gloves, and go as many as twelve rounds until one of you is knocked out, the judges make a decision, or your manager throws in the towel.
- If you are thinking street fight, on the other hand, you show up at his house that morning with a dozen friends, jump him as he walks out the door, and beat him to a bloody pulp. Then you kick him a few more times while he's down, trample his flowerbeds for good measure, and drive away.
- If you are thinking combat, you wait outside his house Monday night and put a .50 BMG caliber bullet through his head with a Barrett sniper rifle from half a mile away.

A bit of disparity between those scenarios, huh? Street fights are much more like combat than sports competition. Slickly choreographed Hollywood films only exacerbate the fantasy of what true violence entails. Beware these misconceptions. Don't confuse sports with combat or misconstrue entertainment with reality.

Never Underestimate the Fighting Intelligence of Your Opponent

He must be able to mystify his officers and men by false reports and appearances, and thus keep them in total ignorance.
— *Sun Tzu*

When you cannot be deceived by men you will have realized the wisdom of strategy.
— *Miyamoto Musashi*

Never underestimate the fighting intelligence, skill, or determination of your opponent. Make this error and you are almost certainly going to be down and out fast. He looks small, sure, but he may have been on the judo mat since he was four years old. He looks slow, sure, and so does a ginormous NFL lineman who can run a 40-yard dash in under five seconds. Your adversary may look stupid, but odds are good that he is not.

Never forget that he's not going to attack you unless he thinks he can win. You really cannot know how tough someone is simply by looking at him.

Ken, a childhood friend of Wilder's, moved to Los Angeles to become a police officer. After a few years on the LA force, he transferred to Las Vegas where he spent the rest of his law enforcement career. They had occasion to see each other a couple of times over the years. During one visit, Wilder asked his friend, "What was the toughest encounter you ever had as a police officer?"

The six-foot-two-inch tall law enforcement officer said, "A big hooker I cornered in an alley. She bounced my ass up and down that alley before my partner got there. I got in trouble fast."

Stunned by that revelation, Wilder asked the logical question. Was she really a "he," a transvestite? Ken shifted his eyes over to

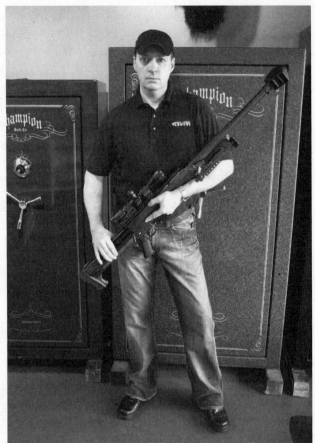

Barrett .50 caliber sniper rifle. This puppy can hit targets as far as 1,800 meters (approximately 2,000 yards) away with pinpoint accuracy.

him without turning his head and replied in a monotone, "No, no she wasn't."

Never, under any condition, underestimate the fighting intelligence, or physical skill of your adversary. The fight that Ken nearly lost with the prostitute is a great example. He had a simple goal, to get her off the street. He was trying to get her into the car and down to the station. She, on the other hand, had flipped into combat mode. Her mindset was something along the lines of, "This psycho 'John' is trying to slit my throat."

The prostitute did not have a restrictor that said, "Oh, it is a police officer. I'd better be quiet, pay attention, and follow his orders." Her experience was working against her logic and common sense. It said, "Fight! Get it over with now. Hurt him fast before he kills you!"

The officer and prostitute had two totally opposing perspectives—one planet, two different worlds.

"Fighting intelligence" is a special kind of intelligence that comes from experience, intensity, and the root desire of the body to survive. It is not intellect or brainpower as we commonly think of when we hear the word "intelligence." Fighting intelligence does not ponder, test, or audit. It instinctually acts and instantly responds to stimuli. There is no committee, no sleeping on it. It happens here and now.

The adage goes, "Don't judge the book by its cover." This is true. There is a reason this guy is attacking you. He has conducted an interview and you passed. To him you're a victim. Unless he is delusional, drunk, or drugged out of his mind, he not only thinks he can win, but has done so before. Never underestimate the fighting intelligence or physical skill level of your opponent.

> Never underestimate the fighting intelligence, or physical skill of your opponent. There is a reason this guy is attacking you. Unless he is delusional, drunk, or drugged out of his mind, he not only thinks he can win, but has done so before.

Size and Intensity Are Not the Same Thing

Other conditions being equal, if one force is hurled against another ten times its size, the result will be the flight of the former.
— *Sun Tzu*

Small people must be completely familiar with the spirit of large people, and large people must be familiar with the spirit of small people. Whatever your size, do not be misled by the reactions of your own body.
— *Miyamoto Musashi*

There is a famous saying, originally attributed to author Mark Twain, that goes, "It is not the size of the dog in the fight, but the size of the fight in the dog." Often quoted, this maxim is absolutely true.

For example, in 1942 Audie Murphy (1924–1971) tried to enlist in the military at the outset of World War II. He was turned down by both the United States Marines and the Paratroopers for being too small, underweight, and slightly built. When the Army finally accepted him, they tried to make him serve as a cook… until he reached the battlefield.

In two years of service at the European front during WWII, Murphy killed 240 German soldiers in documented firefights. He won the Medal of Honor, the Distinguished Service Cross, the Legion of Merit, the Silver Star (twice), and the Bronze Medal (twice). He was also awarded the Purple Heart three times for combat injuries plus a variety of other honors totaling some thirty-two medals. This made him America's most decorated WWII combat veteran.

How did a scrawny eighteen-year-old boy, named "Audie" from Texas do it? Despite his small stature, he was one tough SOB. His father deserted the family when he was a small child. Only nine of his twelve brothers and sisters lived past the age of eighteen. His mother died when he was sixteen, leaving him in charge, and he gave the three remaining kids up to an orphanage.

He had a rough life that might have broken a lesser man, yet it forged a mental toughness that far outweighed his physical build. He was resilient too, tough enough to jump up on a burning tank and use a .50 caliber machine gun to hold off advancing German troops, killing fifty, all while bleeding from a leg wound.

Next time you equate size to intensity, remember the guy you are about to square up with might have had a rougher life than Audie Murphy. If so, you are about ready to find out what intensity really means up close and personal…

> Before he enlisted in the Army, Audie Murphy was turned down by two other branches of the military because he was too small and underweight, yet he went on to become the most decorated United States combat soldier of World War II. Mental toughness often trumps physical size and strength in a fight. As the adage goes, it is not the size of the dog in the fight, but the size of the fight in the dog.

According to the *Guinness Book of World Records*, Lieutenant Colonel Matt Urban (1919–1995) surpassed Murphy's feat to become the most combat-decorated soldier in American history. He was born Matty Louis Urbanowitz. We doubt either man would care who had more medals. They both served their country with honor, distinguishing themselves with a mental and physical toughness that superseded everything else. The honors simply followed their deeds.

Audie and Matty, while not exactly endowed with manly monikers such as Killer or Spike, were definitely guys you wouldn't want to cross. When it came to a fight, they both proved that size and intensity are not the same thing.

Take Nothing for Granted

He wins his battles by making no mistakes. Making no mistakes is what establishes the certainty of victory, for it means conquering an enemy that is already defeated… Hence, the skillful fighter puts himself into a position that makes defeat impossible, and does not miss the moment for defeating the enemy.
— Sun Tzu

In large-scale strategy, the area to watch is the enemy's strength. "Perception" and "sight" are the two methods of seeing. Perception consists of concentrating strongly on the enemy's spirit, overseeing the condition of the battlefield, fixing the gaze strongly, seeing the progress of the fight and the changes of advantage.
— Miyamoto Musashi

Kane was driving home from work on an arterial road through a mixed residential/industrial district one afternoon when he noticed flashing lights in his rear-view mirror. He took a quick glance at the speedometer, gave a sigh of relief that he was not exceeding the 35 MPH speed limit, and pulled over to the right to let the officer pass. Since the officer was not coming for him, Kane gave the incident little additional thought until he came upon a stoplight at a four-way intersection a few blocks later.

Although there were half a dozen cars between him and the light, Kane's truck cab was high enough up that he could see across the intersection to where the officer who had recently passed by had pulled over to the side of the road in front of a small apartment building halfway down the next block. As the policeman exited his vehicle, Kane noticed that he was wearing a helmet and ballistic vest, not the normal concealed vest that all officers wear on daily basis, but rather a bulky, riot-style over-garment that is rarely seen on the street. Furthermore, he was carrying an assault rifle, not exactly standard gear for a traffic control officer.

While Kane was waiting at the signal, seven more police cars arrived—one more from behind his vehicle, three from the opposite direction on the same roadway, and three from one of the cross streets. They came in quickly with lights flashing but no sirens and parked on both sides of the street in front of the apartment. Although not all the officers had exited their vehicles by the time the light changed, Kane noticed that they were all wearing ballistic helmets and bulletproof vests.

This developing situation was definitely concerning him. It's not an everyday occurrence, at least not in Seattle, for that many police cars to converge on any given location, particularly not with officers dressed for battle. While Kane had previously participated in a stadium drill that included the Seattle Police Department SWAT team, National Guard, and various other emergency services personnel, he had never seen officers dressed in this manner on the street. And, frankly, even though they were more than half a block away, he wasn't all that excited about seeing them quite so up close and personal.

Despite whatever danger had drawn law enforcement's attention, however, fully six cars that were on the road in front of Kane's vehicle failed to react to anything out of the ordinary. Perhaps they never even noticed a developing problem. Regardless, all of those drivers continued forward along the main arterial through the light, passing the gathered officers who were pulling an assortment of impressive-looking ordinance from their vehicles, clearly oblivious to the danger that this scene presented. Kane, on the other hand, turned right at the light choosing a safer path. As he went around the corner, he noticed in his rearview mirror at least three or four other vehicles behind him also continuing along the main arterial through the light instead of detouring along a safer but longer path as he had chosen to do.

Perusing the newspaper the next day, it was evident that nothing dramatic had happened during this event. There was only a routine drug arrest—no shootout, no body count. Regardless, there easily could have been. Driving between heavily armed officers and their intended target is foolhardy behavior. While a car door has some chance of stopping a stray bullet, windows most definitely do not. Despite this fact, everyone else was either unaware or unconcerned about the danger. If you watch the portrayal of police officers on television enough, it is easy to become disassociated from such events, never realizing that you may be placing yourself in imminent danger merely by proximity.

Since the best way to avoid injury in a fight is not getting into one in the first place, your prime strategy must be to become aware of and steer clear of the danger before it is too late. If you miss the cues or the situation spins out of control too fast to avoid, you have blown your self-defense. Good situational awareness means paying attention to the details, particularly those things that stand apart from the norm as the officers' presence certainly did on this occasion. Sometimes, though, it is not quite so obvious, perhaps only a feeling that something is wrong. Listen to your internal radar. If it pings off of something unusual, pay extra attention, look for avenues of escape, and be prepared to take action.

Whenever you are in public, it is important to pay attention to the subtle and not-so-subtle cues around you. Watch for people who look out of place or act in an unusual manner. Things like making too much or too little eye contact, hiding one's hands from plain view, moving stiffly or awkwardly, or dressing in an unusual manner might be of particular concern. Similarly, a group of toughs trying to look casual or a crowd that has gathered for no apparent reason might also be causes for concern. Look not only for what you can see, but also for what others are reacting to as well. Body language is important. They may very well have spotted something important that you missed. Pay attention to sounds and smells as well visual cues.

Being prepared and alert for trouble can stave off most attacks before they begin. Put yourself in a potential attacker's shoes, taking note of locations where you might lurk if you wanted to get the jump on someone. A few extra precautions near these potential ambush sites can add an extra layer of safety. The sooner you spot a potential attacker, the more time you will have to react. Keep your hands free to the extent possible so that you are ready to use them at a moment's notice.

Do your best to avoid potentially dangerous locations, times, and people. Be particularly cautious when traveling in fringe areas between populated and isolated areas such as when you go from a shopping mall to a parking lot, particularly at night. Plan ahead and take precautions. For example, if you need money from a cash machine during a night out, choose one inside a well-lit, busy store rather than using an isolated, freestanding parking lot kiosk or bank side ATM. Better still, use a credit card and avoid carrying large amounts of cash altogether.

When it comes to awareness and avoidance, the cornerstones of self-defense, it's the little things that matter. Take nothing for granted.

Little Things Are Often Important

The sight of men whispering together in small knots or speaking in subdued tones points to disaffection amongst the rank and file.
— *Sun Tzu*

Know the smallest things and the biggest things, the shallowest things and the deepest things. As if it were a straight road mapped out on the ground.
— *Miyamoto Musashi*

See the knife clip in the right front pocket of his blue jeans? Right there—you know he has a knife. Turning his right hip slightly away from you is a tiny little motion, yet it is going to get real significant in a moment. Once he turns a bit, you can no longer see that knife. Now you need to watch his right hand, yet he has dropped that back too. Suddenly you see his arm begin a slight upward movement. Is he innocently scratching an itch, or pulling out that knife in order to gut you with it?

It all takes place in a fraction of a second—little time, little movements. Unfortunately, these little things can snowball into a serious crisis in a very short period of time too. What about the quiet guy in the corner? You're discussing politics, religion, or some other emotional topic with your buddies when you notice movement in your peripheral vision. That guy in the corner suddenly sits up straighter. As he gets up out of his chair, you notice that he has lowered his shoulders and slowed his breathing. He then moves purposefully toward you with a serious look on his face. Does he need to take a pee real bad or is he about to attack?

> When it comes to awareness and avoidance, it's the little things that matter. Pay attention to the subtle and not-so-subtle clues around you. Watch for people who look out of place or act in an unusual manner. Look for other people's reactions to things you may have missed that might become important. Pay attention to unusual sounds and smells too, taking nothing for granted.

Little things that become important aren't limited to threat indicators that help you know when someone's gunning for you. They also include environmental considerations such as terrain, weather conditions, escape routes, sources of cover or concealment, bystanders, impromptu weapons, and so on; another reason, yet again, why situational awareness is so important. If you want to take best advantage of these factors, it is important to pay attention to the details you're given before trouble starts. You'll be far too busy defending yourself afterward.

Terrain, for example, can help or hinder you. If you can take the high ground in an uneven environment such as a hill, stairwell, or pile of debris, it becomes much more difficult for your opponent to reach you or prevent your escape. Spilled blood, oil or foodstuffs, loose gravel, wet grass or leaves, mud, and other hazardous conditions may affect your footing. If you are aware of these surroundings, you can adjust your stance, find a stable place, or maneuver your opponent onto slippery ground to gain an advantage.

Similarly, weather conditions may help or hurt. It is hard to fight with the sun in your eyes. Heat, humidity, and dehydration can sap your stamina, increasing the urgency of ending a fight quickly. Conversely, it is tough to grapple in powdery snow, icy conditions, or pouring rain, making it easier to get away if you can control your balance, posture, and speed.

Little things are particularly important when it comes to weapons. Obviously if you do not realize that the other guy is armed until after he attacks you, you are in serious trouble. It's more than just that, though: Bullets that miss or pass through their target continue to travel down range, potentially striking innocent bystanders. Self-defense sprays such as Mace or pepper spray don't work very well in windy, rainy, or enclosed areas where they might dissipate or blow back in your face. Grappling with a Mace-covered adversary can be extraordinarily problematic; that stuff is both extremely slick and highly irritating to your eyes, nose, and throat. Impromptu weapons like bottles, bricks, boards, rocks, pool cues, fire extinguishers, flashlights, hammers, and wrenches might be lying around in close proximity for you or your adversary to pick up and use. You need to pay attention to these details.

Be wary of bystanders too. People who oversee a confrontation can be good, bad, or neutral. Unless they are people whose job it is to get involved such as bouncers, security personnel, or law enforcement officers, you really don't know what they might do. They

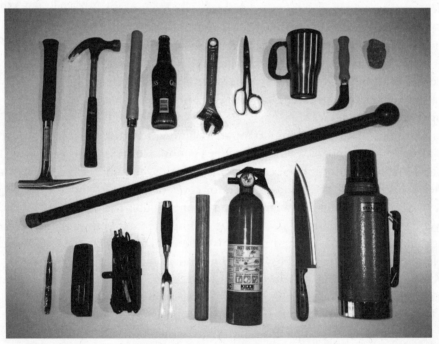

Almost anything can be a weapon if you know how to use it properly. Pay attention to little things such as objects lying around that may be utilized as impromptu weapons by you or your attacker during a fight.

may be inclined to help you, of course, but they could just as easily ignore your plight in favor of their own safety or for fear of legal repercussions.

The "bystander effect," a sociological phenomenon where the more witnesses present the less likely it is that any individual person will intervene has been studied extensively since the infamous murder of Catherine "Kitty" Genovese in 1964. In a more recent example, when a 22-year-old college student was attacked and severely beaten near the University of Washington campus on January 8, 2008, the assault was witnessed by at least half a dozen individuals who responded to the police investigation afterward, yet none of them intervened or called for help at the time of the attack. Afterward, the heavily bleeding victim managed to make it to her car and drive several blocks to the north campus entrance where she found a parking lot attendant who dialed 9-1-1. Authorities later reported that she had suffered severe head injuries and a broken jaw, but was expected to make a full recovery.

> Little things are often important—little time, little movements. Through good situational awareness and keen observation, you might spot a weapon or discover hostile intent before it is too late to react. During a fight, you might be able to take advantage of terrain, weather conditions, escape routes, sources of cover or concealment, bystanders, or impromptu weapons if you pay attention to those important details ahead of time.

Bystanders may even be inclined to hurt you, especially if they are friends or associates of the other guy. Knowing whether or not people hanging around the scene are part of the same group can be important. Even if bystanders do not get directly involved, witnesses may be called upon to testify to your actions in court, so in addition to fighting off your adversary you need to be cognizant of how witnesses might perceive whatever you choose to do. Once again, details count.

Little things are often important. Good situational awareness and keen observation can help you spot dangerous situations before it is too late to react. During a fight, you might be able to take advantage of terrain, weather conditions, escape routes, sources of cover or concealment, bystanders, or impromptu weapons if you paid attention to those important details ahead of time.

Know Your Territory

The art of war recognizes nine varieties of ground: (1) dispersive ground; (2) facile ground; (3) contentious ground; (4) open ground; (5) ground of intersecting highways; (6) serious ground; (7) difficult ground; (8) hemmed-in ground; (9) desperate ground.

– Sun Tzu

First see the distance timing and the background timing. This is the main thing in strategy. It is especially important to know the background timing; otherwise your strategy will become uncertain.

– Miyamoto Musashi

How many ways are there in and out of the office you are working in, the bar you're drinking at, the restaurant where you eat, or the house you are visiting? Can you see the front door? Do you know who is coming and going? Where are the exits, both front, back, and emergency? Which exits can you see and monitor and which ones are hidden from your view? Are there windows you can fit through that may be opened or broken out? How far away are you from these exits? If you want to get out quickly, who and what stand in your way? If you leave the building by a side or back door, where does exiting that way place you once you get outside? What can you expect to find there?

It is very important to understand your territory regardless of where you are, maintaining awareness of all entrances and exits as well as what you might expect to find should you take one of them. Know all the various routes by which you might escape should something bad start to happen. Violence can happen anywhere. It does not matter whether you are sitting in a building, walking down the street, or driving in traffic; you must always be aware of avenues for escape.

Be aware and leave any area where trouble seems to be brewing. The way you came in is usually a safe way to retreat. Nevertheless, it's more important to move to safety than to move away from danger. Slinking off quietly is generally best. Rash or aggressive movements might make you the target of violence that was meant for someone else. Here are some general guidelines to follow.

- Walk away normally if you only have a feeling that things are not right. Listen to your intuition. It is better to be embarrassed and safe than seriously injured if you don't take heed of your internal warnings.
- Evade potential or developing threats by crossing the street, turning, and walking back the way you came from, turning down another street, or otherwise moving toward a safer location. Whenever possible, moving toward heavily populated areas is best.
- If actual trouble becomes apparent, move away from it quickly but calmly. If the bad guy(s) starts after you, run away swiftly.
- Call attention to your predicament by yelling for help as appropriate. Pointing out an attacker's weapon or shouting "fire" or some other attention-getting phrases tends to work better than a generic cry for help.*

Wilder once had an instructor who, when going to a restaurant, would always ask the wait staff to reseat him. Without exception, he would choose a different table from the one where he was originally placed by the host. When Wilder noticed this behavior, he found it rather odd, asking his teacher why he always did that.

---

* Don't shout "fire" if he's got a gun though. That'd be somewhat counterproductive...

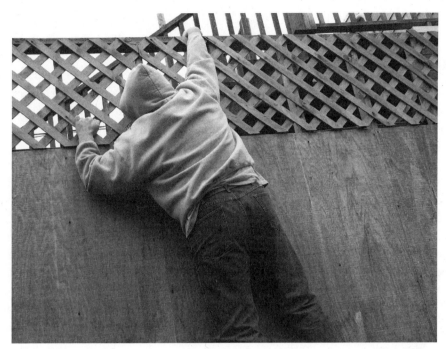

Hopping fences can be a good way to escape, but be sure you have a good lead on your pursuers before you try it. Getting dragged off a fence and slammed onto the ground is absolutely no fun.

The explanation was interesting. His teacher wanted to see as much of the restaurant as he could. He did not like having his back to a window and always wanted to be able to see the front door. That way nobody could come up behind him and nobody could come in the restaurant unobserved.

Paranoid behavior? In today's world, maybe not. After all, restaurants have been shot up, crashed into, and even blown up on numerous occasions. Case in point: On July 18, 1984, James Oliver Huberty walked into the San Ysidro, California McDonald's restaurant and murdered 21 people, including five children and six teenagers, and wounded 19 more victims before being killed by a police officer. That incident was one of the worst mass murders in the United States at that time.

Choose your friends wisely. Knowing your territory also means understanding the proclivities of the people with whom you spend time. Hang out with people who like to cause trouble, and it will eventually catch up with not only them but also with you.

If you are part of a group and find yourselves in a hazardous situation, the best policy is that you either all run at once or everyone stays to fight. There should be some pre-arranged signal to ensure that you are all on the same page. Running away together, even if you flee in opposite directions, leaves no one in a tight spot. If the person you were counting on to cover your back flees, on the other hand, you could be in serious trouble.

Similarly, you should not leave your friends to the wolves either.

With or without a group, if something bad happens you will need a way out. The way in which you escape is dependant upon how many attackers there are, how bad they want to catch you, and the tactical situation you encounter. Most people you will encounter on the street will not be motivated to chase you beyond a certain distance. If, for example, you encounter a couple of thugs looking to make a quick buck, they should be relatively easy to distract and escape from, especially if you throw a few dollars their way before you run.

Bad guys do try to go after you on occasion though. The longer you keep out of an adversary's hands, the more likely they will be to give up. Dragging stuff into a pursuer's way, dodging around obstacles, over fences, or through hedges, or otherwise slowing them down is a good way to string them out, facilitating your ability to escape successfully. Your goal is to get enough of a lead to lose your pursuers completely, find somewhere safe to hide, convince your opponents to give up, or otherwise gain safety. In the meantime, however, you need to ensure that as few opponents as possible are in striking distance to engage you. After all, if one opponent can tie you up by engaging in combat, the others may have time to join in before you can end the battle.

> If something bad happens, you will need a way out. Knowing your territory gives you a significant advantage whenever you need to escape from trouble. This not only means having an awareness of entrances, exits, and avenues for escape, but also understanding the proclivities of the people you hang out with as well. Hang out with people who like to cause trouble, and it will eventually catch up with not only them but with you as well.

You may find shops you can duck through, fences you can climb over, gaps in hedges you can worm through, and other bottlenecks where only a single person can slip through at a time. Be careful about climbing anything though. Unless your pursuers are a good distance behind you, slowing your forward progress long enough to overcome an obstacle may let them close too much of the gap you have created. Getting dragged off a fence and slammed into the ground is too easily the outcome.

Hopping fences can provide an extra level of safety if you are friendly with a neighbor's dog and have enough of a lead to do so successfully. This assumes that the dogs will leave you alone and harass your pursuers, of course. If you have a choice, going over a fence at the corner where four yards meet is an excellent location. That way, if you choose unwisely and the dog or neighbor is not as friendly as you expected, it is just a short hop into a safer yard.

In areas that are less familiar to you, you must be especially cautious about what is on the other side of a fence, however. If you cannot see through the fence, you may wish to choose an alternate route. After all, it would not do to hop over a fence only to discover an angry Rottweiler, land in an empty pool, become entangled in thorny rosebushes, or break your ankle from an unexpectedly long drop.

Crossing a busy street is another good, albeit dangerous, way to escape pursuers. To be most successful, run parallel to traffic, choosing your best moment to act before crossing. If there are multiple lanes, you can implement this "run parallel then cross" method for each lane.

If someone is chasing you in a car, he can travel a whole lot faster than you can. He can also use it as a weapon to squash you. Vehicles can cause a whole lot more damage than firearms. Be sure to cut 90 degrees at your first opportunity, bolting between parked cars, through any convenient business, housing complex, narrow alley, or other area that the pursuing vehicle cannot easily pass through. Travel a couple of blocks then change directions again so that your pursuers cannot simply go around the block and catch sight of you all over again. Be cautious if you see or hear some of your pursuers leaving the vehicle because they may be able to split into more than one search party. Knowing that they have done so will influence which directions remain available for escape.

Knowing your territory gives you a significant advantage whenever you need to escape from trouble.

Restrain Impassioned Friends

There are five dangerous faults which may affect a general: (1) recklessness, which leads to destruction; (2) cowardice, which leads to capture; (3) a hasty temper, which can be provoked by insults; (4) a delicacy of honor which is sensitive to shame; (5) over-solicitude for his men, which exposes him to worry and trouble.

— Sun Tzu

When you opponent is hurrying recklessly, you must act contrarily, and keep calm. You must not be influenced by the opponent. Train diligently to attain this spirit.

— Miyamoto Musashi

You know him affectionately as "no-shirt guy." You know, the one who's always bouncing up and down, screaming, shouting, cheerleading, and generally making an ass of himself in the stands while you watch the game. A few beers and some harsh words later and, predictably, your buddy Mr. No-shirt is fighting with some other fan. Now, instead of enjoying yourself you're trying to drag him off the other guy, calm things down, and make sure no one is seriously hurt when suddenly the police arrive. A few hours later, you are bailing him out of jail. Again.

Or perhaps you know him by some other name such as "chip on his shoulder guy." Regardless, it's always the mouthy friend who gets things going, isn't it? These guys come in many different flavors—small and mouthy, big and arrogant, crazy, or just plain dumb.

Whatever your friend's demeanor or intelligence level, you needn't let him and his big fat mouth write a check that you need to cash.

This is even more important if the situation is already ongoing. If the monkey dance is underway, it is very difficult to get things back under control before things get violent. This is where your impassioned friend will invariably want to throw the proverbial match into the gas-filled room. Stop him from doing so.

Here's a good example. It was late in the third quarter of an exciting college football game. Fans from both teams had packed the stands in the east end zone. Throughout the game, there had been all the typical taunts and insults you might expect in that sort of environment, but nothing horribly serious had occurred despite the fact that one group of home team fans from the northeast side kept running in front of the predominantly visitor fans on the southeast side and bopping around in a little victory dance with each big play or touchdown that was scored.

As illicit alcohol flowed and tempers ran hot, Kane and his crew took increasingly stricter measures to keep the rowdy fans apart. They drew an imaginary line between the two sections, telling rowdies on both sides that so long as they stuck to their own section, they could rabble-rouse to their hearts' content. Cross the line to taunt the other team's fans, however, and they'd be thrown out of the stadium. Guess who the first person was to cross the line? Why, no-shirt guy, of course.

Actually, there were several guys without shirts, but it was one of that bare-chested crew who took it upon himself to test the limit. He got in an argument with the security guard who tried to prevent him from reaching the opposing fans. No-shirt's friends, slightly smarter or more sober, were trying to hold him back without success. Kane, realizing what was about to happen from a few yards away, grabbed a few additional guards, radioed the police, and moved to intervene.

> Restrain impassioned friends. It's always your big-mouthed buddy who gets things going. These guys come in many different flavors—small and mouthy, big and arrogant, crazy, or just plain stupid. Whatever your friend's demeanor or intelligence level, don't let his big fat mouth write a check that you need to cash. If he insists on behaving immaturely, find someone else with whom to hang out.

Unfortunately, by the time he got there, the security guy already had a bloody nose and Mr. No-shirt was beating his chest in glee, doing his best Tarzan imitation with the injured guard lying at his feet. He even elbowed one of his friends who was still trying unsuccessfully to hold him back, cracking him hard enough in the cheek to make his teeth snap together.

Fortunately, the police showed up at the same time. Since they had seen everything that occurred before they arrived, they were able to take direct action. Seconds later, Mr. No-shirt was in handcuffs. While the police led him off to jail, Kane escorted No-shirt's friends out of the stadium, took their tickets, and ordered the gate guards not to let them back in. Despite the fact that they had not directly participated in the

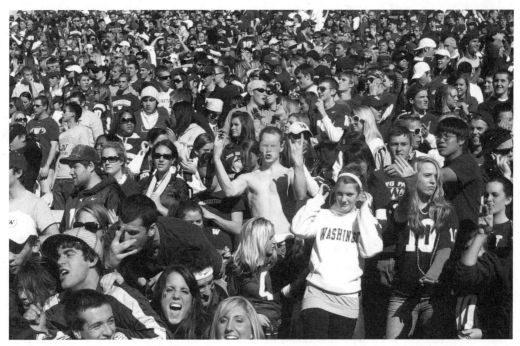

"No-shirt guy." Don't let his big fat mouth write a check that you need to cash right along with him. Restrain impassioned friends… or find new ones.

altercation, they got thrown out too. They'd already been warned twice and the third time was the charm.

Collectively, they missed one of the most exciting games of the year, an affair that was decided by a clutch field goal in the waning seconds of the first overtime period. No-shirt guy wrote a check that his friends had to cash along with him. While they were not injured and, fortunately, did not have to cool their heels along with him in jail, they still paid a price. It could have been far worse and, if they keep hanging out with him, undoubtedly will be in the future. Restrain impassioned friends. If they insist on behaving immaturely, find new ones.

When it Comes to Violence, Girlfriends Can Be Helpful… but Generally Not

The skillful tactician may be likened to the shuai-jan. Now the shuai-jan is a snake that is found in the Chung mountains. Strike at its head, and you will be attacked by its tail; strike at its tail, and you will be attacked by its head; strike at its middle, and you will be attacked by head and tail both.

– Sun Tzu

Fright often occurs, caused by the unexpected.
                                              — Miyamoto Musashi

Some girlfriends think it's pretty sexy for you to fight over them. They will go out of their way to set up situations where you can prove your manhood by doing so. The fact is that this is ancient, tribal thinking. There was a time in the world where that type of behavior was essential to choosing a mate. The biggest and strongest male ensured her survival in a hunter-gatherer society, and for that matter, in an early agrarian one as well.

This type of behavior has no place in modern society. If your girlfriend thinks that getting you to bash some guy upside the head in fighting for her honor is cool, you are with the wrong woman. You need to take a deep look at where that behavior is coming from, why you are attracted to it, and consider how it is going to get you in trouble. And then you need to leave.

If you are in public and your girlfriend is setting you up to fight in front of her or her friends, you need to disassociate yourself right away from her and the situation she is creating. She is walking trouble. She will not just get you into one fight, but many. This is because she thinks that violence is cool at some deep-rooted level. If you are hanging out with this type of person, you truly are playing with fire.

"Baby, that guy over there just called me a bitch," she might say. "Go over there and demand an apology from him!" Are you going to walk over to that big, bald, tattooed guy with the pool cue in his hand, the one who is glaring at you with an unblinking eye? Most likely not. At least not if you are smart. Does the scenario change if he is a short guy with a pocket protector and thick glasses held together with athletic tape? It probably will but it shouldn't.

> If your girlfriend (or boyfriend for that matter) thinks that violence in defense of the woman's honor is cool, you are playing with fire. She will not just get you into one fight, but many. Sooner or later, she will get you seriously hurt, maimed, or killed… or sued or thrown in jail. Dump her (or him) now!

In 1984, four young men accosted Bernard Getz on a New York subway. A self-employed electrical repairman running a small business out of his city apartment, Getz could be described as a classic nerd. Whatever version of the story you may have heard, despite guilt or innocence of all involved, four people wound up being shot in about one and a half seconds during the encounter.

Getz, who carried a concealed weapon, had practiced speed shooting and was very good with the gun. Because of all his practice, his gun was more than an equalizer; it gave him the advantage. How many other nerds might you run across who carry a weapon? Knife, gun, pool cue, baseball bat, or beer bottle, it makes no difference—dead is dead, maimed is maimed—whatever the cause.

If you are thinking "fight" and the other guy is thinking "combat," you are in for a world of hurt. A fight implies a rules-based event, something like a boxing match or mixed martial arts competition. In a fight, you might punch, kick, and/or throw each other

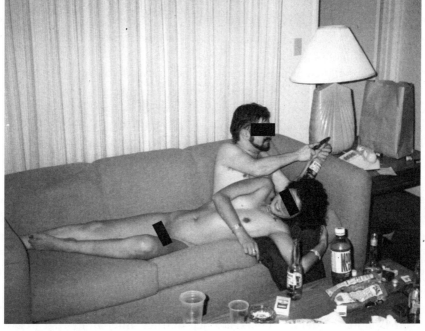

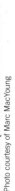

Photo courtesy of Marc MacYoung

If your girlfriend thinks that violence in defense of her honor is cool, you are playing with fire. She will not just get you into one fight, but many.

down, but you are not likely to kick the other guy's head in or stomp on his throat once he is down. Combat, on the other hand, is a no-holds-barred struggle for survival. That's where weapons come into play, eyes are gouged out, ears are bitten off, testicles are torn loose, and serious repercussions can be expected.

So, the bottom line is that if your girlfriend wants you to fight for her honor, if she just thinks it is cool for you to fight, don't. Get another girlfriend. For women who are reading this book, our recommendation for you is the same as when the genders are reversed. This guy is trouble; you need to look real hard at what is happening to you. Dump him now and find someone else to hang out with.

Live to Fight Another Day

If the enemy has occupied them before you, do not follow him, but retreat and try to entice him away.
— Sun Tzu

In single combat, you can win by relaxing your body and spirit and then, catching on to the moment the enemy relaxes attack strongly and quickly, forestalling him.
— Miyamoto Musashi

"That's f%&king b%$#sh*t," growled the tattooed, goateed guy at the bar, berating the waitress with a string of invectives that could make a drunken sailor blush. The waitress walked away, but Wilder, who overheard the argument, could not. From his table across the room he felt compelled to say, "You're a tough guy."

The tattooed guy leaned back in his chair, turned his head toward Wilder, and snarled, "You wanna see how tough?" He crossed his muscular arms across his broad chest and glared dead-eyed across the room, waiting for a response.

Okaaaay, now Wilder had a decision to make. Would he escalate the issue to a fight? He suddenly realized that he had fallen into an interview. He had foolishly thought he was going to point out the other guy's rudeness and get an apology while the other guy was ready to fight and looking for an excuse to do it.

Realizing instantly that he needed to send a different message, Wilder looked into the other guy's eyes, gave a nod toward the football game playing on the bar's TV, and asked, "Who do you like, Vikings or Lions?" The tattooed guy smirked and shifted his gaze back up at the television without a saying another word. Wilder had answered his question… His query about the football game stated, in essence, "No. I really don't want to find out how tough you are."

Does such a response make Wilder a wimp? Was he a loser for not wanting to fight for the waitress' honor? After all, he's a black belt in three different martial arts. Shouldn't he have taught this rude guy a lesson in manners? Of course not. He understood the consequences of such actions and chose the better part of valor. Win or lose, if it came to physical blows Wilder would have been in serious trouble.

If he beat the other guy down, the fact that Wilder was a black belt would undoubtedly have come out in court, dramatically increasing the odds that he would lose a criminal and/or civil trial. Not only does he have a *dojo* Web site, but he's also a published author with several martial arts books under his name. Lawyers and prosecutors can Google too. If, on the other hand, he got beat down himself, the consequences could have been just as dire if not worse. Would it have been worth being sued for everything he owned, accumulating thousands of dollars in legal fees while having his reputation dragged through the mud, or becoming crippled, maimed, or even killed over a few rude words? Definitely not!

Know what is worth fighting for and what is not. That's the purpose of the questionnaire in Appendix A. It will help you dispassionately identify what is worth the risks of a physical confrontation before you need to make such choices under fire. Unless your life or the life of another is on the line, it's almost always best to swallow your pride and walk away. Live to fight another day.

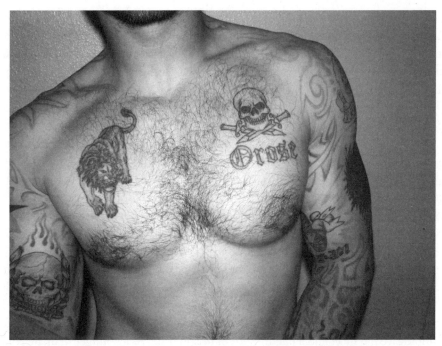

From his table across the room he felt compelled to say, "You're a tough guy." The tattooed guy leaned back in his chair and snarled, "You wanna see how tough?"

When You Think You Are a Good Fighter, You're Not

There are five dangerous faults which may affect a general: (1) recklessness, which leads to destruction...
— *Sun Tzu*

If you study a Way daily, and your spirit diverges, you may think you are obeying a good way, but objectively it is not the true Way. If you are following the true Way and diverge a little, this will later become a large divergence.
— *Miyamoto Musashi*

Self-assurance is not demonstrated with slumped shoulders, hanging head, a shuffling walk, or weak voice. Quite the opposite, these clues tell predators, bullies, and thugs that you are an easy mark. Being the doormat or the mouse in the corner often makes you a target for the bully. Holding your head high, walking deliberately, and making eye contact, on the other hand, are good signs of confidence.

Puffing your chest out and sneering is no way to make friends though. Being over-confident can also make you a mark, somebody who has something to prove. That means that you are easy to provoke. Arrogance is not a good look on anybody. Giving everybody a hard stare is not too beneficial either.

Being at either end of this spectrum is a bad idea, yet being overconfident is a great way to find the fast path to a good beating. You are more likely to go "hands on" than an under-confident person is. Knock that chip off your shoulder. Truly tough guys don't need to prove it. Smart guys don't try to find out.

> Violence always has consequences. Know what is worth fighting for and what is not, dispassionately evaluating your priorities and values before you need to make such judgments in the heat of the moment. It is far better to live to fight another day than to make rash choices you may live to regret.

Do you think you are pretty tough, a good fighter? Maybe you did a little boxing in the neighborhood and took some martial arts for a couple of years a while back. Or maybe you were a Golden Gloves champion or a big league tournament competitor with a display case full of trophies. Perhaps you're even a black belt. Big deal! You're nothing compared to the guy standing across from you, the one with the dead-eyed stare who wants to rip your arm off and beat you to death with it.

This guy, to paint one possible scenario, used to get pummeled by his mother's boyfriend at least once a week… for twelve years. He learned fast and early how to bully, intimidate, and get his way by physical force. He knows what pain is—inside and out. And he revels in it. He is well known to the police too, compiling an impressive rap sheet and a fair amount of prison time. As a younger man, he got passed around among the prisoners yet nowadays he's the one putting the hurt on. In and out of the joint, he has had to fight. He is familiar with both ends of the knife, gun, brass knuckles, and bludgeon, and has some pretty impressive scars as well to prove it. Violence is an everyday occurrence to him; it means little other than a tool that is used to satisfy his wanton desires. You, my friend, are nothing but a blip on the chart of his evening's events. He can throw you to the ground, stomp on your neck, and walk away without a second thought. You live, you die; it makes no difference to him.

Perhaps he's a contractor for Blackwater Global Security. After three tours, half a dozen Purple Hearts, and a Bronze Star or two, he mustered out of the service but found that he couldn't adapt to civilian life. An adrenaline junkie, he loves to fight and got more than his share of action in Iraq, Afghanistan, and a host of Third World countries with unruly populations and acute violence problems. He used to keep a mental log of how many people he has killed but lost track somewhere around 80. He not only has the best training that money can buy, but he's got more than fifteen years of hard-earned, hands-on experience that has helped him refine how to use it. He's killed with a knife, gun, and his bare hands, not counting various and sundry pieces of heavy artillery. He loves the smell of napalm in the morning; blood and mud, sh*t and sweat are nothing new to him. He may not look much like Rambo, but he's a real life, snake-eating SOB who can take you and all your friends apart without breaking a sweat. You are not even a road bump along his path but rather a slug to be salted, a bug to be squashed, or a fish to be gutted.

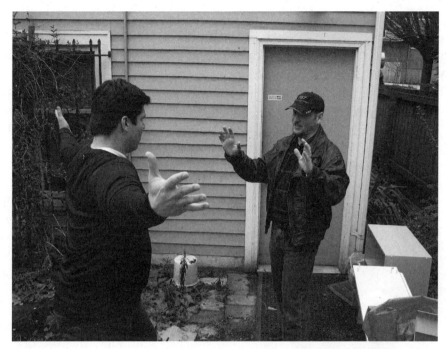

Violence always has consequences. Know what is worth fighting for and what is not, dispassionately evaluating your priorities and values before you need to make such judgments in the heat of the moment.

Or, maybe he looks like a little old man, but he's spent a lifetime studying traditional karate. He learned old school in Japan, starting at the age of four where his father trained him five hours a day year-round, beating him with a rattan stick whenever he made a mistake. He spent years just perfecting a single stance and has since mastered every aspect of his art. His form is so good that you can punch him in the solar plexus as hard as you like and he'll just laugh and tell you to hit harder. By the time he reached his late teens, he was *dojo* busting, dueling with local *sensei* * who paid him protection money for the privilege of continuing to run their martial arts schools after he had beat them down. In his early twenties, he beat down a *yakuza*† member in the blink of an eye, crushing him so severely that the rest of the gang was too terrified to seek revenge. His body mechanics are so flawless that at the age of sixty he can still perform *ikken hissatsu*,‡ killing with

---

* *Sensei* means teacher, literally "one who has come before." In this case, it refers specifically to martial arts instructors.

† *Yakuza* means "violence group." Criminal gangs, they are more-or-less the Japanese equivalent of the Italian mafia. While semi-legitimate in many cases, they tend to be heavily involved in extortion, blackmail, racketeering, drug trafficking, arms smuggling, prostitution, and similar illicit activities.

‡ Roughly translated, *ikken hissatsu* means "one blow one kill." It is the rare albeit very real ability to deliver fight-ending power, breaking bones, disrupting internal organs, or literally killing an opponent outright, with every single punch or kick

a single blow. Throw a punch at this guy and if you're lucky he'll laugh in your face and walk away. If he's in a bad mood, however, he'll crush you like a grape.

All three of these aforementioned characters are based on real people, guys who know violence inside and out. Will you always run across a "heavy hitter," such as we have described, every time you get in a fight? Odds say that you won't, yet just like a nuclear bomb it takes only one to screw up your whole day. No matter how tough you are, there is always someone out there who's tougher. No matter how good a fighter you are, there is always someone out there who's better. Walk away; you are not that good.

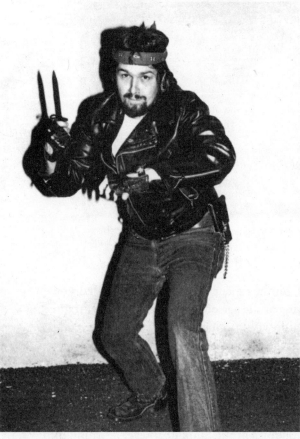

Do you really have what it takes to tangle with a heavy hitter, a career criminal, mental case, or a seasoned street fighter in a live-fire situation? You're not that good. And even if you are, it doesn't pay to find out.

Here's a chilling, real life example of what tangling with a "heavy hitter" is actually like. On March 7, 2003, Sgt. Marcus Young, an 18-year veteran of the Ukiah, California Police Department received a seemingly routine shoplifting call at a Wal-Mart store. He had a 17-year-old police cadet named Julian Covella riding along with him at the time. They met briefly with store security to understand the situation, collected the suspect, and then proceeded to bring her out to the patrol car. No big deal, right?

Wrong. As Sgt. Young and Wal-Mart security guard Brett Schott put the shoplifting suspect Monica Winnie, 18, into the back seat of the patrol car, her 35-year-old companion Neal Beckman tried to intervene. A dangerous looking individual with small devil horns tattooed on his forehead, he approached the group with his hands hidden from view in his pockets. As Beckman approached, Sgt. Young commanded, "Take your hands out of your pockets," but received no response. He repeated his command to which Beckman responded, "I have a knife," drew his blade, and began to attack.

It only takes a highly trained police officer a second or two to draw his weapon and fire an aimed shot. Regrettably, Young didn't have that long. Since he was caught flat-footed, we've suddenly got an open-hand battle against a committed, competent, and downright psychopathic knife-wielding attacker. But it gets even worse yet; what Young did not see was Beckman's gun, a .38 caliber revolver, held in his other hand.

Utilizing both his police training and the skills he developed as a 2nd *dan* black belt in karate, Young quickly wrenched the attacker's arm into a lock but was unable to force him to let go of the knife. As the two of them slammed into the side of the car, Beckman began firing, hitting Young in the face, body, and arm.

Schott, the unarmed security guard, leapt into the fight, wrenching the revolver away from Beckman. He aimed it at the suspect and pulled the trigger. Before Schott realized that the gun had already been emptied into Sgt. Young and would no longer fire, the suspect stabbed him in the chest with his knife, collapsing a lung. Weakened by this massive chest wound, Schott disengaged, trying to find cover.

While this occurred, Sgt. Young had a brief moment and a little space to even the odds, bringing his own weapon on line. He regained his feet and tried to reach for his gun. Unfortunately, he quickly discovered that his humerus (upper arm bone) had been shattered by the Beckman's bullets, paralyzing his gun arm from nerve damage. He tried to draw with his left hand instead, only to find that it had been ripped apart during the struggle with the knife, its separated tendons visible through the opened skin.

Deprived of his weapons as well, Beckman dove into the front seat of the police car, closed the door, and frantically began searching for the hidden switch that would release the loaded Remington shotgun and HK sub-machine gun locked therein. As the suspect tried to free the heavy weapons in the vehicle, Young turned to his cadet Covella and said, "Take my gun out and put it in my hand." The boy quickly released the safety strap and placed the firearm into Young's mangled left hand.

> No matter how tough you are, there is always someone out there who's tougher. No matter how good a fighter you are, there is always someone out there who's better. Do you really want to find out if you have what it takes to tangle with a heavy hitter, a career criminal, mental case, or a seasoned street fighter in a live-fire situation? You're not that good. And even if you are, it doesn't pay to find out. Will you always run across a "heavy hitter" every time you get in a fight? Odds say that you won't, yet just like a nuclear bomb it only takes only one to screw up your whole day.

Kneeling to steady himself, Young tried to shoot the suspect through the closed door to no avail. His bullets did not penetrate all the way through. Re-aiming through the closed window instead, he managed to place two rounds into the suspect, dropping him. Young then asked Covella to call for assistance and began deliberate, controlled breathing exercises to keep himself calm, conscious, and alive until medical personnel could respond.

Schott, the security guard, recovered from his horrific injuries. Both he and police cadet Covella received numerous awards for valor from their roles in the incident. These included heroism citations from the Veterans of Foreign Wars and the American Legion, and dual Citizen of the Year awards from the California Narcotics Officers' Association. Covella has since been accepted as a cadet at the United States Naval Academy at Annapolis.

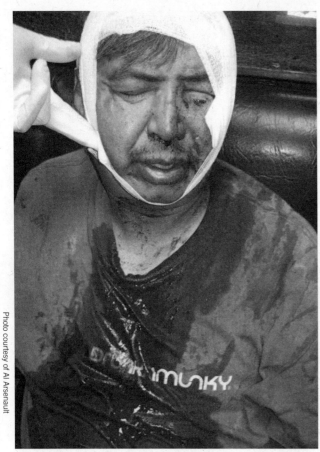

Real-life violence isn't horribly romantic.

As of late 2004, Sergeant Young was on light duty, still recovering from his severe physical injuries and facing more surgery. He was awarded the National Rifle Association's honor as Police Officer of the Year for 2003, as well as the Mayor's Medal of Valor. He was also nominated for the Presidential Medal of Valor and the California Attorney General's Office Medal of Valor. He retired from the Ukiah PD after 20 years in law enforcement in August 2006 and was subsequently hired by the Mendocino Community College as a Coordinator for the Administration of Justice Program

The Young/Beckman incident has been included in fear and anger management classes at the California Police Standards and Training council. Young reported that he felt he owes his survival not only to Schott and Covella, but also to the many instructors who trained him over the years. "They taught me to shoot from awkward positions if I was wounded," he related, "and they taught me to be resourceful and keep thinking and keep fighting no matter how I might be injured. They taught me to never give up."

Real violence isn't so romantic, huh? How would you fare in Young's place? If you were shot, stabbed, and mangled with the kinds of horrific injuries that he suffered, would you truly have the fortitude to fight on, or would you lie down and die? Most people wouldn't make it, even most soldiers and police officers. It's not just mental and physical toughness that let him survive but also a bit of luck as well. Had Schott and Covella not intervened, Young almost certainly would not have survived. Beckman would have been able to free one of the heavy weapons and then finish him off.

Do you really want to find out if you have what it takes in a live-fire situation? As combat veterans have come to realize, you never hear the one that hits you, only the near misses. You're not that good. And even if you are, it doesn't pay to find out.

Don't Claim Your Turf

When a chieftain is fighting in his own territory, it is dispersive ground.
— *Sun Tzu*

Musashi does not address claiming and holding ground in The Book of Five Rings.

Claiming your turf is about as tribal an act as you can commit. When you claim turf, you are no brighter than a caveman. Wilder once sat on the couch listening while his friend described a co-worker's son who was shot dead at the age of twenty-two, outside of a rural bar. He had heard about the tragic incident on the news, but now he was getting the full story. And it was about claiming turf.

The twenty-two-year-old, David, had gotten into a bar fight with another guy. When the fight was broken up, the other guy was 86ed from the establishment. As he was leaving, shouting and challenges ensued, and threats were made, yet David chose to stay in the bar for the rest of the evening. He was having fun with his friends. It was his turf, he'd claimed it, and he wasn't about to give it up. He did not want to go home until closing time.

As he left to go to his car, he found himself suddenly confronted by the other guy who had returned with a gun. Seconds later, David was dead in the dirt from a bullet to his brain. For extra measure, the other guy put a bullet in his eye too. The other guy then fled the country back to Taiwan or possibly mainland China. The end result of that evening was a promising life cut short with no possibility of justice.

It's only common sense; if you get in a fight and win you need to leave soon afterward so that you cannot be found again that night. Revenge happens… a lot. It is not your turf; you don't live there. No matter how much you like the place it's still just a bar. If you really want to keep drinking, go find another establishment a long way away. Or, better yet, call it a night.

Turf mentality means that someone has to win and someone else must lose. It almost guarantees violence because the other guy has no face-saving way to back down. He leaves or you make him leave, there's no in-between. That's unnecessary, juvenile, and dangerous.

If you are mature, you don't fight unless you have to. When your life or that of a loved one is on the line, when you face grave bodily injury or death without fighting, then you pour it on with all you've got. When you don't have to fight, however, you walk away. It's the smart, mature thing to do.

Maturity means being confident in who you are. Taunts, threats, and name-calling will not injure your ego bad enough to make you feel a need to strike out. Swallow your pride and walk away. There is no good reason to stake your turf. Turf is for gangs to fight over because it is their livelihood. That's where they deal drugs, sell guns, manage prostitutes, and commit other crimes to earn their living. Turf means nothing to you, at least not if you are smart.

Invading Your Opponent's Territory Means One of Two Things

When an invading force crosses a river in its onward march, do not advance to meet it in mid-stream. It will be best to let half the army get across, and then deliver your attack.

— *Sun Tzu*

You must push down his thrust, and throw off his hold when he tries to grapple. This is the meaning of "to hold down a pillow." When you have grasped this principle, whatever the enemy tries to bring about in the fight you will see in advance and suppress it.

— *Miyamoto Musashi*

Humans are by nature territorial. We all have a concept of personal space, an invisible barrier surrounding us through which only intimate relations are welcome. Anyone who else who gets too close makes us uncomfortable. The exact distance varies by culture, of course, yet that boundary exists just about everywhere. Beyond our personal space, we often claim other territory as well, things like parking spots, concert seats, or chairs at our favorite bar. Whenever someone encroaches on what we believe is ours, it generates an emotional response and, oftentimes, a physical reaction as well.

Invading an opponent's territory means one of two things: Either you are fighting or the other guy is retreating. If you have studied martial arts, you know that when fighting correctly there is no backing up. You may dodge, evade, or shift off the line of your opponent's attack, but you never move straight backwards. As Wilder's old football coach used to say, you should "be rolled on the balls of your feet." This means that whoever is attacking is forcefully invading the other person's territory, moving very aggressively.

> Whenever you claim turf, you put yourself in a win-lose mentality. It's yours now, so it cannot be his. That type of thinking frequently leads to violence. No matter how much you like the place, a bar is just a bar. You don't own it; you don't need to defend it. Do the smart thing and walk away.

Wilder had a karate instructor in the 1980s named Kevin who, when sparring, would push students around the *dojo* instead of hitting them. Each time the student tried to close distance to strike, he would find himself pushed backward or to the side. *Sensei* would say firmly, "You're in my space." It made no difference to this instructor where the student was, only that the student was in his space. Insofar as sparring was concerned, the entire *dojo* was his space. He had the skills and ability to take over his opponent's territory with impunity.

If you assume the other person is automatically going to retreat when you move in on him, you have made a mental mistake. Expect a fight; be thankful if you find retreat instead, but be prepared for the alternative. Whenever you invade the other guy's territory, expect a fight like the karate students discovered when sparring with their *sensei*.

If invading the other guy's space often leads to a fight, the important question becomes whether or not that space is really worth fighting for. Is a pool table worth it? What about a parking space, a place in line, or good spot at a concert near the stage?

Let's use the pool table example. It's pretty simple; if you are willing to fight over a table in a bar that you don't even own, you are operating at a tribal level. You are behaving like a monkey who is willing to fight over one fruit tree when the jungle is full of perfectly good fruit trees that are just a swing and a hop away. A monkey doesn't own the fruit tree and you don't own that section of the bar. Fighting for such things is dangerous and stupid.

Here are a few behaviors to watch for when looking at people who may be trying to establish their territory, especially in a bar. Understanding these behaviors can help you avoid inadvertently crossing someone you did not intend to insult.

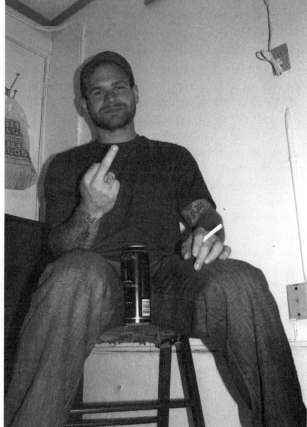

- Moving a coaster or ashtray that is not in their way after a person sits down is, in essence, a way of saying that it is now their space and the object serves as a border. This is done not only in bars but also in restaurants and business environments too.

- Placing an object of status on the table such as a wallet, cell phone, file folder, or expensive fountain pen can serve the same purpose. It says, "This is my space and I am brandishing power or prestige to prove it." By displaying an object of status this person is trying to show the world that he is in some way better than everyone else.

- Sitting with your back to the wall tells others that you are careful, prepared, and ready to defend yourself. Perhaps

Invading someone's space causes confrontation, forcing him to either retreat or fight.

you're a bit paranoid too, yet keeping one's back protected is a sign of a hardened target.

- Sitting at the head of table tells others, "I am the top dog." Want to cause a problem without saying a word? Go to somebody else's house and sit at the head of the table without first being invited to do so. See how far that gets you. It is a fast way to becoming very unwelcome.

- Sitting with legs wide apart and/or leaning back tells others, "I am surveying my domain." Add a chair tipped back against the wall, particularly when on the higher level of a split-level floor, and you have a message that is loudly broadcast. It's an attempt to convey authority. This is your space, and no one else's.

The same thing happens in other venues too. Take jail, for example. Although he has never committed nor been convicted of any crime, Wilder has, unfortunately, spent a few days in jail when he was falsely accused of wrongdoing. Sitting at the wood and metal table in a jail cell that weekend, Wilder calmly watched the television mounted up on the ceiling. Another inmate walked up to him and waved a plastic bag in front of him, shaking it down low by his waist. The bag contained scraps of paper, green and white. Wilder looked at the bag and then glanced down at the counter, suddenly realizing that it was a game table. A checkerboard had been carved into the surface.

> Humans are by nature territorial. We have a concept of personal space, something found in most every culture throughout the world. We often claim other territory as well, staking claim on something we believe is ours by right or by might. Whenever someone encroaches on our territory, it generates an emotional response and, oftentimes, a physical one as well. Invading someone's space almost always guarantees a confrontation, forcing him to either retreat or fight.

Without an exchange of words, Wilder got up and went back to his rack. What happened? The man with the paper scraps wanted to play checkers, but asking Wilder to move would have meant invading Wilder's territory. A potential refusal to move would have opened the possibility of a fight, or at least an escalation. A shake of a bag, on the other hand, was not a threat. It was not a real question either, yet the implication was clear. In this way, they both got what they wanted without an overt invasion of the other's territory.

Wilder got up and went to his bunk and the other guy sat down at the game table. No invasion, no issue. If you invade another guy's territory, you force him to either retreat or fight. Odds of violence vary by circumstance, of course. While jailhouse confrontations are pretty common, aggressive behaviors can occur just about anywhere. Keep this in mind next time you think of invading someone's territory.

Darn Near Everybody Has a Knife... And it Changes Everything in a Fight

Rapidity is the essence of war: take advantage of the enemy's unreadiness, make your way by unexpected routes, and attack unguarded spots.
– Sun Tzu

When you take up a sword, you must feel intent on cutting the enemy.
– Miyamoto Musashi

Do a little drill for the next few days. Carefully look at people's pants pockets, especially guy's pockets. You will see metal clips for securing folding knives within the pocket and bulges or outlines of pocketknives that are bouncing around freely therein. On their belts, you will see holsters for multi-tools, fixed blades, and other types of knives too. Knives, knives everywhere… so many knives, in fact, that about 70 percent of the adult male population in the United States carries one on a regular basis.

After the tragedy of 9/11, stadium security has dramatically increased across the country. Nevertheless, walking through security at Qwest Field (Seahawks Stadium in Seattle) Kane and Wilder spotted 22 people illegally carrying knives before they got to their seats. It's not that these people were a bunch of hardened criminals, mind you, but rather that knives are so common and carried so habitually that people bring them darn near everywhere. Even the heightened security had not stopped them because there were no metal detectors and no pat-down searches, only bag checks and visual inspections.

Knives are supposed to be tools, but more often than not, they are seen as weapons. If you are looking at young men when you do the drill, you will see more knives: older men less, women fewer still. Young men often carry a knife as a security blanket, a subtle way of saying, "I am dangerous." Here's the kicker. They are… even if they don't know it.

There are two kinds of people who carry knives—those who know what they are doing and the vast majority of others, those who don't. It doesn't really matter though. Skilled or unskilled, nearly any person can cripple or kill you with any knife he chooses to wield.

We have a mutual friend named Jeff who works as an emergency room physician. In addition to being a doctor, he is an accomplished martial artist as well. Wilder once asked him, "Have you ever looked at a person bleeding on your operating table and thought to yourself, 'the guy who did this really knew what he was doing'?" Dr. Jeff answered, "No. Violence is violence."

You need to remember that statement. Violence is violence! The end result of contact with a knife, whether in the hands of a pro or the hands of a punk, is the same. It's all bad.

From time to time Kane teaches a seminar on the realities of knife fighting. It is primarily designed to scare the crap out of people who don't fully appreciate what a blade can actually do to a human being and subsequently enhance students' awareness of how to avoid running afoul of one and not get cut if they do. Among other things, he shares stories like the Young/Beckman incident and autopsy photos of unfortunates who did not learn those important lessons.

While the graphic pictures have made more than one student lose his lunch, the demonstration that really hits home goes like this: To show just how dangerous a knife truly is, Kane hangs a large hunk of meat, something that comes on the bone such as a leg of lamb, from a rope. He then takes a legal-length,* two-and-a-half-inch-blade folding knife and makes three cuts—a horizontal slash, a vertical slash, and a stab. After slicing up the meat, he whips out a measuring tape to show the damage. He can consistently make five- to six-inch-long by two-inch-deep gashes in the meat. It's actually quite easy to do with a sharp knife; most students can duplicate that feat when given the opportunity to try. Kane can also reliably strike the bone with the stab, even when it takes two to four inches of compression to do so, providing that he hits hard and fast enough. The noise of the blade hitting the bone is particularly chilling. After showing what a legal-length blade can do, he duplicates the experiment with a larger weapon. That can get really scary indeed.

If you are thinking feet and fists only to discover a knife or other weapon in the middle of a fight, you are more than likely doomed. The stark reality is that most victims of weapon attacks do not recognize the severity of the threat in time to react properly. Imi Sde-Or, the founder of the martial art *Krav Maga*, wrote, "Victims who survived a violent confrontation against a knife-wielding assailant consistently reported that they were completely unaware of the existence of the weapon until after they had suffered stab or slash wounds. In essence, these survivors of edged-weapon attacks state that they believed they were engaged in some sort of fist fight; only later, after sustaining injuries, did they realize that the assailant was armed."

While we are on the subject of knives in the hands of an aggressor, you really needn't think knife at all; any old weapon will do. To illustrate the point, Wilder knows a guy named Ben who was hit so hard in the face with a beer bottle that it shattered. Unlike Hollywood movies, real bottles are pretty tough to break. That strike not only knocked him out, but he still bears the scars on his nose today. That fight ended right then and there—one blow, one weapon. Done.

Near everybody has a knife and it changes everything in a fight. Consider this carefully before you throw the first blow.

Know When He's Armed, You'll Live Longer That Way

Warriors who lived in the times of Sun Tzu and Miyamoto Musashi fought life and death battles using various weapons from swords to spears, halberds, arrows, and more. These fighters were rarely, if ever, unarmed; even the fans that *samurai* carried in their belts could be used as impromptu weapons. Every comment these authors made was against the backdrop of armed opponents. You would do well to assume the same environment. Bad guys cheat to win, frequently employing weapons on the street. The major difference is that nowadays you rarely see them coming.

---

* In most jurisdictions.

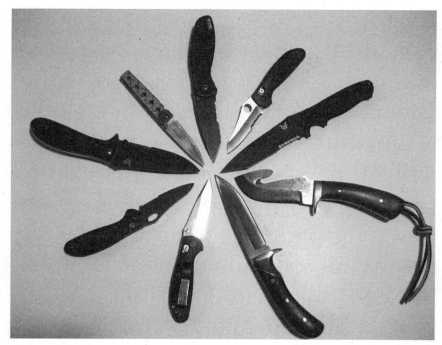

Nearly anyone can cripple or kill you quite easily with a blade. It takes no special skill or training.

Despite what you may have learned in martial arts class, unarmed civilians who tangle with weapon-wielding attackers invariably get hurt. Often quite badly. Armed assaults are far more dangerous to the victim than unarmed ones. While crimes of non-lethal violence committed with or without weapons were about equally likely to result in victim injury, armed assaults are three-and-a-half times as likely as unarmed encounters to result in serious injuries. In fact, some 96 percent of all homicides involve a weapon.

The best way to defend yourself against an armed aggressor, of course, is to avoid the altercation completely, using good situational awareness to spot the bad guy before he attacks you and find somewhere else to be. Otherwise, your only options are either to run like hell, respond with a better weapon, or both—clearly not the best choice but an effective one nevertheless. It is important, therefore, to learn how to spot a weapon before it is used against you.

With few exceptions, civilians who carry a weapon need to do so in a manner where it cannot be seen by those around them yet can be drawn in very big hurry should the need arise. If you are legally carrying a weapon for self-defense, you will not want

An estimated 70 percent of adult males carry a knife on a regular basis in the United States. While most are law-abiding citizens who use these knives as the tools they are intended to be, the presence of any knife changes everything in a fight. The end result of contact with a knife, whether in the hands of a pro or the hands of a punk, is the same. Anyone can cripple or kill you quite easily with a blade. It takes no special skill or training.

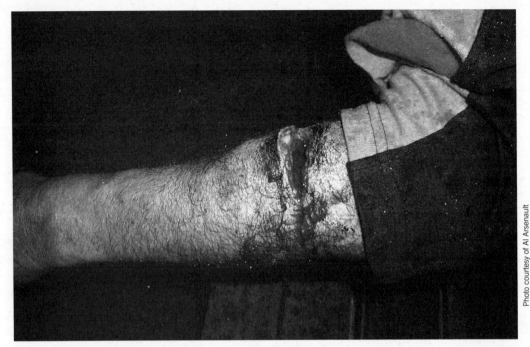

A sharp knife can do tremendous damage. A big, sharp knife can get downright scary. Even a cheap blade can easily mutilate or kill you.

to be stopped every twenty feet by a police officer summoned by some frightened by-stander who spotted and reported your weapon. Further, you will not want to forewarn possible aggressors of the fact that you are armed. Bad guys also conceal their weapons not only for the reasons listed above but also to increase the chances of a successful ambush when they attack you or whomever they have chosen as their victim.

Since you will not generally see a weapon carried openly, it is really important to know how to spot when someone is armed with a concealed device. This is especially important when you consider the aforementioned fact that an estimated 70 percent of adult males carry a knife. While that statistic includes multi-tools that may have dubious value as weapons, even a cheap blade can easily mutilate or kill you.

The vast majority of weapon concealment strategies have one thing in common—accessibility. After all, a weapon does you no good if you cannot get to it rapidly when you need it. Blades, handguns, batons, and just about anything else concealable can be hidden in similar ways, most of which are centered on or around the waist.

Most law-abiding civilians who own a gun use a holster to carry their weapon. Holsters make the most reliable carry systems because they rigidly affix the weapon to a specific spot on the body. That way it can always be found when it is needed, even under extreme stress. There are varieties of holsters that can be attached to one's belt either inside or outside of the pants. Shoulder and ankle holsters also exist, of course, but are far less common than other types. Many folding knives come with belt clips designed to hold them firmly against the side of your pocket where they are easily located by touch. Knives can be carried in holsters too, of course.

Criminals, on the other hand, rarely use a holster. The most common ad hoc carry position for firearms is inside the pants, either in the front alongside the hipbone or in the small of the back. Because the weapon has a tendency to move around when carried in this fashion, you can often spot a bad guy touching himself to assure that it is in the proper place or adjusting the weapon to get it back into the proper carry position.

Pants or jacket pockets are always a handy choice as well. Like the inside-the-pants carry, they are not as reliable or easy to get to as a holster when you need rapid access since the weapon may become repositioned as you move about during the day. For example, a pistol slid into your pocket may flip around such that the handle cannot be grasped without moving the gun first. If you pull it out by the barrel, it will not do you much good until you change your grip. Similarly, knives carried in a pocket take longer to orient and open then when a holster or belt clip is used. In a fast and furious encounter, you may not have enough time to free, orient, and deploy the weapon before it is too late.

Weapons can also be palmed, hidden behind an arm or leg, or held out of sight beneath a covering object such as a folded jacket or newspaper. These systems facilitate rapid access but can be easier to spot than other methods and preclude the use of the hand that carries the weapon for anything other than deploying the device in combat. If the weapon is already drawn and held in a concealed position, you will be in extremely serious trouble if you do not spot your adversary's intent. He has already decided to attack and is maneuvering into position to do so.

Weapons, can also be "hidden" in plain sight too. A hot cup of coffee tossed into a bad guy's face can make an effective deterrent. A solidly built pen can operate much like a martial arts *kubaton** or even like a knife. A cane, walking stick, heavy purse, or laptop computer can be used as a bludgeon. Heavy keys on a lanyard can work much like a medieval flail, albeit far less effectively. A beer bottle, pool cue, baseball bat, or mug can be just as effective in a pinch as a weapon designed for combat. Almost anything can be a weapon if you know how to use it properly.

Pay particular attention to a person's hands and midsection, looking for unusual bumps, bulges, out-of-place items of clothing, or odd movements. Look for clips that indicate a knife, heavy belts that may indicate a holster, and other visible signs of something hidden from plain view. Watch for subtle touches or patting movements as someone

---

* Invented by Takayuki Kubota the kubaton is a hard plastic or metal cylinder about 5 to 6 inches long that can be used for striking, pressure point manipulations, and control techniques. It is frequently sold with an attacked key ring as a "self-defense key chain."

validates that his weapon is still in place or adjusts its position. Even when a holster is used, without a sufficiently sturdy belt to go along with it the weapon may still slide around and need to be repositioned.

Most people wear their watch on their weak-hand side. That means that if the watch is on the left hand, odds are good that he's right-handed. It does not always work out that way, but can be a good indicator. Regardless, people tend to carry their primary weapon on their strong side, so if you think that someone is right-handed look there first.

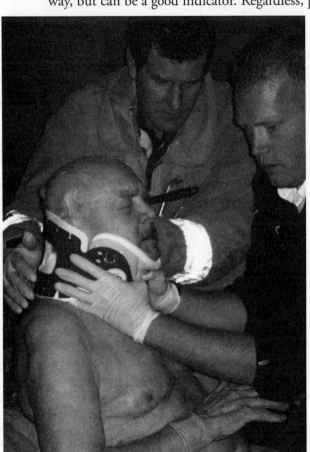

Also, look for concealing clothing that may be covering a weapon. Examples include a jacket worn in hot weather, a vest that covers the waistline (especially the hips/lower back), or a loose shirt that is only buttoned high. Anyone who wears his or her outdoor wear indoors may well be concealing a weapon under it. If the weapon is carried in a pocket or secured using a specially designed piece of concealment clothing, it might cause the garment to appear off-balanced, hanging lower on the side where the weapon is carried.

Pay special attention to the person's hands. After all, that's what deploys the weapon. Hands buried in pockets, hidden under a jacket or shirt, or simply held out of sight may be holding a weapon. Or the person could simply have cold fingers. It never hurts to be prudent yet can hurt an awful lot if you are not cautious. Be wary of stiff fingers, clenched fists, and other odd hand movements as they could be used to conceal a lethal device or indicate a general precursor of violence.

Armed assaults are 3.5 times as likely as unarmed encounters to result in serious injuries. Worse yet, some 96 percent of all homicides involve a weapon.

Just because a weapon is not in use at the beginning of a fight doesn't necessarily mean that it won't be by the end, particularly if the other guy thinks he's in danger of losing. Before, during, and even after a fight, watch for the upward or sideways motion of withdrawing a weapon from its sheath, holster, or hiding place; a weapon cannot be used until it is deployed. While you will frequently rely on your eyes to spot a concealed weapon, you can use your ears too. Listen for the sound of

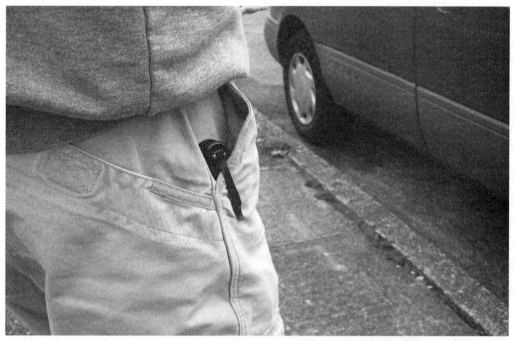

An estimated 70 percent of adult males in the U.S. carry some type of knife or multi-tool on a regular basis.

a weapon being drawn or readied for action, especially when you cannot clearly see a potential adversary such as when you are in a crowd, where someone is behind you, or when it is very dark. Audible indicators can include

- Click (such as releasing mechanical safety on a handgun, racking the slide to chamber a round, or locking open a folding knife blade).

- Snap (such as unlocking a retention device such as a holster safety strap).

- Rustle (such as moving clothing aside to facilitate drawing the weapon).

- Velcro* (such as opening a pouch or removing a retention device such as a holster safety strap).

---

* Is Velcro a noise? We are referring to the ripping sound that Velcro makes when unfastened.

Armed assaults are about three-and-a-half times more likely to result in serious injuries for the victim than unarmed ones. In fact, some 96 percent of all homicides involve a weapon. Consequently, it is really important to be able to spot hidden weapons before they can be used against you. The vast majority of weapon concealment strategies have one thing in common—accessibility. After all, a weapon does you no good if you cannot get to it rapidly when you need it. Blades, handguns, batons, and other concealable weapons tend to be hidden in similar ways, most of which are centered on or around the waist. Weapons can also be palmed, hidden behind an arm or leg, held out of sight beneath a covering object, or even "hidden" in plain sight. Know how to detect when he's armed and practice your skills regularly; you'll live longer that way.

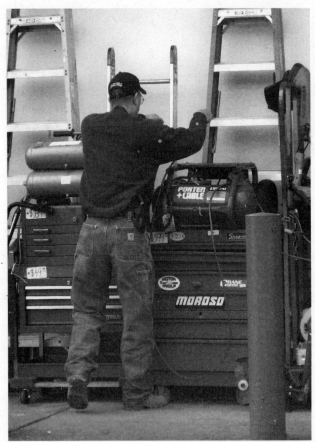

Most law-abiding civilians who own a gun use a holster to carry their weapon. Criminals, on the other hand, rarely use one. Either way, the most common carry positions are centered on or around the waistline.

Don't worry about being confused by cell phones, pagers, PDAs, MP3 players, or other harmless devices. It is far better to be overly cautious than injured or dead through ignoring warning signs. Just because you believe that someone is armed does not necessarily imply that you will take immediate action, but you should be prepared to do so as necessary. Trust your instincts.

Feeling is important too, both psychologically and physiologically. Pay attention to your intuition. Though we are often conditioned to ignore it, everyone has a biologically built-in danger sense. Use it.

Weapon awareness is relatively easy to practice. Take an outdoor seat at a restaurant in a high foot-traffic area, hang out in a mall, or take a walk through a public place and carefully watch passersby. Count how many knives, guns, and other weapons you can spot. Who is carrying them? How are they concealed? What subtle clues did you notice that helped you spot the weapon? Once you get good at consciously finding these devices, you can begin to pick them up subconsciously as well. Honing your intuition in this manner builds solid survival skills.

Gangs Are Not Your Friend

The skillful tactician may be likened to the shuai-jan. Now the shuai-jan is a snake...He will win whose army is animated by the same spirit throughout all its ranks.

— Sun Tzu

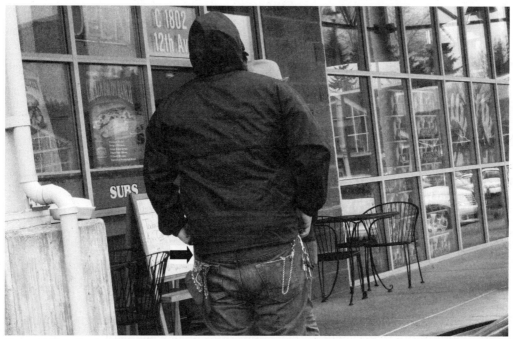

Pay particular attention to a person's hands and midsection to spot a weapon, looking for unusual bumps, bulges, out-of-place items of clothing, or odd movements. Note the tip of the holster peaking out from under this guy's jacket.

In large-scale strategy, if you have a strong army and are relying on strength to win, but the enemy also has a strong army, the battle will be fierce. This is the same for both sides.

– Miyamoto Musashi

Gangs are groups of people who share a group name and identity, interact among themselves to the exclusion of others, claim a territory, create a climate of fear and intimidation within their domain, communicate in a unique style, wear distinctive clothing, and engage in criminal or antisocial activities on a regular basis. We're not talking about a Little League team here. Gang members frequently utilize tattoos, scars, or cigarette burns to announce their affiliation. These markings are usually obvious, seen on the arms and/or chest, but can also be discreet such as wearing a tattoo on the inside of the lower lip. Even their vehicles may be distinctive, with lowered frames, neon, excessive chrome, or tinted windows.

Gang members hold three things preeminent—respect, reputation, and revenge. Consequently, if you cross a gang member in any manner, things will get ugly fast. For example, even looking at one with the wrong facial expression (commonly called "mugging" or "mean-mugging") can get you seriously hurt or killed. Imagine a gang banger's reaction to a more obvious sign of disrespect such as a derogatory comment, push, kick, or punch.

Unlike what you may have been led to believe, gang membership crosses all racial, ethnic, social, and economic lines. It is not just a ghetto thing. There are Asian gangs, black gangs, white gangs, Hispanic gangs, skinhead gangs, outlaw motorcycle gangs, and so on. These gangs include both umbrella groups and associated sets with names like 18th Street Gang; .45 Crew; Almighty P Stone Nation; Black Gangster Disciples; Bloods, Border Brothers; Crips, Dykes Taking Over (DTO); Friends Stand United (a.k.a. FSU or F*ck Sh*t Up); Hells Angels; Hispanic Norteños; Hispanic Sureños (Sur-13); L.A. Death Squad; Latin Kings; Mara Salvatrucha (MS-13); Outlaws, Pagans; Banditos; Texas Syndicate; and Vice Lords.

Both male and female gang members instigate violence, carry weapons, deal drugs, participate in crimes, and take leadership roles within the organizations. They carry the marks of violence with pride, comparing knife scars, bullet wounds, burns, and various disfigurements to prove how tough they are and augment their reputations. Gangs get involved in everything from drug trafficking and manufacture to robbery, auto theft, carjacking, burglary, felonious assault, rape, murder, kidnapping, weapons trafficking, arson, prostitution, fraud, identity theft, vandalism, money laundering, extortion, and human trafficking.

According to the Office of Juvenile Justice and Delinquency Prevention, a branch of the U.S. Department of Justice, as of 2007 there are an estimated 21,500 active youth gangs in the United States with some 731,500 members. These gang members account for roughly ten percent of all violent crimes as well as ten percent of homicides in the country. This does not include prison gangs, motorcycle gangs, or adult gangs, which would drive these percentages up even higher. Furthermore, according to the Bureau of Justice Statistics less than half of all gang-related crimes are reported to the police, so you can see that violence and gangs not only go hand-in-hand, but also that the levels of violence they create are significant.

While some youths seek gang affiliation to make up for parental abuse or neglect at home, others simply crave the lifestyle which is popularized in music, videos, movies, and television shows. Sex, drugs, money, and weapons can be quite glamorous to young people, especially young males. Some people live in the wrong neighborhood or spend a bit of prison time and are forced to join a gang in order to survive. Regardless of how they get involved, the gang becomes the member's surrogate family so if you mess with one gang member, you have messed with all of them. This can result in anything from a severe beat down to a homicide.

However much "respect" you might feel you want or deserve, the average gang member craves it tenfold. Gang bangers will do everything they can to disrespect others

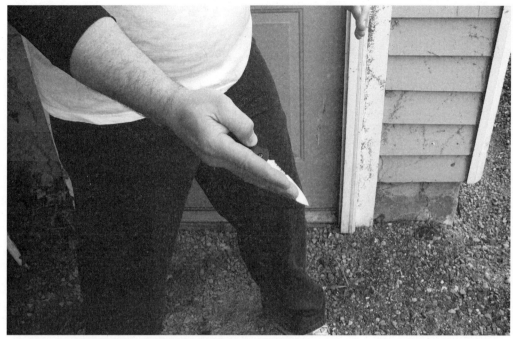

Be wary of stiff fingers, clenched fists, and other odd hand movements as they could be used to conceal a lethal device or indicate a general precursor of violence.

while propping up themselves. Graffiti, hand signs, verbal challenges, stare-downs, and physical assaults are common in gang culture. While it is typically targeted at rival gang members, innocent civilians can easily become targets and/or get caught in the middle.

New gang members must pass through some form of violent initiation, such as being beaten to a pulp by other members, in order to join. This process is called "getting jumped in." It instills a sense of toughness and pride by those who survive. New members are frequently required to commit a violent crime such as an assault, rape, or murder. As you can see, this is not your average club. Gang reputations are made through crimes, violent antisocial actions that strike fear into the hearts of others.

Reputation is so important that gang bangers will even brag to the police, admitting crimes or even making them up on occasion in order to boost their status. For example, when a 25-year-old gang member was arrested after a 2005 club fight where a 36-year-old victim was beaten to death, he told the responding officers, "I got good elbows. People don't know about my elbows." He later pled guilty to negligent homicide when it was determined that an elbow to the head had caused the victim's fatal trauma.

Because gang bangers often do not expect to have a long-term future, they live in the moment, doing whatever they feel like without regard to consequences. Many do not expect to live past the age of twenty-five. That can seem like a pretty long time if you get initiated into the gang at the age of thirteen or fourteen.

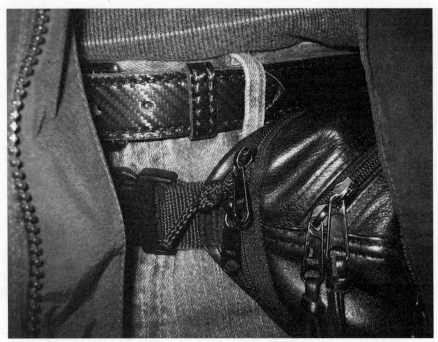

This ain't no geekwad fanny pack. The cord sticking out between the two zippers gives away the fact that it's a concealed holster.

Revenge is a huge deal with gangs. If a gang member feels disrespected or thinks that his reputation has been harmed, retribution will certainly follow. If it doesn't, he'll get knocked down a peg or two, beaten, disgraced, or potentially even killed by his associates. Consequently, no assault or insult can be left unanswered, no matter how small.

Wearing the wrong colors, traveling in the wrong area, or gazing with an unsuitable expression can bring about the same type of murderous retribution such as a rape, murder, or physical assault. While this vengeance is often swift, that is not always the case. Asian gangs, for example, sometimes talk about the "100-year revenge," patiently waiting for the right opportunity to strike. If you think you are "bad" enough to take on a gang member, you are downright stupid.

Listen to the Subtle (and Not-so-Subtle) Warnings You Get

Without subtle ingenuity of mind, one cannot make certain of the truth of their reports.

— Sun Tzu

An individual can easily change his mind, so his movements are difficult to predict. You must appreciate this.

— Miyamoto Musashi

We've spent much time writing about awareness on the street. It's important in relationships too. Don't turn your brain off when you walk into your home. After all, according to the Bureau of Justice Statistics, more than half of all homicides are committed by someone known to the victim. That means that your wife or husband, girlfriend or boyfriend, sister or brother, friend, relative, or acquaintance might just do you in someday.

The song *You Don't Love Me Anymore* by "Weird Al" Yankovic leads into the first chorus with the lyrics:

> *Why did you disconnect the brakes on my car?*
> *That kind of thing is hard to ignore*
> *Got a funny feeling, you don't love me anymore*

After several verses describing increasingly horrific behaviors from his no-longer-in-love girlfriend, including things like telling all her friends that he's the antichrist, pushing him down an elevator shaft, and slamming his face onto a hot BBQ grill, Yankovic drops the line:

> *You're still the light of my life*
> *Oh darling I'm begging, won't you put down that knife*

Yankovic is a world-class comedian, a truly funny guy. As with most of his material, this song is hysterical, at least for people who haven't lived through domestic violence. Sadly, what he jokes about in the song is all too true in some relationships. Little hints become bigger hints; small behaviors turn into larger ones. And if you don't pay attention to the clues, something bad inevitably happens.

Case in point: "She took a fishing knife out of his tackle box and stabbed him seven times in the chest. Killed him," Wilder's business partner, Rick, told him over the phone. "What, you mean your painter, Jeff?" Wilder asked. "Yep," Rick replied, "Stabbed him last night while he slept."

Jeff was a good employee. He was on time, had a talent for painting cars, and he loved the outdoors. Jeff's girlfriend, on the other hand, was wild. She was a real knockout but had little control over her emotions. In fact, the police had been to their home several times, especially on the weekends. She had even been sentenced to jail for assaulting him before.

Sadly, Jeff never stood a chance that night. While he peacefully slept, she went into his tackle box and pulled out a boning knife, symbolically taking her weapon from his favorite pastime: fishing. The blade was sharp and light with a long, tapered point, and a keen edge. She crept into their bedroom, held the boning knife high over his chest, and thrust it downward into his heart with both hands. Then she pulled it out and slammed it in again… and again, and again, and again, and again, and then once more for good measure. And then she left the house.

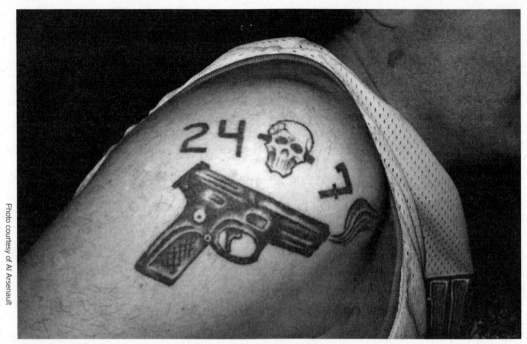

Photo courtesy of Al Arsenault

Gang tattoo. Respect, reputation, and revenge are the hallmarks of gang culture. If you think you are tough enough to take on a gang banger, you are just plain stupid.

Respect, reputation, and revenge are the hallmarks of gang culture. If you think you are tough enough to take on a gang banger, you are just plain stupid. Mess with one and you've messed with them all. No disrespect, challenge, or assault will go unanswered. Since most gang members care little for societal norms, there is little they will not do to avenge a perceived slight. Most do not expect to live past the age of twenty-five; consequently their "living in the now" mentality makes them capable of just about anything. You have a lot more to lose than they do. That's an equation that's heavily weighted against you.

Everybody who had ever met Jeff liked him. He was pleasant, easy to know, and honest. Anybody that met the two of them, however, had difficulty understanding their relationship. While everyone was saddened by what had happened, it didn't really take anyone all that much by surprise. In fact, not too long before the incident someone had joked, "I hope she's really good in bed man, because you know she's gonna do you in one day." All the hints were there, the warnings loud and clear, yet Jeff did not heed any of them. Now he's dead.

Domestic violence can go both ways, yet more often than not it's the guy who is the abuser. In fact, between 1976 and 2004, more than thirty percent of female murder victims were killed by their husband or boyfriend, a rather substantial number when you realize that less than ten percent of male victims were killed by an intimate over that same period. That's why we have so many battered women's shelters, victim advocates, and community resources that focus on helping women and children move away from hazardous relationships.

It might not happen as often, or at least not be reported as

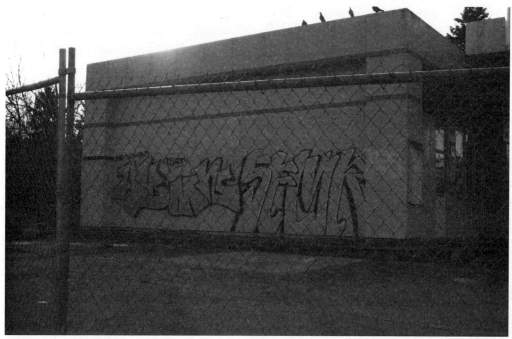

Graffiti, hand signs, verbal challenges, stare-downs, and physical assaults are common in gang culture. While it is typically targeted at rival gang members, innocent civilians can easily become targets and/or get caught in the middle.

much, but men are definitely abuse victims too. More than 100,000 men are violently assaulted or killed by their wives or girlfriends each year in the United States.

Here are some warning signs of abusive relationships that apply to both sexes, reliable predictors of eventual violence or murder.

- Your partner frequently yells at you, reprimands you, or demeans you in public. You have cause to fear his/her temper or are concerned about what kind of mood he or she is in on a regular basis.

- Your partner isolates you, prevents you from getting or keeping a job, keeps you from seeing friends or family, or otherwise alienates your friends or family so that they feel uncomfortable being around that person. This is another method of cutting you from the herd, eliminating your support group.

- Your partner keeps you from leaving your house or apartment from time to time, or conversely, occasionally locks you out of your home.

- Your partner threatens to hurt or kill you, your children, your family, your friends, or your pets. All such threats, even ones given in jest, should be taken seriously.

- Your partner hits, slaps, pushes, or shoves you, pulls your hair, or inflicts unwanted physical injury on you in any way, even during sex. The first time your significant other strikes you should be the last. Screaming and yelling might be tolerated on occasion but physical abuse never should be.

- Your partner exhibits extreme jealously, checking in on you frequently, following you around or hiring someone else to do so, going through your mail, or installing monitoring programs on your computer. He or she becomes angry when you talk to or look at people of the opposite gender even when you have a legitimate reason for doing so.

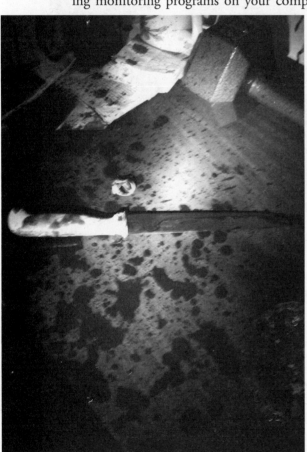

Since female-on-male violence can be harder to predict than vice-versa, subtle warning signs must be heeded.

One of the most important things a domestic abuse victim can do is get away from the perpetrator before things get worse. Danger to the victim and any children or pets they might have, however, is likely to increase at the time of separation so you have to be careful about how you do it. Nevertheless, if you feel threatened in a relationship it is essential to take action right away. It is easy to rationalize or procrastinate, hoping that things will get better. Most of the time, however, they won't.

It can be tough to leave but you must do it. You can work around economic issues such as loss of housing, income, health insurance, or transportation. It's a bit tougher, but you can work through emotional, cultural, religious, or family issues too. You might even have heard horror stories of health care providers, law enforcement officers, social workers, or even the courts blaming the victim, particularly when he's a guy, but those things are rare and a good lawyer can help you work through them.

Don't be embarrassed to death. Leave. There are plenty of resources to help you do the right thing and keep yourself safe. In most communities, there are both government and private agencies that can help you work through these issues, providing relocation, temporary housing, medical assistance, and attending to other needs as appropriate.

There are some very interesting differences between men and women when it comes to fighting that can also become important in dysfunctional relationships. For the most part, men have "hot" rage. If they're going to lash out violently, it will be in the heat of anger. Women, on the other hand, tend to have "cold" rage. They're the ones who will take revenge long after the incident that inflamed them has passed, quite possibly after you've forgotten all about the argument, indiscretion, or whatever it was that occurred.

Since female-on-male violence can be harder to predict, subtle warning signs must be heeded. Women are more likely than men to get you while you sleep, stabbing you in the chest, setting you on fire, or putting a bullet in your head. They are the ones who might cut off your penis and throw it out the window of a moving car (Lorena Bobbitt, 1993) or flush it down the toilet (Kim Tran, 2005). If you are truly unlucky, she might become enraged, tear off your testicle with her bare hands, and try to eat it (Amanda Monti, 2007).

One of the factors that may influence these differences between men and women is in the way in which adrenaline affects the genders. When men are confronted with extreme emotional or violent situations, their adrenaline kicks off like a rocket, surging quickly and dissipating rapidly afterward as well. In a home invasion situation, for example, when the male homeowner shoots the suspect, the killing is likely to take place near the front door. When police officers arrive, they will typically find that the suspect has been shot perhaps two or three times, just enough to make sure he's no longer a threat.

> Listen to all the little warnings you get, not only around strangers on the street, but also in relationships as well. Little hints become bigger hints; small behaviors turn into larger ones. And if you don't pay attention to the clues, something bad is bound to happen. While women are often on the receiving end of domestic abuse, men can be victims as well (for example, John Wayne Bobbitt). The most important thing you can do if you are in an abusive relationship is to get away from the perpetrator immediately before things get worse.

Women, on the other hand, get a much slower, longer lasting adrenaline surge. It takes longer to get going and dissipates a lot more slowly than you find in men. In that same home invasion scenario, police often find the dead robber in a back bedroom where he had chased and cornered the female homeowner. But here's the kicker. Rather than shooting him a couple of times she's emptied the gun into him, perhaps even reloading and doing it again. Interesting difference, huh?

Listen to all the little warnings you get. Intimates can be just as hazardous to your health and wellbeing as strangers. Little hints can become bigger hints; small behaviors can turn into larger ones. Pay attention and be safe.

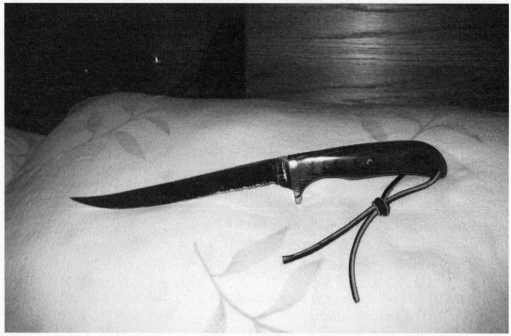

She thrust the knife downward into his heart with both hands. Then she pulled it out and slammed it in again… and again, and again, and again, and again, and then once more for good measure. And then she left the house.

Summary

The following is a brief recap of the content you have read in this section.

- Self-defense begins with the concept of situational awareness, the ability to spot trouble before it can reach you. Any time you are near others it pays to be vigilant. Bad guys want easy prey, oblivious folks who never see them coming and can't or won't fight back. As a result, tough, prepared targets are usually left alone in favor of easier victims. You cannot, however, walk around in a constant state of hyper-vigilance or paranoia. It's neither healthy nor prudent. Consequently, self-defense experts often use a color code system that defines appropriate levels of awareness to help you strike the right balance, pay attention to what's important, and keep yourself safe. The colors themselves are far less important than the overall concept—different levels of awareness are appropriate for different situations.

- No matter how aware you might be, it still takes two to tango. Sometimes your worst enemy when it comes to self-defense is yourself. If you've got a chip on your shoulder or an ego that you simply can't keep in check, you're pointing a loaded gun at your own head. Escalato is the cycle of one-upmanship that inevitably leads to physical violence unless one party is willing to lose face and back down. While it's a game that's really easy to get caught up in, it's also one that you really don't want to play if you're smart. Even if the other guy is a complete ass, it is far better to walk away than it is to fight to prove that you are right.

- Criminals, bullies, and thugs do not want to fight—they want to win. And they're downright eager to cheat their way to victory because they don't want to get hurt in the process. They prey on the naïve and unobservant, weaklings and fools who make easy, profitable targets. Before they strike, these guys look you over to be sure that they have a pretty darn good chance to succeed. The less you look and act like a victim during this interview process, the safer you will be.

- There is always some type of escalation that precedes physical violence, even a really short one. Sometimes it is obvious while other times it takes place solely in the mind of the aggressor. Nevertheless, some sort of clue precedes the attack. By understanding these threat indicators, you will have a better opportunity to avoid confrontations altogether, or where necessary, defend yourself effectively. If you miss these signs, you will have a tough time responding to sudden violence. While you are still trying to wrap your head around what is happening, you will find yourself getting hurt. Once you have been injured, it's pretty tough to respond effectively.

- While predators need a good size pool of victims from which to choose, they cannot operate in highly public places for fear of getting caught. Consequently, fringe areas adjacent to public places are where the majority of violent crimes occur. This includes areas such as parking lots, alleyways, bus stations, subways, bathrooms, stairwells, ATM kiosks, and the like. In order to initiate an attack, the adversary must be close enough to strike. It is important to understand how the bad guys, bullies, and thugs might close distance, recognizing their tactics before their trap is sprung.

- Calling in support might preclude the need to fight. The imminent arrival of law enforcement officers or a large group of your friends changes the equation in your adversary's eyes. Suddenly you are no longer a hopeless victim, but rather a well-protected target.

- Self-defense requires more than just physical skills. What you say can be even more important than what you do when confronted by a potential adversary. Clever words can de-escalate a tense situation, stave off bloodshed until help arrives, or momentarily distract an opponent to facilitate your counterattack and escape. On the other hand, having to be right at any cost, reacting indignantly in the face of a threat, or insulting an adversary often guarantees that a conflict will escalate into violence. It goes both ways. Words cannot be used against you unless you give them power. If you let insults or name-calling make you angry, they knock you off your mental equilibrium, leaving you vulnerable.

- If you are in error about something, admit it. Honesty is a much better way to de-escalate a bad situation than lying or stubbornly refusing to acknowledge a wrong. You can usually tell when someone knows they are wrong because they begin to make the argument personal. It is tough on the ego to admit fault, but it sure beats eating through a straw because you got your jaw busted when your face was pounded in. Similarly, giving the other guy a face-saving way out affords him the opportunity to back down gracefully too. Put his back up against the wall and he may feel forced to lash out.

- A clear intent to defend yourself can oftentimes cut short a fight before it begins. Your words and demeanor must convince your adversary that he's picked on the wrong guy. It is critical that you take steps to ensure that your message is heard, particularly when emotions are running hot.

- Don't be anxious for a fight. It's all well and good to dream about how tough you are, yet the ferocious brutality of a street fight is light years beyond any boxing match or martial arts tournament you may have won. Slickly choreographed Hollywood films only exacerbate the fantasy of what true violence entails. Beware these misconceptions. Don't confuse sports with combat or misconstrue entertainment with reality.

- Never underestimate the fighting intelligence of your opponent. There is a reason this guy is picking on you. He not only thinks he can win, but has done so before. Either that or he's a delusional head case, drug addict, or drunk, a trait that in certain circumstances may be even worse. Nevertheless, mental toughness often trumps physical size or strength in a fight. For example, Audie Murphy was turned down by two other branches of the military because he was too small and underweight. After finally enlisting in the Army, Murphy went on to become the most decorated United States combat soldier of World War II. Don't underestimate the fighting intelligence of your opponent.

- When it comes to self-defense, it is critical to pay attention to the subtle clues around you. Watch for people who look out of place or act in an unusual manner. Look for other people's reactions to things you may have missed as well. Pay attention to sounds and smells as well as visual cues. Take nothing for granted.

- Little things are often important—little time, little movements. Through keen observation, you might spot a weapon or discover hostile intent before it is too late to react. During a fight, you might be able to take advantage of terrain, weather conditions, escape routes, or impromptu weapons if you pay attention to those important details ahead of time.

- If something bad happens, you will need a way out. Knowing your territory gives you an important advantage whenever you need to escape from trouble. This not only means having an awareness of entrances, exits, and avenues for escape, but also a good understanding of your friend's proclivities as well. Hang out with people who like to cause trouble and it will eventually catch up with not only them but also with you too.

- Restrain impassioned friends. Don't let your buddy's big fat mouth write a check that you need to cash. If he insists on behaving immaturely, find someone else to hang out with. The same goes for intimate relations. If your girlfriend thinks that violence in defense of her honor is cool, you are with the wrong type of person. She will not just get you into one fight, but many. Sooner or later, she will get you seriously hurt, maimed, or killed… or thrown in jail and sued for everything you own.

- Violence always has consequences. Know what is worth fighting for and what is not. Dispassionately evaluate your priorities and values before you need to make such judgments in the heat of the moment. It is far better to live to fight another day than to make rash choices you may live to regret.

- No matter how tough you are, there is always someone out there who's tougher, faster, or just plain better. Do you really want to find out if you have what it takes to tangle with a heavy hitter, a career criminal, mental case, or a seasoned street fighter in a live fire situation? You're not that good. And even if you are, it doesn't pay to find out. Claiming turf puts you in a win-lose mentality. It's yours now, so it cannot be theirs. That type of thinking frequently leads to violence. Do the smart thing and walk away.

- Whenever someone encroaches on our territory or violates our personal space, it generates an emotional response. Oftentimes this leads to a physical response as well. Invading someone's space almost always guarantees a confrontation, forcing him to either retreat or fight. Know this before you invade someone else's territory.

- The presence of a knife, something carried by roughly 70 percent of adult males in the United States on a regular basis, changes everything in a fight. Anyone can cripple or kill you quite easily with a blade; it takes no special skill or training. In fact, all forms of armed assaults are far more dangerous to the victim than unarmed ones, about three-and-a-half times as likely to result in serious injuries. Worse yet, some 96 percent of all homicides involve a weapon. Consequently, it is really important to be able to spot hidden weapons before they can be used against you.

- Respect, reputation, and revenge are the hallmarks of gang culture. If you think you are tough enough to take on a gang banger, you are just plain stupid. Mess with one banger and you've messed with them all. No disrespect, challenge, or assault will go unanswered. Since most gang members tend to live for the moment and care little for societal norms, nothing is off the table when it comes to avenging any perceived slight.

- Listen to all the little warnings you get, not only around strangers on the street, but also in relationships as well. Little hints become bigger hints; small behaviors turn into larger ones. If you don't pay attention to the clues, something bad is bound to happen to you. While women are often on the receiving end of domestic abuse, men can be victims as well.

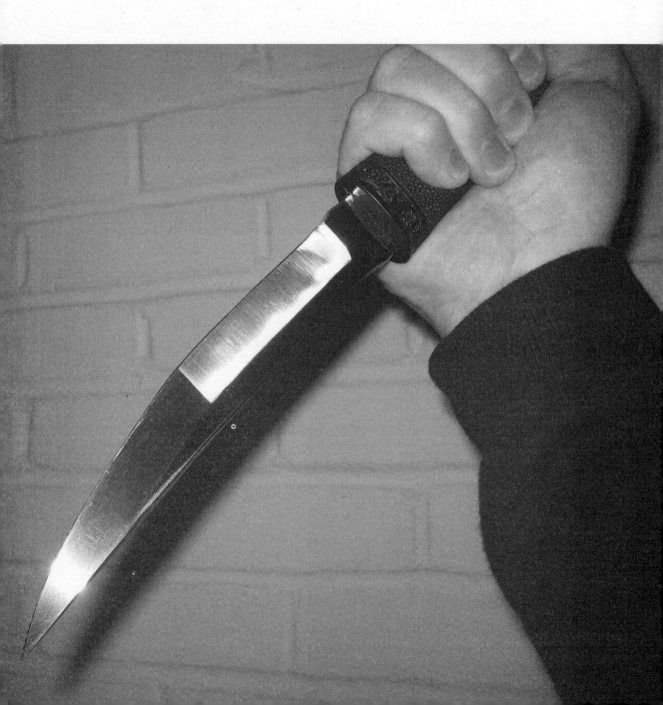

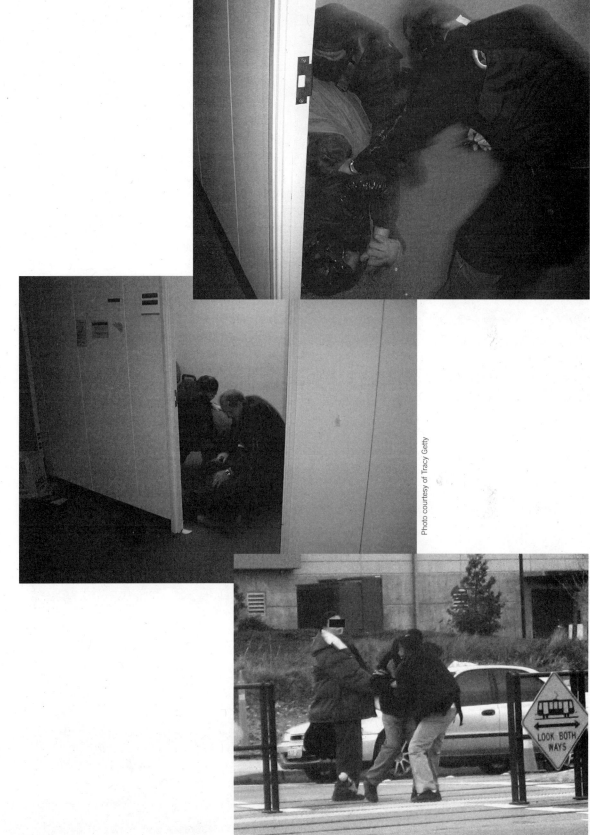

LOOK BOTH WAYS

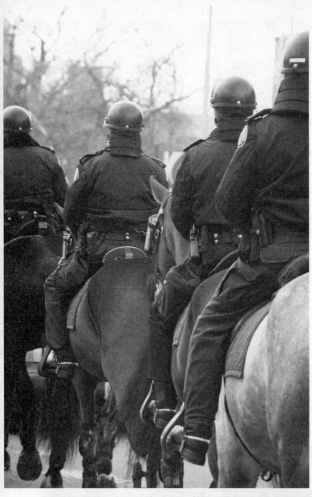

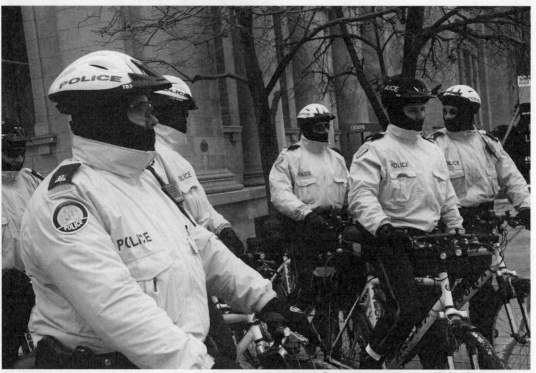

Photos on these pages courtesy of BigStockPhoto.com

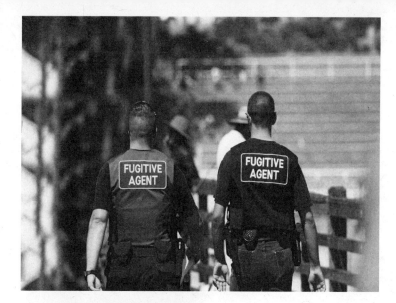

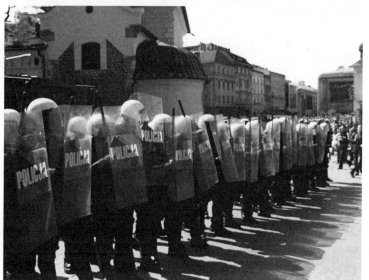

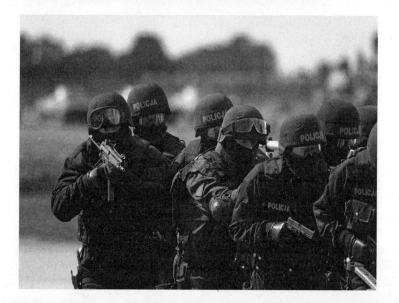

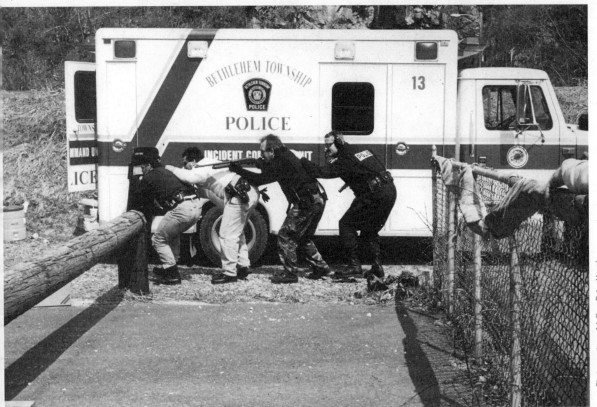

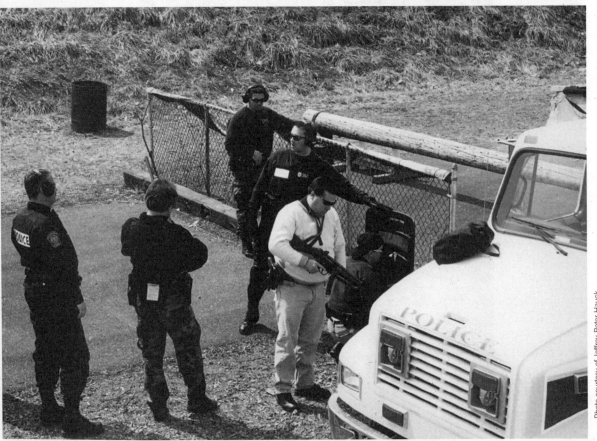

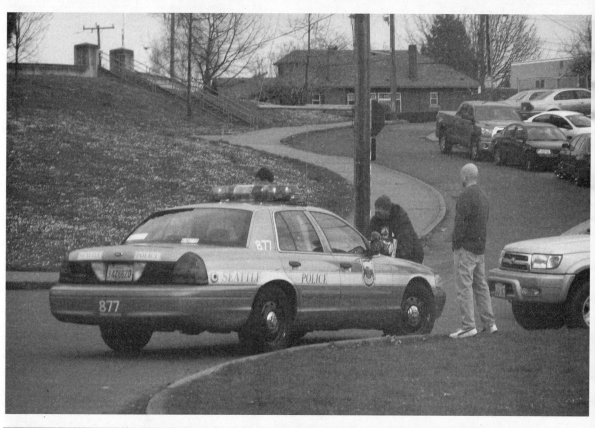

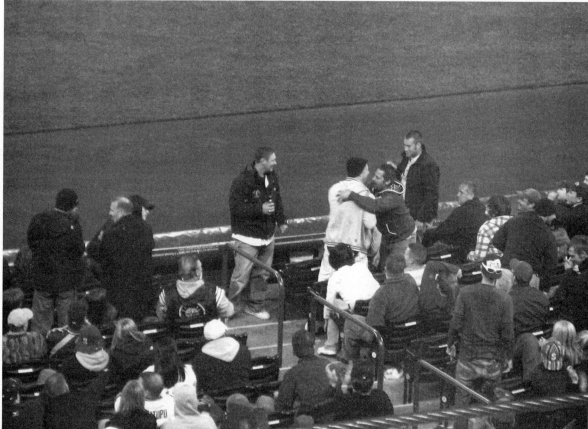

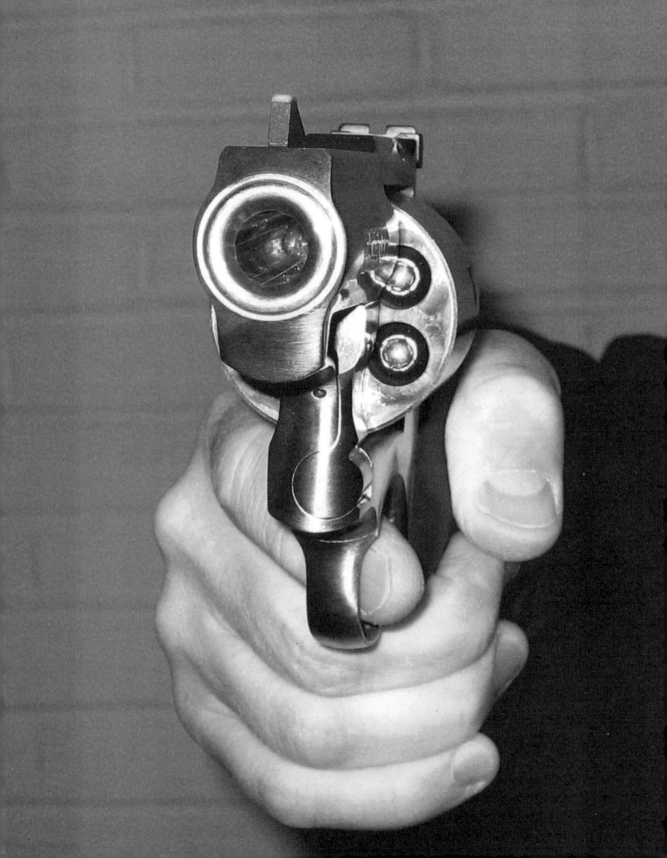

During A Violent Encounter

Lotus seeds
Jump every which-way
As they wish.
  — Sosen (1694–1776)[5]

Unfortunately, there are instances when you have no choice but to fight and others where it is prudent to do so. If you've gotta fight, you need to know how to do it effectively. This section is about what actually happens during a violent encounter, helping you understand clever things you might want to try and dumb things you should attempt to avoid when things get rough.

If you do have to fight, you must avoid being injured long enough to give yourself a reasonable chance to strike back, so the awareness you have already learned about remains important. It's pretty hard to battle effectively when you're disoriented, bleeding, and reeling in agony. Further, to remain safe, your response must at least knock your adversary off his game plan, if not disable him straightaway. Having a variety of reliable techniques to draw from can give you a leg up if your initial response is thwarted by the other guy as it often will be. He's not going to attack you unless he thinks he can win, so odds are good that he has at least a little experience at doing it right. He will be doing his damnedest to pound your face in, pulling out every dirty trick he can think of in an effort to mess you up.

While this book largely focuses on the principles of violence, we offer a variety of practical applications in this section that you can use to give yourself reasonable odds of surviving a violent encounter. Unfortunately, no book, no matter how well written, can substitute for professional hands-on training when it comes to handling violence. If you are interesting in learning how to defend yourself effectively, we suggest you seriously consider taking up martial arts classes. At the risk of making a crass, commercial statement, our book *The Way to Black Belt: A Comprehensive Guide to Rapid, Rock-Solid Results* is a great resource to get started along that path.

Fighting should never be your first choice, but sometimes it's your only choice to keep yourself or someone you care about safe. In addition to learning some solid fighting techniques, you will discover some important principles that help you understand when you can legally get away with going physical. Unfortunately countervailing force is not a yes/no equation. What you can and cannot do under the eyes of the law can be highly nuanced. Consequently, this section identifies appropriate levels of force that you might be able to employ while keeping yourself out of jail whenever you have to get hands on.

He Who Strikes the First Blow Admits He's Lost the Argument

Whoever is first in the field and awaits the coming of the enemy, will be fresh for the fight; whoever is second in the field and has to hasten to battle will arrive exhausted.

– *Sun Tzu*

The first is to forestall him by attacking. This is called ken no sen (to set him up).
– *Miyamoto Musashi*

There is an old Chinese proverb that states, "He who strikes the first blow admits he's lost the argument." Throwing the first punch can put you on shaky ground legally speaking too. Consequently, most civilians are taught that striking first is a bad thing. If you are already a martial artist, you have undoubtedly heard that karate is first and foremost a defensive art. This tradition is best described by Gichin Funakoshi's* famous saying, "*karate ni sente nashi*" which translates as "there is no first strike in karate."

While this statement is true, it is also commonly misunderstood, often to the detriment of martial artists who find themselves in serious trouble the first time they take their *dojo* training to a real fight on the street. Following Funakoshi's admonishment, they tend to wait until they have already been attacked and very possibly struck with force before taking any action. By then it is often too late. If a trained martial artist has this challenge, imagine how much more difficult it would be for an untrained civilian to survive a fight if he cedes initiative to the attacker.

To be clear, *karateka*, like most martial artists, are taught to avoid seeking conflict. This convention helps practitioners of potentially lethal arts behave in a manner appropriate to interaction within polite society; something we'd all agree is a positive thing indeed. This mindset is so important that it goes beyond mere words and is even reflected in the training methods and physical movements of the art. For example, every *kata*† in *Goju Ryu* karate (which Kane and Wilder practice) begins with a defensive technique.

The challenge is, then, to make that defensive move work to your advantage. What many don't realize is that defensive techniques when executed properly are designed to be just as fight-stopping as offensive ones. *Uke*, in Japanese, means "receive" rather than

---

* Gichin Funakoshi (1868–1957) was the founder of Shotokan karate, a style that is very popular around the world today.

† *Kata* means "formal exercise," a logical series of offensive and defensive movements performed in a particular order during solo training.

"block," an important distinction. Traditional fighting arts were developed long before the advent of modern medicine. In those days, almost any injury suffered in battle could ultimately prove fatal through infection or other collateral impact. Consequently, even the defensive tactics were nasty and highly effective.

The ancient masters understood that if they were to only block an adversary's attack, he would continue to strike until they did something more effective to disable him, or they were beaten into a bloody pulp, or he decided to stop of his own volition. Consequently, all martial applications, including the defensive ones, were designed in such a manner that they could be used to end a confrontation as quickly as possible. Despite advancements in technology, the nature of hand-to-hand fighting remains much the same today as it was in ancient times.

Here is where the confusion lies. To many, "no first strike" implies waiting for an adversary to attack rather than trying to counter successfully when you are already injured or out of position from the force of your attacker's initial blow. After all, once you block the first strike another is inevitably already on its way, so you are effectively behind the count before you begin. No one throws only a single punch in a fight. In order to decipher the true intent of Funakoshi's statement, we must understand a bit about initiative and how it is used in a fight.

- Late initiative (*go no sen* in Japanese) means blocking and counterstriking after an adversary has already attacked. This is the method that new martial artists are initially taught. It means to receive or block a blow and then to strike back. It is a great learning method because it breaks advanced techniques down into small movements, but it is not practical on the street where you are likely to become overwhelmed by a determined aggressor. This is elementary stuff, abandoned quickly once any significant level of skill has been achieved.

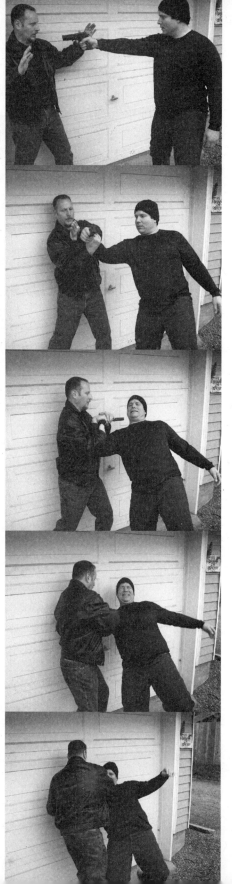

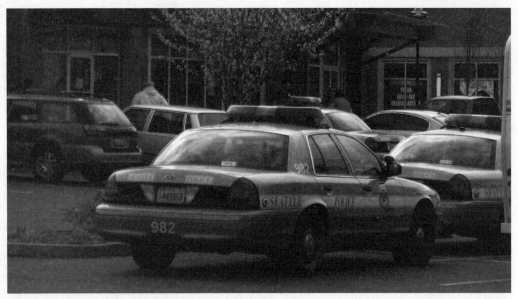

Whenever you fight, you run the risk injuring, maiming, or killing another human being, even if only by accident. If you are seen as the aggressor in the eyes of the law, you will be facing serious jail time and/or crippling civil liability.

- Simultaneous initiative (*sen no sen* in Japanese) means intercepting the adversary's blow just after it begins. This is an intermediate form of martial arts, using quickness and power to simultaneously attack and defend, cutting off the opponent's strike before it makes contact. This is where we begin to find street-worthy application. With dedicated training and a bit of practice, this is very achievable.

- Preemptive initiative (*sen-sen no sen* in Japanese) means cutting off a blow before it even starts. Practitioners sense that an attack will be forthcoming and then cut it short before the aggressor has the chance to transform the mental desire to attack into the physical movement necessary to execute that desire. This is the ultimate goal of martial training insofar as self-defense is concerned, advanced martial arts. It's also really tough to learn.

Preemptive initiative, or *sen-sen no sen*, cuts off an attack before it is fully in play, looking an awful lot like a first strike yet is still a defensive movement. This is what Funakoshi really meant: Striking to cut off an impending attack is okay while instigating unwarranted violence on your own volition is not. If you can walk away from a confrontation, you absolutely should do so. It is not only morally the right thing to do but it also allows you to avoid potentially serious repercussions as well. Most rational people would agree that picking fights on the street is a bad idea.

To clarify further, Funakoshi wrote, "When there are no avenues of escape or one is caught even before any attempt to escape can be made, then for the first time the use of self-defense techniques should be considered. Even at times like these, do not show any intention of attacking, but first let the attacker become careless. At that time attack him concentrating one's whole strength in one blow to a vital point and in the moment of surprise, escape, and seek shelter and help." Notice that he wrote, "at that time attack him" as opposed to "after he strikes launch your counterattack." Preemptive initiative is fully consistent with this approach. He also talks about seeking "shelter and help." Your intent should be to stop the assault so that you can escape to safety or otherwise remain safe until help arrives, not to beat down your adversary.

Clearly martial artists should only engage in physical violence if there is no other choice. Sometime around 506 B.C. Sun Tzu wrote, "To win one hundred victories in one hundred battles is not the highest skill. To subdue an enemy without fighting is the highest skill." There are many peaceful ways to settle a disagreement, any one of which is preferable to a physical confrontation. If you cannot escape from danger, however, that does not mean that you must stand around waiting to get hit before you can act in your own defense. This is especially important in multiple attacker and armed aggressor scenarios where hesitation will most likely get you mutilated or killed.

> Never start a fight. If you can walk away from a confrontation, by all means do so. It is not only morally the right thing to do but it allows you to avoid serious repercussions as well. A preemptive strike as you sense an imminent threat, on the other hand, is a legitimate and street-worthy defensive technique so long as your intent is to stop the assault so that you can escape to safety or otherwise remain safe until help arrives rather than to beat down your adversary. You'll need to be able to clearly articulate why you knew he was going to assault you before you clobbered him when you talk with the police though.

This same perspective is expressed in a famous quote from the Bible, though once again it is commonly misunderstood. A common translation of Matthew 5:39 reads: "But I say unto you, that ye resist not evil: but whosoever shall smite thee on thy right cheek, turn to him the other also." A more accurate translation according to many biblical scholars would be, "But I say to you, do not resist evil with evil."

There is a huge difference between a command to "not resist evil" and a command to "not resist with evil." Turning the other cheek is a metaphor for not seeking vengeance for or responding violently to insults. While very sound advice, it is not a literal requirement to stand there and let someone beat you down without offering even token resistance. Evil must be resisted—evil impulses in yourself as well as evil actions from others.

Whoever is attacking you has almost certainly assaulted someone before. The more times he gets away with it, the more dangerous he is likely to become. If you successfully defend yourself against an assailant, you not only save your own life or well-being but likely that of the bad guy's next victim as well.

While there truly is no first strike in karate (or any other martial art for that matter), there should be proactive defense in situations that warrant it. Good and moral people ignore insults and avoid seeking revenge, yet that does not mean that they should be passive and allow themselves or others to be slaughtered. If confronted with unavoidable danger, it is perfectly all right to offer a vigorous response. Your intent, however, must be to escape to safety, not to kill your attacker, humiliate him, or otherwise teach him a lesson. Throwing the first blow not only means that you've lost the argument, but also that you're the bad guy as well… unless it's preemptive initiative in your defense.

You've Got a "Stay Out of Jail Free" Card if You Use It Wisely

Soldiers when in desperate straits lose the sense of fear.
– Sun Tzu

There is the spirit of winning without a sword.
– Miyamoto Musashi

Countervailing force, or physical self-defense, is violence applied against an aggressor to keep him from hurting you. In the process, you may intentionally or unintentionally injure, maim, cripple, or even kill your adversary. Even if you give the other guy a bloody nose or a minor bruise, it can still have serious repercussions, such as a night in jail or nice fat, juicy lawsuit. Imagine what would happen if you killed him… As the old saying goes, "The bigger the crime, the bigger the time." Because of this possibility, it is important to understand how your actions might be scrutinized under the law.

A legitimate case of self-defense and a good lawyer can get you off the hook most, but not all, of the time. Consequently, it is really important to know when you're on solid legal ground. We're martial artists, not attorneys, so nothing in this book constitutes a legal opinion nor should any of its contents be treated as such. While we have done our due diligence and believe these guidelines are true and correct, it is prudent to check with an attorney in your local jurisdiction to understand how the laws work where you live and frequently travel. The law is very nuanced, so such things are never universal.

The Doctrine of Competing Harms. The doctrine of competing harms, or doctrine of necessity, as it is often called, is a very important point of law when it comes to self-defense. This concept has been around a very long time. It stems from English Common Law. Here's an example of that language from Maine's Criminal Code:[*]

§103. **Competing harms:**
  1. Conduct which the actor believes to be necessary to avoid imminent physical harm to himself or another is justifiable if the desirability and urgency of avoiding such harm outweigh, according to ordinary standards of reasonableness, the harm sought to be prevented by the statute defining the crime charged. The desirability and urgency of such conduct may not rest upon considerations pertaining to the morality and advisability of such statute.

---

[*] Title 17-A, Part 1, Chapter 5 (Defenses and affirmative defenses; justification).

2. When the actor was reckless or criminally negligent in bringing about the circumstances requiring a choice of harms or in appraising the necessity of his conduct, the justification provided in subsection 1 does not apply in a prosecution for any crime for which recklessness or criminal negligence, as the case may be, suffices to establish criminal liability.

In plain terms, this means that, under the right circumstances, you have a legitimate excuse for breaking the law and will not be held criminally liable for your actions. For example, while murder is clearly illegal, killing someone in self-defense is acceptable in certain conditions. In essence, you are not held accountable for your actions because your conduct was necessary to prevent some greater harm to yourself and/or your loved ones.

You've probably never had to kill someone in self-defense so it's most likely a bit hard to wrap your head around what that truly entails. Sure, you've seen it on TV, but we've already pointed out the fallacy of relying on Hollywood when it comes to real violence. For the moment, let's use a different example that most people can relate to since there is a good chance that you've either done something just like this or can easily imagine doing so yourself:

Pretend that you're driving your car along a winding, two-lane road with a double yellow line down the center. Your entire family is riding along with you. It is raining heavily, you are traveling at a prudent pace somewhat below the regular speed limit, and there are no cars in the opposite lane.

Clearly, the law states that you cannot cross the center line, even to pass another vehicle. That's why it's marked with the double-yellow line. Most of the time it is prudent to follow that law, driving in your own lane for everyone's safety. What happens, however, if as you round a corner the rain-soaked ground gives way and a tree suddenly falls into your path or a rockslide covers your lane?

You have microseconds to make a decision. There is a potentially lethal barrier looming right in front of you, so close that you know you would crash into it even if you slammed on your brakes the moment you saw it. The law, on the other hand, says you've got to stay in your lane. So, what would you do? Why, you'd temporarily break the law to cross the centerline and move out of harm's way, right? Not a hard choice to make in this example. It's perfectly acceptable to avoid the greater harm that a crash would cause by illegally changing lanes until you get around the obstacle.

The doctrine of competing harms is why police officers break the speed limit when racing to a crime scene too. If they were to travel at the posted speed, someone could very well die before they got there. More importantly, this same reasoning is why you can apply potentially lethal countervailing force to defend yourself from harm when you are attacked by a predator on the street.

Most jurisdictions recognize the doctrine of competing harms only under limited circumstances, however. It is usually considered an "affirmative" defense. That means that it shifts the burden of proof from the prosecutor to the defendant since you are admitting that you broke the law but arguing that you should not be held liable for doing so. Normally, it's the prosecutor who has to prove his case, not the defendant. Consequently, you need a really good attorney on your side if you're going to use this approach, someone who's skilled at defending innocent parties in self-defense situations.* Generally, to prove your case successfully, you must show evidence that

> Whenever you tee off on another person, you run the risk injuring, maiming, or potentially even killing him, even when you were not actively trying to do so. If you are seen as the aggressor in the eyes of the law, you will be faced with the very real possibility of spending time in jail and/or losing a ton of money in a civil lawsuit. Consequently, you need a way of knowing when it's prudent to strike. If the four criteria—ability, opportunity, jeopardy, and preclusion (AOJP)—are all met, you have a pretty good legal case for taking action. If one or more of these conditions are absent, however, you are on shaky legal ground should you decide to fight with the other guy.

1. The harm you sought to avoid outweighed the danger of the prohibited conduct you were charged with.
2. You had no reasonable alternative but to engage in the prohibited conduct in order to avoid that harm.
3. You stopped doing the prohibited conduct as soon as the danger passed.
4. You did not create the danger you sought to avoid.

In our driving example, crossing the centerline was definitely less harmful than crashing into the potentially deadly obstacle so you're good on the first criterion. You had no reasonable alternative (criterion number 2) and immediately moved back into your lane once you passed the danger (criterion number 3). You most certainly did not cause the danger (criterion number 4), so it's all good. Were you pulled over by a police officer for a moving violation after crossing the centerline you'd have a near bulletproof defense in court (in the unlikely event that it ever got that far).

This same reasoning works in self-defense cases too, assuming that all four of these elements are in place. While taking a life is clearly illegal, the competing harm (or urgent necessity) of saving your own life outweighs the harm you did to your attacker since he initiated the confrontation. In other words, it can be your "stay out of jail free" card if you play it right.

While the doctrine of competing harms is the legal basis upon which you can make a case for killing someone in self-defense, in practical reality it's not necessarily a clear enough guideline to use on the street. The challenge is that it can be tough to keep all

---

* The wrong legal strategy can blow your case. Many criminal defense attorneys are used to dealing primarily with guilty individuals whose cases may be handled differently from innocent ones. Guilt or innocence aside, self-defense cases typically offer unique challenges not found in other areas of law. You'll need a specialist to guide you through.

these obscure points of law in your head when things get ugly. That's why many defense combatives instructors teach the AOJP principle to their students instead of, or in addition to, the doctrine of competing harms. It's relatively easy to remember, and an extraordinarily useful guideline to keep you out of trouble. Here's how it works.

The AOJP Principle

The AOJP principle is a good way to ascertain whether it makes sense to use physical force in self-defense situation. AOJP stands for Ability, Opportunity, Jeopardy, and Preclusion. If all four of these criteria are all met, you have a pretty good legal case for taking action. If one or more of these conditions are absent, however, you are on shaky legal ground. Clearly, you will want to speak with an attorney to understand the laws in your locale, but this principle is a useful, relatively easy to remember guideline.

Ability. Ability means that an attacker has both the physical as well as practical ability to seriously injure, maim, or kill you. This may include the use of fists and feet as well as the application of conventional or improvised weapons such as knives, guns, bottles, baseball bats, or similar instruments. It also includes the physical ability to wield said weapon (or fists or feet for that matter) in a manner that can actually injure you. A small child with a baseball bat does not have the same ability to cause you harm as a professional ball player swinging the same hunk of wood as a weapon. Similarly, unless there is a massive skill differential, a petite woman has less ability to hurt you with a punch or kick than a muscular man.

Opportunity. While your attacker may have the ability to harm you, his ability does not necessarily mean that he also has the immediate opportunity to do so. Your life and well-being must be in clear and present danger before you can legally respond with physical force. For example, a bad guy with a knife has the ability to kill you only so long as he is also within striking range of the weapon or can quickly move into the appropriate distance from which to initiate his attack. A physical barrier such as a chain link fence may protect you from a knife-wielder but not an assailant armed with a gun, so opportunity relates not only to the attacker and the weapon, but also to the environment within which they are deployed as well.

Jeopardy. Jeopardy or "imminent jeopardy" as the law sometimes requires, relates to the specifics of the situation. Any reasonable person in a similar situation should feel in fear for his life. This is a legal attempt to distinguish between a truly hazardous situation and one that is only potentially dangerous. While you are not expected to be able to read an aggressor's mind, you certainly should be able to ascertain his intent from his outward appearance, demeanor, and actions. Someone shouting, "I'm going to kill you," while walking away is probably not an immediate threat even though he may very well come back with a weapon or a group of friends later and become one should you stick around long enough. Someone shouting, "I love you," while lunging toward you with a knife, on the other hand, most likely is an imminent threat.

Preclusion. Even when the ability, opportunity, and jeopardy criteria are satisfied, you must still have no other safe alternatives other than physical force before engaging an opponent in combat. If you can run or retreat from harm's way without further endangering yourself these criteria have not been met. In some jurisdictions, there is no requirement to retreat when attacked in your home or, in some cases, your place of business. Regardless, it is prudent to retreat whenever you have the ability to do so safely. After all, it is impossible for the other guy to hurt you if you're not there.

Use Only as Much Force as the Situation Warrants

If your opponent is of choleric temper, seek to irritate him. Pretend to be weak, that he may grow arrogant.

– Sun Tzu

Miyamoto Musashi made no comments regarding using only as much force as the situation required. He lived in a time when such things were, for the most part, unnecessary. In his day, nearly all fights were to the death yet there was little fear of legal repercussions.

During the escalation process, there are several force options available to help stave off violence: (1) presence, (2) voice, (3) empty-hand restraint, (4) non-lethal force, and, ultimately, (5) lethal force. This continuum is similar to the approach codified by many police departments. The first two levels can potentially prevent violence before it begins, the third may be used proactively as an opponent prepares to strike, and the last two take place after you have already been attacked.

This continuum of force should be applied sensibly to preserve your safety as the situation warrants. There are no absolutes in self-defense, but your ultimate goal should be to apply sufficient force to effectively control the situation and keep yourself from harm without overdoing it. In general, you may legally use reasonable force in defending yourself. "Reasonable force" is considered only that force reasonably necessary to repel the attacker's force.

Exceeding a reasonable level of force may well turn a victim into a perpetrator in the eyes of the courts. Justifiable self-defense is a victim's defense to a criminal and/or civil charge. The legal reasoning goes like this: If your intent was to defend yourself, than a reasonable person would only do so using reasonable force. Sounds a bit circular but it is very important. Using a higher level of force infers that you had intent to needlessly harm the other guy. This allows the perpetrator turned "victim" to use your defensive actions against you, the victim turned perpetrator. Even if a criminal prosecutor dismisses your actions, a civil court may not do so.

In other words, that means that if you overdo things, you're in trouble. Bad guys sue their victims all the time. They even win too. It just isn't right, yet it certainly happens in this litigious society. Clearly, if you under-do things you'll lose the fight, which is trouble of a whole different kind. Your response needs to be "just right."

1. Presence

If you are a trained martial artist or just a well-conditioned athlete, your presence alone can frequently de-escalate a dangerous situation. Carry yourself with confidence and be prepared to act. Predators who are good at sensing body language may back off simply because they can tell that you are prepared to act. In other words, presence can help you fail the victim interview. Bad guys don't want to tangle with you if they think they are going to get hurt in the process.

2. Voice

Use your verbal skills and tone of voice to talk an aggressor out of attacking you or otherwise get him to back down. Even when you cannot de-escalate a pending conflict through verbal skills, you may still be able to use your words as a psychological weapon to momentarily confuse or disrupt an opponent, giving yourself an opportunity to act. Your voice is a very important weapon in your self-defense arsenal. Don't forget to use it. Furthermore, be wary when the other guy tries to do the same thing back to you.

3. Empty-hand restraint

Restraint, disarm, and control techniques can be employed to keep an aggressor from hurting you and/or themselves until law enforcement professionals arrive. You will generally want to respond with a slightly greater degree of force than is used against you. Pulling a weapon on an unarmed attacker, for example, almost always makes you the bad guy.

> Many confrontations can be resolved without violence. Even when it becomes necessary to go hands on, it is important to exercise a judicious level of force sufficient to control the other guy without overreacting. An excessive response can make you the bad guy in the eyes of the law. Force options you might select from include (1) presence, (2) voice, (3) empty-hand restraint, (4) non-lethal force, and, ultimately, (5) lethal force. The first two options can prevent violence before it begins, the third may be used proactively as an opponent prepares to strike, and the last two take place after you have already been attacked.

Beware of chokes and other violent-looking responses. Pins, locks, arm bars, and similar control techniques are preferable if you can apply them safely and effectively. Be very cautious of going to the ground unless you are absolutely sure that your attacker acted alone and does not have friends who might take advantage of your vulnerability to attack though.

Pinning or holding down the drunken uncle at a family gathering might work very effectively, while the same tactics used on an adversary in a crowded bar will almost certainly not. If you do use a restraint technique, try to hold the other guy face down so that he had less chance of fighting free. Sports like judo require that you pin your opponent face up, giving him a sporting chance, something that's bound to go poorly on the street.

4. Non-lethal force

Non-lethal force is the next step up on the force continuum. This includes striking, kicking, and a whole bunch of other martial arts techniques that cause damage to your opponent. Such strikes should be aimed at non-vital areas of the body. An elbow or knee to the gut is unlikely to kill your adversary while the very same blow to his head could easily result in serious injuries, brain damage, or even death. Certain weapons such as *kubaton*, pepper spray, or Tasers can also be used for non-lethal force or restraint applications. Law enforcement and military professionals have an even wider array of non-lethal weapons (for example, water cannons, stun grenades, teargas) to choose from than civilians do.[*]

If restraint techniques do not work or will put you in danger because your assailant is armed, much bigger than you are, or there is more than one of them, you may have to escalate directly to this level should other options fail. Hit-and-run tactics such as kicking the knee or stomping the foot may slow your adversary down sufficiently to let you get away without needing to seriously damage him.

5. Lethal force

The final level is lethal force. This includes both martial arts applications applied to vital areas of the body that can cause significant damage such as strikes to the head or solar plexus. In some cases, chokes may be considered lethal force too. Similarly, deployment of various lethal weapons such as knives, guns, bludgeons, and the like may also be called for. This level should be avoided unless there is no other way to escape a violent encounter unscathed.

When lethal force is warranted your life is at stake. Consequently, all bets are off. Chances are good that someone won't be walking away from these types of encounters so they must be taken very seriously. You must be mentally and physically prepared to do whatever it takes to survive (see "The Will to Kill" in Appendix C for more information).

Is it really better to be judged by twelve than carried by six? Some self-defense experts throw around the phrase, "It's better to be judged by twelve than carried by six." We do not advocate that sentiment because we feel that it trivializes the seriousness of violent confrontations. Never forget that if you are found guilty in a jury trial, you will be spending a whole lot of quality time in a confined environment with unpredictable, dangerous neighbors who may be less than friendly when you interact with them. You may also suffer consequences with others in the community, facing challenges from family, friends, employers, and those you wish to interact positively with on a daily basis.

Bad things can happen when you fight for your life, but that doesn't mean that you shouldn't fight for everything you're worth if it gets to that point. Under no circumstances should you let fear of legal consequences keep you from living through a violent encounter, particularly against an armed assailant. If you don't survive, everything else is meaningless.

[*] Just because something is designed to be less then lethal does not mean that it cannot accidentally kill someone. Exercise caution when utilizing any type of weapon.

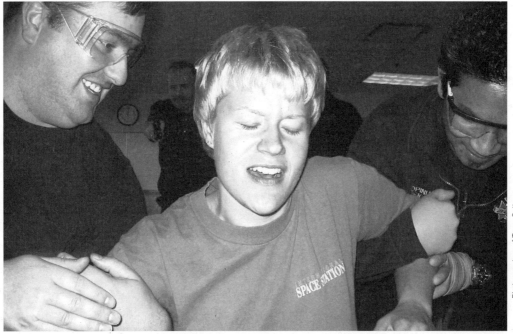

Photo courtesy of Tracy Getty

To pass Taser certification, you must be zapped in training. The paramedics are laughing because she let out an uncharacteristically foul expletive before succumbing to the voltage.

Most confrontations can be resolved without violence. Even when it becomes necessary to go hands on, it is important to exercise a judicious level of force sufficient to control the other guy without overreacting. Use only as much force as the situation warrants.

Know How to Wrangle Drunks

Now, when your weapons are dulled, your ardor damped, your strength exhausted and your treasure spent, other chieftains will spring up to take advantage of your extremity. Then no man, however wise, will be able to avert the consequences that must ensue.

— Sun Tzu

If his rhythm is disorganized, or if he has fallen into evasive or retreating attitudes, we must crush him straightaway.

— Miyamoto Musashi

Not all encounters are deadly. In fact, a few can even be downright comical. Wrangling drunks, for example, is typically light years apart from tangling with armed assailants. It is important to be able to respond appropriately across the entire continuum of

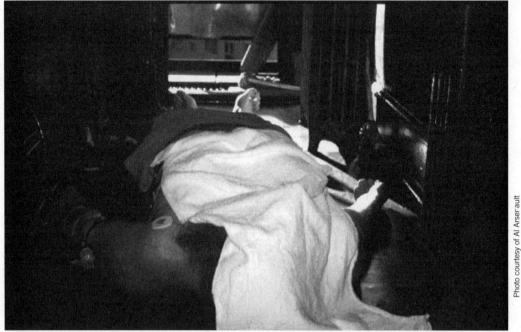

Photo courtesy of Al Arserault

Under no circumstances should you let fear of legal consequences keep you from living through a violent encounter, particularly against an armed assailant. If you don't survive, everything else is meaningless.

violence as we have outlined in the previous section. Since many violent encounters are facilitated by alcohol-induced impairment, we'll spend a little time examining how to deal with such situations.

For your amusement we'll begin with the following true story that was contributed by our friend and fellow martial artist Dave Organ. This incident took place in June 2007. While it is positively humorous, at least in retrospect, there are important lessons that can be gleaned from the event too, which is, of course, why we have included it here.

> **While my diplomatic skills are good, I don't have a lot of experience negotiating with ambassadors from planet Tequila. Drunks, even ones with all the power and grace of an anemic octopus, can be difficult to control without causing injury.**
>
> I work as the manager, bartender, and bouncer of a small restaurant and lounge in the little town of Westerose, Alberta (Canada). In my time, I've had to deal with my share of hostile encounters, but this particular incident ranks as probably the funniest one I've ever experienced.
>
> First, some background. Shortly after our restaurant opened, I hired a new bartender named 'Fred' (all names have been changed to protect the idiotic; it is, after all, a small town). I fired him after the first day for drinking on the job. As it turns out, he's the town

drunk, which just goes to show what happens when you're new to the area and don't know people yet. Despite firing him, I liked the guy—he's warm, friendly, and funny and really is a kick-ass bartender. I had no problems with having him and his friend Dean in the lounge for drinks virtually every night.

The thing is I worried about his heavy drinking. He's one of those guys who seems perfectly normal for a certain amount of drinks, and then descends quickly into total inebriation. It's awfully hard to determine a cutoff point for him. One moment he's fine, the next he's sliding down the walls.

Well, that night I'd had enough, so I cut him off and ordered his waitress not to serve him any more drinks. He became surly and abusive. I tolerated his attitude for a little while and tried to mollify him, but eventually I gave up, banned him from the bar, and ejected him. He began threatening me physically, but his buddy got him out the door and off the premises. End of story.

Or so I thought.

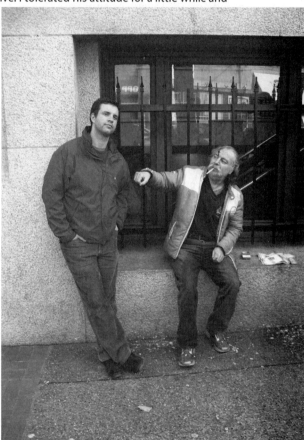

Fred decided I had 'called him out,' so he lumbered around to the kitchen entrance to confront me. One problem: I wasn't there. But, half the kitchen staff was. I had no interest at all in dealing with him, so I didn't bother to go out. What would be the point? I knew that my presence would only inflame the situation so I let those guys deal with it. His buddy Dean finally wrangled him away from the door and led him back to the front entrance where they got into an argument about their treatment with Greg, the restaurant owner.

Greg was arguing right back... bad idea. You don't argue with patrons, ever, especially not drunk patrons you've just kicked out. Finally, after a few minutes, I knew that I had to intervene. I went out into the lobby and said, "No more arguing. You were abusive. I banned you. This is your tab, you signed it. End of story." Surprisingly, it was—they grumbled and left. Last I saw of Fred, he was winding his way through the nearly empty parking lot towards home.

Not all encounters are deadly. In fact, a few can even be downright comical. Wrangling drunks can often be a good example, though you still have to take such incidents seriously.

Once he was gone, I took a few minutes to calm everyone down. Ejecting Fred was high entertainment for the yahoos in the lounge. Things quickly returned to normal. After about half an hour, I stepped out the kitchen entrance for a smoke, lit up, looked up… and here comes Fred!!!

The bugger had waited by the corner of the Laundromat in order to ambush me. As soon as I stepped out the door, he charged…

And charged…

And charged…

Er… perhaps I'd better explain. It wasn't exactly the best-planned ambush in the history of warfare. The Laundromat was over a hundred meters (328 feet) away from me. I looked up, saw him approach, said "Oh, for God's sake!" and waited. And waited… I tried placating him as he approached; tried calming him down but no dice. Fred was on the warpath, the blood singing in his veins, screaming his terrible war chant, "Hey motherf%&ker you think you're so bad! Come on motherf%&ker I'll do ya, I'll do ya, I'll do ya…" Et cetera…

The mighty clash of two forces colliding sounded rather a lot like a feather pillow hitting a concrete wall which is… well… more or less what happened. He pushed his chest into me. I turned him around and pushed him away, hoping he'd get the idea. He came back flailing, but I held him at arms length so he couldn't reach me.

Finally, he tried to kick me, which didn't exactly have the desired outcome either. I pushed down on his shoulders and swept his supporting leg, dropping him gently enough that he wouldn't get hurt on landing. He wound up upside down on his head, legs wrapped around my right leg, with me cradling his ankles with my right arm to keep him from kicking me.

"Hey motherf%&ker you think you're so bad! Come on motherf%&ker I'll do ya, I'll do ya, I'll do ya…"

We were against the stucco wall, unfortunately out of view of the windows, so I was forced to walk backwards about 3 meters (10 feet) to get help—step, drag Fred. Step, draaaaag Fred…

"Hey motherf%&ker you think you're so bad! Come on motherf%&ker I'll do ya, I'll do ya, I'll do ya…"

I tapped on the window until I got a response and one of the lounge patrons—ironically, one I'd already tossed in the past—wandered out to have a look. He stopped for a moment to stare at the ridiculous scene. Fred was still on his head, wriggling around like a worm on a hook and screaming bloody vengeance.

"Hey motherf%&ker you think you're so bad! Come on motherf%&ker I'll do ya, I'll do ya, I'll do ya…"

I calmly said, "James, do me a favour would you? Could you please go inside and get Greg and Dean? Thanks."

"Hey motherf%&ker you think you're so bad! Come on motherf%&ker I'll do ya, I'll do ya, I'll do ya..."

"Oh, shut up."

So, after a few more minutes Dean and Greg came out and they too had to stop to take in the weird tableau. By this time, I'd lit another cigarette with my free hand and was worrying about what Fred's muddy work boots were doing to my nice black satin shirt. Finally using Greg's strength and Dean's persuasion, they unwrapped the mighty warrior from around my leg. I stepped back, and after a certain amount of struggling and cussing, they got him bundled into a car and drove him off home again.

At that moment, all I could do was shake my head and remark, "I think I just got attacked by the Stay-Puft Marshmallow Man," at which point everyone within earshot rolled over laughing. I shrugged, ordered my people back into the restaurant, poured myself a root beer, and began writing my incident report. End of story again.

Or not. Yup, he came back again. He walked the whole two kilometers (approximately 1¼ miles) from his house to visit more mighty destruction upon me. I just rolled my eyes and kept watching the basketball game on television.

Shortly after Fred arrived, his father, a frail-looking old man, came roaring up in his Dodge Caravan, jumped out, grabbed Fred, and gave him what I hadn't at any point—a full-power clobber to the chin—much to the delight of all onlookers. Well, THAT finally took the fight out of him for real. He was bundled, again, into the car and taken away—this time for good.

While my diplomatic skills are good, I don't have a lot of experience negotiating with ambassadors from planet Tequila. Drunks, even ones with all the power and grace of an anemic octopus, can be difficult to control without causing injury, at least to one with my limited experience. While I had all sorts of nasty ways of finishing the encounter earlier if I'd wished, all I wanted to do was hold him in one place until the 'cavalry' arrived. I didn't want to take the chance and hurt him accidentally. All, in all, it turned out they way you want these things to, with little injury and peace quickly restored.

You will undoubtedly recognize several themes in this story that we've covered previously, such as using good situational awareness, avoiding ambushes, knowing that most attacks occur in fringe areas like parking lots, taking revenge, staking one's territory, and so on. While it is a good refresher on these subjects, we'll focus on handling drunks effectively rather than rehashing old material.

Effects of Alcohol

Let's begin by describing some of the effects of alcohol. Alcohol is a drug that depresses your system. If you and/or the other guy imbibe, it will affect both your body and your behavior. It impairs your judgment, limits your inhibitions, and tends to exacerbate your moods. This can spell trouble in a confrontation.

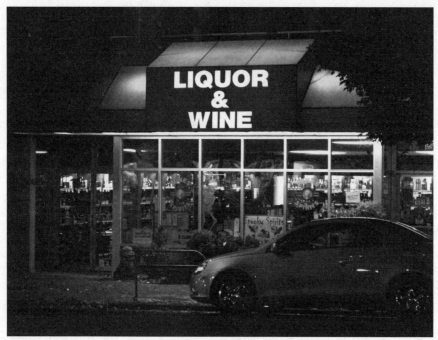

Alcohol is a drug that depresses your system. It will affect both your body and your behavior. It impairs judgment, limits inhibitions, and tends to exacerbate your moods. This can spell trouble in a confrontation.

Interestingly enough, however, if two people consume the exact same amount of alcohol, the effects on each person may be quite different. How fast you drink, what type of beverage you consume, your weight, your body fat percentage, what you have or have not eaten, the presence of other drugs (for example, prescription medications, narcotic substances), the social situation, your mood, and why you have chosen to drink on a particular occasion can all determine how alcohol affects you. Prolonged drinking over time increases your tolerance, yet it can also cause you to become physically and psychologically dependant.

The type and concentration of alcohol consumed also affect your rate of intoxication. Most people can only metabolize about one drink per hour; that's somewhere between one half and one ounce of alcohol. Consequently, the faster you drink, the greater the effect of the drug. One drink is generally considered to be 12 ounces of beer, five ounces of wine, or one ounce of hard liquor, so tossing back shots will hit you a lot harder than nursing a beer. While as little as one drink can affect certain individuals, anything more than one ounce of alcohol per hour will cause some level of impairment.

The Washington State Liquor Control Board advises that a typical 180-pound man can consume about three drinks in an hour before surpassing the legal limit of 0.08 Blood Alcohol Level (BAL). The level of impairment at this point can be quite severe. A

110-pound woman, on the other hand, can consume only one or two glasses of wine or beer in an hour and get the same adverse effects. The following table illustrates what different levels of drink can do to you. Since everyone is different, these can only be rough guidelines.

Blood Alcohol Level (BAL)	Effects of Alcohol
0.02	Slight mood changes.
0.06	Lowered inhibition, impaired judgment, reduced mental capacity, and poor decision-making ability.
0.08	Legally drunk in most jurisdictions. Deteriorated reaction time, reduced control.
0.15	Impaired balance, movement, and coordination. Difficulty standing, walking, and talking.
0.20	Decreased pain, reduced sensation, erratic emotions, and diminished reflexes.
0.30	Severely degraded reflexes; semi-consciousness. There are many recorded instances of individuals dying from alcohol poisoning at levels as low as 0.30.
0.40	Loss of consciousness, very limited reflexes, and extreme anesthetic effects. Potential coma or death. Roughly 50 percent of people die at this level.
0.50	Almost certain death.

After you drink alcohol, it passes through three stages as it becomes metabolized: (1) absorbing, (2) transporting, and (3) changing.

- Absorbing: To begin this process, once the alcohol is consumed, it is absorbed into your system. This does not work quite like digesting regular food, however. A small amount of alcohol is absorbed directly into the bloodstream by the mucosal lining of the mouth while the rest is absorbed through the lining of the stomach and small intestine. Food, water, and fruit juice help to slow this process, while carbonation works to speed it up.

- Transporting: Next, once the alcohol has gotten into your bloodstream, it must circulate throughout your body, in order to affect all of your organs. In most people, this process only takes 90 seconds or so after absorption. That's how fast blood circulates throughout your entire body.

- Changing: Once the alcohol hits your system, it must then be changed into a non-harmful substance so that you will not be poisoned by it. About ten percent of it is eliminated through sweat, breath, and urine. Your liver must detoxify the

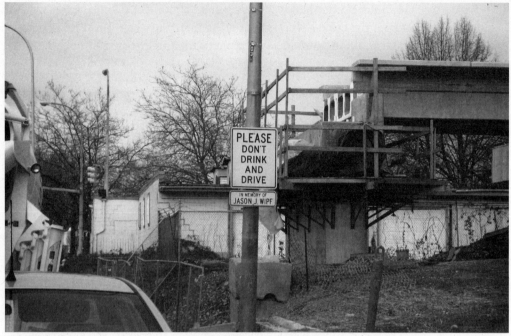

A typical 180-pound man can consume about three drinks in an hour before surpassing the legal limit. Violence and drinking go hand-in-hand—forty-one percent of violent offenders are intoxicated when they commit their crimes.

rest. The liver breaks down alcohol at a rate of about half an ounce per hour. Some people can detoxify more, others less. Regardless, nothing will speed the natural rate for any given individual. When the rate of alcohol consumed exceeds the liver's detoxification rate, the amount of alcohol in the bloodstream begins to increase. That's how you get drunk.

As you drink, alcohol impairs judgment, reduces inhibitions, and makes it much easier for you to commit violence. Impairment won't cause you to do something you would never consider when sober, however. For example, in 2007 Dr. Peter Giancola, a psychology professor at U.K. in Lexington, conducted a study of male social drinkers aged 21 to 33 years old. He found that in hostile situations, drunks who were already inclined toward violence tended to focus on provocative, aggression-facilitating stimuli rather than on inhibitory cues, whereas drunks who were not inclined toward violence tended toward the opposite. "Alcohol doesn't make you do different things," he reported. "It just allows what is already inside you to come out. It takes the brakes off."

Alcohol muddles your mind so that you don't fully think things through. It also relaxes your inhibitions so that you're more likely to act out while giving you a more-or-less socially acceptable excuse for your behavior (or at least portions of it). That's a really dangerous mix. According to the Bureau of Justice Statistics, about 36 percent of all criminals and 41 percent of violent offenders are intoxicated with alcohol when they commit the crimes for which they are convicted. These numbers get even higher if you add drugs into the mix (we'll address that more in a bit).

This was certainly the case in the drunk-wrangling story you just read. Although he was never charged with a crime, Fred was most certainly drunk off his ass. And he became very aggressive. Fortunately, Dave was not ever in any real danger during this encounter though he certainly could have been had Fred come back with some sort of weapon rather than using his fists.

Drunks can be unpredictable, violent, and very difficult to corral. Tangling with one when you're sober gives you a significant advantage. When you're drunk too, it only exacerbates the situation. Either way, you need to do your best to keep a cool head.

To begin, never argue with a drunk. As the old saying goes, "Reason goes into the bottle faster than the alcohol comes out of it." If you can get away with it, just smile, nod, and say "Yes" or "No" as appropriate. Oftentimes, however, liquid courage will lead the other guy to take a swing at you. That's when you'll undoubtedly be tempted to strike back.

Unfortunately, hitting a drunk doesn't work nearly as well as you might think. It's not necessarily that they don't feel pain, but rather that they don't feel it as much or as immediately as sober people do. Having run up against hundreds of rowdy, intoxicated fans at the stadium, Kane has a bit of practice wrangling drunks. In his experience, two strategies work the best: drunk dodging and drunk spinning.

Drunk Dodging

Drunk dodging focuses on the goal of escape yet it is not quite as defensive as it sounds. For example, because stadium seats are built on tiers, many encounters occur in the stairway between the rows. On several occasions when a drunken fan has taken a swing at him, Kane has neatly sidestepped the blow and then calmly watched his overbalanced adversary tumble down the stairs. This is a nice strategy since he does not even have to lay hands on the other guy to put him out of the fight.

Even if the other guy is not on an uneven slope, any drunk's reactions are impaired. It can be relatively simple to set him up to punch a wall or similar object by dancing out of the way at the last moment when he strikes. Similarly, you can simply dodge and dash to safety or even play "matador" until help arrives. Our

> Never argue with a drunk. As the old saying goes, "Reason goes into the bottle faster than the alcohol comes out of it." Drunks can be unpredictable, violent, and very difficult to corral. Tangling with one when you're sober gives you a significant advantage, however. Unfortunately, when you're drunk too, it only exacerbates the situation. Hitting a drunk really doesn't work all that well most of the time. It's not necessarily that they don't feel pain, but rather that they don't feel it as much or as immediately as sober people do. A better strategy is to either dodge his blows in order to let him overbalance himself and facilitate your escape or spin him to cause disorientation and make him fall. Once he's down you can control him or move to safety.

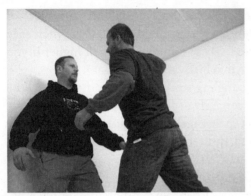

Drunk Dodging, step 1

main point here is that you don't always have to fight a drunk; you may very well be able to use your unimpaired reflexes and better coordination to get away without throwing a blow.

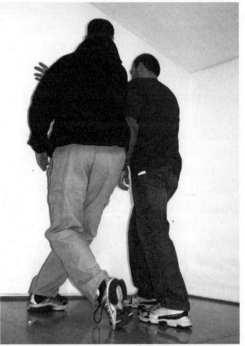

Drunk Dodging, step 2

Drunk Spinning

If you do have to fight, the goal is generally control the other guy unless he's got some sort of weapon or is exceedingly large and/or excessively violent. It may not be sufficient to simply get away in situations where the other guy is out of control and may hurt others if you do not intercede. Or, perhaps, you must fight in order to get away. Either way, in these circumstances spinning the other guy often works better than just about anything else. When a sober person spins around quickly it can be slightly disorienting, yet for a drunk it can often be debilitating, particularly when done unexpectedly with sufficient force.

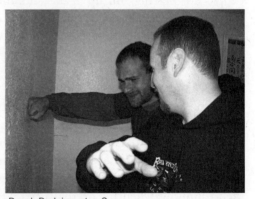

Drunk Dodging, step 3

Self-defense expert Marc "Animal" MacYoung postulates that the reason for this is that alcohol acts as a diuretic. As the person gets dehydrated, the fluid in his inner ear begins to dry out as well. This reduces his sense of balance and makes him more susceptible to being spun. Here's how this works.

The vestibular system of the inner ear is responsible for our sensations of balance and motion. The inner ear is made up of a complex series of fluid-filled tubes that run through the temporal bone of the skull. This bony labyrinth is filled with a fluid called perilymph. Within this structure is a second series of tubes made out of delicate cellular material called the membranous labyrinth. The fluid inside these membranous structures is called endolymph. If the level or viscosity of these fluids is impaired through drink, the sense of balance is reduced. Further, as the head spins around, the fluid sloshes quickly thus increasing the sense of motion. This combination can be severely dizzying to the drunk, rendering him much easier to control. It works faster and easier than trying to beat him to a pulp, and plays much better in court afterward too.

It's easiest to spin a person by using his head. While the neck is very strong front-to-back or side-to-side, it is rather weak when pulled both ways at once. Neck cranks take advantage of this fact by stretching and twisting simultaneously. If you can control the other guy's head, his body has to follow. You can grab a hold of his hair, ears, jaw, or neck to pull and twist with. If you don't get the opportunity to do that, you might also be able to arm whip or shoulder check the other guy to get him to spin.

You really don't want a circular motion, however; it's far better to corkscrew him in a downward spiral. That's not only harder to ward off, but also much more effective in disorienting a foe. And it almost always dumps him onto the ground facilitating your ability to control him or get away.

Effects of Other Drugs

Unfortunately, alcohol is not the only drug you might encounter. People who use drugs are roughly twice as likely to engage in violent behaviors as people who do not. In general, it is best to avoid tangling with anyone who is under the influence drugs because such confrontations can become extraordinarily ugly. Leave such things to law enforcement professionals whenever possible. For example, it can take as many as a dozen officers to restrain someone effectively in a drug-induced frenzy without accidentally killing him because non-lethal weapons such as pepper spray and Tasers can prove ineffective in such cases. There is a good chance that many, if not all, participants will be injured in the process when those types of situations occur.

According to the Bureau of Justice Statistics, more than half of violent criminal offenders are under the influence of drugs and/or alcohol at the time of their offense for which they are subsequently convicted. The drugs of choice are most often marijuana, cocaine/crack, or heroine/opiates. Stimulants such as cocaine/crack are most linked to violence. Similarly, about 30 percent of victims are intoxicated with drugs at the time they are attacked.

It is useful to understand (at least in general) the effects that various drugs may have on a person's nervous system. There are five main drug groupings: (1) narcotics, (2) depressants, (3) stimulants, (4) hallucinogens, and (5) cannabis.

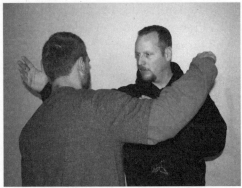

Drunk Spinning, step 1

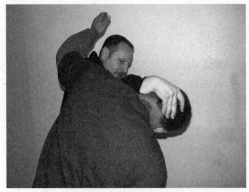

Drunk Spinning, step 2

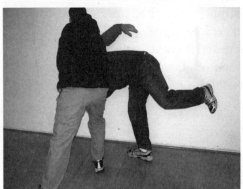
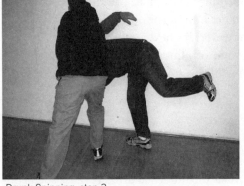

Drunk Spinning, step 3

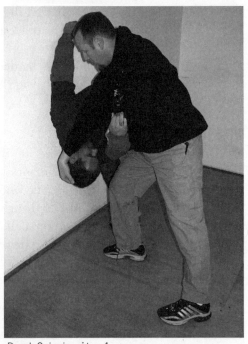

Drunk Spinning, step 4

1. Narcotics: Narcotics can include drugs such as heroin, methadone, opium, and morphine, which can cause euphoria, drowsiness, respiratory depression, and constricted pupils among other things. These drugs may be injected, snorted, or smoked. Symptoms of withdrawal include sweating, cramps, and nausea.

2. Depressants: Depressants include substances such as barbiturates, methaqualone, solvents, and alcohol, which cause disorientation, dizziness, slurred speech, delusions, hallucinations, and, of course, euphoria. Symptoms of withdrawal include tremors, delirium, and convulsions. These substances decrease dexterity and increase the users' potential for accidental injury by five to fifty times.

3. Stimulants: Stimulants include drugs such as cocaine, crack, amphetamines, and methamphetamines, which can cause hyper-alertness, excitation, euphoria, and insomnia. Symptoms of withdrawal include irritability, depression, and disorientation. Crack, a popular street drug, frequently causes rapid, intense euphoria followed by a sharp crash, often accompanied by violent impulses. Methamphetamines, also popular on the street, can cause intense euphoria, tremendous energy, heightened sexual potency, paranoid impulses, and violent behavior. People in this condition frequently have decreased pain sensitivity and can be very difficult to restrain, much more so than people who are merely drunk.

4. Hallucinogens: Hallucinogens can include substances such as LSD (lysergic acid diethylamide) and phencyclidine, which can cause users to experience time dilation, delusions, and illusions that can be linked with suicide and self-mutilation as well as accidental trauma. Hallucinogens cause their effects by disrupting the interaction of nerve cells and the neurotransmitter serotonin. Distributed throughout the brain and spinal cord, the serotonin system is involved in the control of behavioral, perceptual, and regulatory systems, including mood, hunger, body temperature, sexual behavior, muscle control, and sensory perception. Some hallucinogens such as LSD can cause intense emotional swings.

5. Cannabis: Cannabis can include such drugs as marijuana and hashish, which can cause increased appetite, relaxed inhibitions, and euphoria. Marijuana is the most commonly used illicit drug, used either solo or in combination with other substances by about three-quarters of people who take drugs. Withdrawal symptoms include insomnia and hyperactivity.

Wrangling drunks is a unique, albeit quite common, form of fighting. It's important to know how to do it well. It is also useful to be able to identify the presence of other types of drugs so that you can either avoid encounters with impaired individuals or be prepared to deal with them effectively.

Never Hit a Girl... Unless She's Armed

Sun Tzu and Miyamoto Musashi made no distinctions regarding gender. To them all adversaries were defined as combatants. In today's world, distinctions of gender are made by friends, family, police, and the courts. The role of combatant is, oftentimes, secondary.

While experienced bouncers, bodyguards, law enforcement officers, soldiers, jail guards, and martial artists know that women can be just as dangerous, or possibly even more so than men,* the courts don't often see it that way. If the "big, burly man" strikes the "tiny helpless woman," even in a case of legitimate self-defense, judges and juries will

---

* Such as instinctively going for the eyes during an attack.

naturally see the size, gender, and strength differential, and take that into account. Stuff like that usually ends badly. Who goes to jail and/or loses the lawsuit, or whatever? Most often, it is the guy. Not always, of course, but commonly enough to be worrisome.

Gender differences can become particularly challenging if you are caught by surprise, reacting instinctively to the situation. Because of your "fight-or-flight" reflex, it can be normal to lash out responsively, yet plays poorly in the court of law as well as the court of public opinion. If you have an occupation that deals with violence on a regular basis, you may be somewhat better prepared from long experience. Regardless, excess caution in such instances is almost always prudent. Act as if you are on live television. Who knows, with all the camera phones, video cameras, closed circuit televisions, and recording technology out there—perhaps you are.

For example, Kane, who supervises security personnel at a football stadium, is much more careful when tangling with females at the games than he is with males. In the last few years, incidents of intoxicated, out-of-control female fans have been on the rise rather dramatically. While Kane and his team are not supposed to use countervailing force against the fans, as that is what the police are there for, in practical reality there are many times that law enforcement does not arrive in time to keep security personnel from needing to use hands-on contact for the safety of all involved.

In those instances, he does his best to verbally control the situation. Further, he tries to bring along enough other staff so that the aggressive individual will feel outnumbered and, hopefully, become more compliant. If that does not work, or if he does not have time to gather his crew, he does his best to use open-hand techniques—nothing that will draw blood or, hopefully, lead to visible or lasting injuries. Lawyers can wreak havoc with that sensational sort of stuff.

> While women can be just as dangerous as men, the courts don't often see it that way. When a big strong man strikes a small weak woman, even in a case of legitimate self-defense, judges and juries will naturally see the size, gender, and strength differential and take that into account. When you beat someone down, it is awfully hard to prove you acted reasonably if the other guy is a girl... unless she's armed with some sort of weapon. Then all bets are off.

He does that with guys too, of course, but takes greater care with women due to the perceived inequities in size and strength. When you are operating in a public venue packed with witnesses, cameras, and various recording devices, you really have to watch your step. All in all, however, he'd much rather eat a punch from most women without responding with force than take a hit from most men. As a martial artist, he has a decent chance of controlling aggressive people without hurting them, but there really are no absolutes when it comes to self-defense. Simple things like pushing someone over can cause a fatal accident if his head hits something hard like a stair or a curb.

This is an important concept on the street too. As stated previously, a continuum of force should always be applied judiciously to preserve your safety as the situation warrants. Your ultimate goal should be to apply sufficient force to effectively control the situation and keep yourself from harm without overdoing anything.

Reasonable force in legal terms is generally considered only that force reasonably necessary to repel an attacker's force.

Unfortunately, "reasonably necessary" is a vague term usually associated with what a "reasonable person" would think necessary. This so-called reasonable person is a fictitious composite of all the reasonably prudent people in a given cross-section of life. Whether the ordinary person acted reasonably will likely be judged against the reasonably prudent, similarly situated ordinary person in the appropriate geographic area. Everyone starts out at this level, but other personal attributes may heighten their required standard of prudence. Trained martial artists, professional fighters (for example, MMA fighters, boxers, or wrestlers), military, and law enforcement personnel are almost always held to a higher standard than ordinary people.

The cornerstone of a legitimate claim of self-defense is the innocence of the claimant. You must be entirely without fault. If you initiate the conflict, you cannot claim self-defense. If you allow a conflict to escalate into a lethal situation when it could have been avoided, you share some degree of culpability and, once again, cannot claim self-defense.

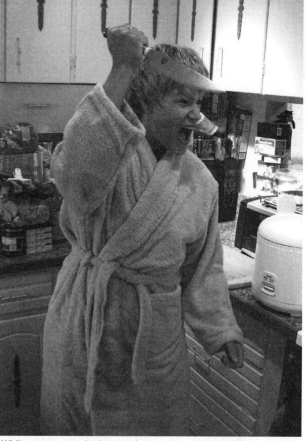

While women can be just as dangerous as a man, the courts don't often see it that way. Never hit a girl unless she's armed.

Depending on the circumstances, almost any form of physical assault can be considered deadly force. In Washington State, deadly force is defined as "The intentional application of force through the use of firearms or any other means reasonably likely to cause death or serious physical injury."* Other jurisdictions will have similar definitions. In general, any blow delivered powerfully and deliberately to a vital part of the body may be construed as deadly force so long as it can be shown that it was struck with the intention, or predictable likelihood, of killing. That means that simply smacking someone upside the head could conceivably be considered deadly force.

The courts are more likely to interpret a blow as deadly force if the person delivering

---

* Revised Code of Washington, RCW 9A.16.010.

it is physically much stronger than the victim, a professional fighter, a trained martial artist, or an assailant who attacks with extreme savagery.* Unfortunately that "physically stronger than the victim" part is rather hard to avoid if you are a male fighting a female unless you are fairly small or she is unusually large.

Equal force doctrines require law-abiding citizens to respond to an attack with little or no more force than that which he perceives is being used against him. In some places, the law clearly specifies that equal force must be exactly equal. The attacked can respond with no more force than that by which he is threatened—slap for slap, punch for punch, kick for kick, or deadly weapon for deadly weapon. Once again, that's pretty tough if you're a guy and your adversary is a girl. Whatever you do may easily be perceived as figurative or literal overkill. Everything changes when weapons are involved, however. An armed opponent clearly has the advantage, so you have much more leeway in your response.

Disparity of force between unarmed combatants is measured in one of two ways. It exists if (1) the victim is being attacked by someone who is physically much stronger or younger or (2) the victim is being attacked by two or more assailants of similar or equal size. In such cases, you may legitimately be able to exert potentially lethal force to defend yourself. Regardless, nowhere can a person legally respond to an assault of slight degree with deadly force.

A great majority of states, in fact, require that law-abiding citizens avoid conflict whenever possible. It is best to withdraw, leaving the scene entirely. It is always a good idea to retreat from a belligerent party who threatens you, unless the attack is so savage that there is not sufficient time to escape or unless withdrawing (or leaving cover in the case of a gunfight) would increase your vulnerability.

The only exception to this rule is within the confines of your own home (or in some places your place of business). In most cases if someone breaks into your home and assaults you, you do not legally need to attempt to retreat. In many cases, it may be prudent to do so anyway, however. This is not true in all jurisdictions, though, so check your local laws carefully. This statute is often called a "castle doctrine."

The bottom line is that in the eyes of the court, you must also be in reasonable fear for your life or someone else's prior to applying countervailing force. That's awful hard to prove if the other guy is a girl, unless she's armed with some sort of weapon. If you are cornered and have to fight, you clearly do whatever you have to in order to assure your safety and well-being. It is essential, however, to make a commitment to yourself to use physical force wisely. Never hit a girl… unless she's armed.

---

* An example of "extreme savagery" in the eyes of the law would be gratuitously raining blows upon a fallen opponent who has obviously given up the conflict, even if he started the fight in the first place.

When He Stops, You Stop

When you surround an army, leave an outlet free. Do not press a desperate foe too hard.

– Sun Tzu

"In One Timing" means, when you have closed with the enemy, to hit him as quickly and directly as possible, without moving your body or settling your spirit, while you see that he is still undecided. The timing of hitting before the enemy decides to withdraw, break or hit, is this "In One Timing"

– Miyamoto Musashi

There is a hilarious scene in the movie *Monty Python and the Holy Grail* where the legendary King Arthur battles the dreaded Black Knight. Wielding Excalibur, Arthur is an invincible warrior, easily cleaving off his adversary's arm. Thinking the battle has been won, Arthur begins to celebrate his victory yet the Black Knight responds, "'Tis but a flesh wound," and continues to battle. This continues until Arthur has hacked off both of the Black Knight's arms as well as his legs and subsequently begins to ride away, leaving his defenseless adversary behind. Unwilling to yield, however, the Black Knight screams, "Come back! I'll bite your knees off!" Clearly, this is a comedic fantasy yet it has some bearing in real life.

If one's heart is truly in a fight, strikes to non-vital areas can have very little effect. Obviously, no one can fight without any arms or legs, yet it is very tough to stop a determined foe. Loren Christensen, a retired military policeman, civilian law enforcement officer, and martial artist who has survived numerous violent confrontations wrote, "I've had to fight guys even after they have been shot and they still fought like maniacs. I know of two occasions where suspects had been shot in their hearts and they fought the officers for several seconds before they crumpled dead to the ground... I saw two cases of people shot in the head—one person took five rounds—and they were still running around screaming and putting up a fuss." In the heat of battle, it is very, very difficult to stop a determined, committed opponent.

Unless you are a master martial artist who can deliver hydrostatic shock that disrupts internal organs with each blow, something that takes a good ten to twenty years of dedicated training to learn let alone perfect, it is really hard to beat somebody down without resorting to a weapon. Either you need to shock the brainstem into shutting down with a knockout blow or you need to break darn near every bone in his body, delivering such extensive physiological damage that it is physically impossible for him to continue fighting. The vast majority of opponents, however, will give up long before you get to that point. Once they stop, you need to stop too. Remain wary in case the other guy changes his mind, of course, but break off your attack and move to a safer location.

One master of strategy, Sun Tzu, tells you to leave a way out for your enemy, saying, "When you surround an army, leave an outlet free. Do not press a desperate foe too hard." This is sound advice because most people who find themselves with their back to the wall, faced with no options but to die or die fighting, will choose to fight and fight hard. You really don't want to mess with a fully committed foe. It's a good way to get hurt.

Another strategy master, Miyamoto Musashi, tells you to be swift and relentless, to "Hit him as quickly and directly as possible." This is excellent advice on the battlefield, but in a civilian context, it can get you into serious legal trouble if you take it too far. Gratuitously reigning down blows on a fallen opponent, for example, makes you the bad guy. When he stops, you've got to stop too. When the clear and immediate threat to you or your loved one is over, it is no longer self-defense. That's the law.

Here is the way it breaks down. If a punk decides to fight with you, whatever the reason, you have right to defend yourself—to a point. If you beat the punk down to the point where he has stopped fighting with you, you have to stop as well. Wilder knows a guy covered in tattoos, James, who wound up in that very situation. He didn't stop and was subsequently charged with felony assault, and found himself facing serious prison time.

> When they stop, you stop. The classic rule is that self-defense begins when deadly danger begins, ends when the danger ends, and revives again if the danger returns. Neither a killing nor a beating that takes place after a crime has already been committed, nor a proactive violent defense before an attack has taken place is legitimately self-defense in the eyes of the law.

Wilder never found out how or why the fight started, but that is really not important here. Our tattooed friend beat the other guy down, the fight was over, sort of, yet the loser of the fight kept running his mouth. Lying on the floor spitting out blood, he continued to yell epithets at our tattooed friend who took offense to his words. The price for running his mouth was more beating.

Dominance had been established and he was clearly the loser, but he kept running his mouth. Unfortunately, James had a record; he had already done three years in a Texas prison. He wouldn't put up with the verbal abuse so he applied more fists to the loser. You see, there were two different codes at work here—the prison code of dominance and submission on one side and the law on the other. As the song states, the law won. The courts decided that James needed to be put back in jail, while the other guy went into intensive care at Harborview hospital.

The classic rule is that self-defense begins when deadly danger begins, ends when the danger ends, and revives again if the danger returns. Neither a killing nor a beating that takes place after a crime has already been committed, nor a proactive violent defense before an attack has taken place is legitimately self-defense in the eyes of the law.

You can only resort to deadly or potentially deadly force in order to escape imminent and unavoidable danger of death or grave bodily harm. An attacker must not merely have made a threat to attack you (by words and/or actions), but must also be in a position where he or she is obviously and immediately capable of carrying out that threat and/or has begun to do so. A common test is that the attacker must demonstrate intent to attack and have both the means and opportunity to do so. Once he breaks off his assault, you must stop yours too.

Be Prepared to Fight Until It Stops

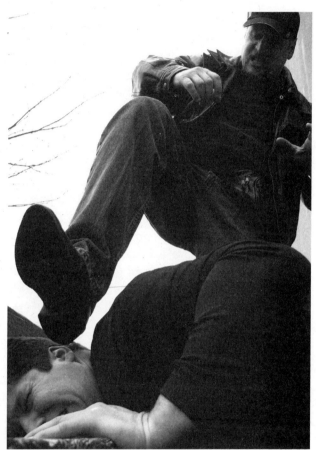

Hence, the skillful fighter puts himself into a position that makes defeat impossible, and does not miss the moment for defeating the enemy.

– Sun Tzu

Whenever you parry, hit, spring, strike, or touch the enemy's cutting sword, you must cut the enemy in the same movement.

– Miyamoto Musashi

Hitting someone and then pausing to ask them, "How was that? Did it hurt?" is ridiculous, yet we do that sort of thing all the time on the practice floor. Tandem drills in the *dojo* are great learning tools when approached correctly, but you cannot forget that you are working with a partner rather than dueling with an opponent. Out on the street your question would sound a lot like, "How wa …" POW, as his fist slams into your face. Once you start fighting, you don't stop until the other guy does. And then you keep your guard up until you're sure he's not faking it.

The classic rule is that self-defense begins when deadly danger begins, ends when the danger ends, and revives again if the danger returns. Stomping the other guy when he's down is not generally considered self-defense.

Hollywood loves to show the bad guys who can take a full power shot to the face and keep on smiling. It proves how tough they are, foreshadowing a kick-ass fight that'll take up five or ten minutes of screen time with the audience cheering enthusiastically all along the way. As we've stated previously, the movies portray a fantasyland. It's fun but not realistic. In real life, there is no pause until he gives up or breaks off the fight. It is critical, however, that when he stops you stop. Even if he started it and you're really pissed off that you got ambushed or sucker punched, you need to stop too.

Be mentally and physically prepared to fight or continue a fight at a moment's notice, however, always keeping your opponent in sight until you can escape to safety. Even if your blow knocks an adversary to the ground, remain alert for a possible continuation of his attack. Remember that most fistfights end when one guy gives up rather than when he can no longer physically continue.

No matter what, you must be prepared to fight until it stops. For example, on January 1, 2008 Meredith Emerson, a 24-year-old University of Georgia graduate, managed to fend off both a knife and a baton attack, holding her own until her assailant tricked her into giving up. Gary Michael Hilton, a burly 61-year-old drifter, subsequently tied her up and carried her to a remote location where he raped and eventually killed her three days later.

Hilton reportedly told police interrogators that his petite victim nearly overpowered him when he first accosted her on an Appalachian hiking trail. According to published reports, Hilton stalked the 5 foot 4 inch tall, 120-pound woman on the trail but was unable to keep up so he laid in wait and intercepted her on her way back down. He pulled a military-style knife and demanded her ATM card. Emerson recognized the threat and immediately fought back.

"The bayonet is probably still up there," Hilton told investigators. "I lost control, and she fought. And as I read in the paper, she's a martial artist." Emerson, who held middle *kyu* ranks (blue belt and green belt) in two different martial arts, ripped the knife out of his hands. He countered with a baton that she was also able to pull from his grasp. As the struggle continued, they fell down a steep slope, leaving both weapons behind.

"I had to hand-fight her," Hilton said. "She wouldn't stop fighting and yelling at the same time so I needed to both control her and silence her." He kept punching her, blackening her eyes, fracturing her nose, and breaking his own hand in the process. He figured that he had worn her down as they moved farther off the trail, but suddenly she began fighting again. He finally got her to stop by telling her that all he wanted was her credit card and PIN number.

Once she relaxed her guard, he restrained her hands with a zip tie, took her to a remote location, and tied her to a tree. He kept her captive in the wilderness for three terrifying days before telling her that he was ready to let her go. Then he beat her to death with a car-jack handle and cut off her head.

Hilton made a plea deal with prosecutors, leading investigators to his victim's remains so that they would not seek the death penalty for his crimes. He was subsequently sentenced to life in prison with the possibility of parole after 30 years.

Never believe anything an assailant tells you. His actions have already demonstrated beyond any doubt that he's a bad guy. Do not relax your guard and get caught by surprise;

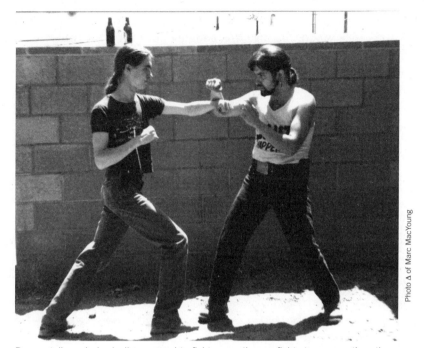

Photo △ of Marc MacYoung

Be mentally and physically prepared to fight or continue a fight at a moment's notice, always keeping your opponent in sight until you can escape to safety.

that is a good way to die. If the other guy thinks that he's losing, he might be more inclined to play possum or pull out a weapon in order to cheat to win. Worse yet, street attacks often involve multiple assailants many of whom are seasoned fighters who know how to take a blow and shrug off the pain. Be mindful of additional assailants and be prepared to continue your defense as long as necessary. Once you have removed yourself from the danger and are absolutely certain that you are no longer under threat, you can safely begin to relax your guard.

Dealing with multiple attackers is extraordinarily challenging. Avoidance is obviously the best and most preferable alternative. If you are forced to fight, you can realistically engage only one opponent at a time. Once the first adversary has been defeated, you may have a chance to flee successfully or you may have to move on to defeat the next attacker, and then get away.

Unfortunately, despite what you may have seen in the movies, the other guys won't line up and wait for you to attack each one in turn. They're going to swarm and overrun, so you are very likely to get hit… a lot. Defense against a large group is generally handled by strategically engaging one person at a time in a manner that confounds the other's ability to reach you. Without a lot of training that's very tough to pull off effectively.

Your response is a form of triage, striking for the greatest impact or taking on the most dangerous threat first. If you can instantaneously and dramatically disable someone, blowing out his knee, shattering his nose, gouging out his eye, or otherwise leaving him huddled in a pool of his own blood, the psychological advantage will be enormous.

If you show no fear in the face of overwhelming odds, your attackers may hesitate giving you the few seconds you need to disengage and escape. If all your adversaries are equally dangerous, take out the easiest target first. This might be the nearest aggressor, smallest guy, or the person with no cover. Once you get away, do not relax your guard until you are absolutely sure you are safe. After all, they could easily change their minds and decide to come after you.

Remain vigilant until you are absolutely certain that your adversary is no longer a threat and that no one else is prepared to take up the battle on his behalf. Once you have escaped to safety, you can relax your guard. As the Chinese proverb states, "Dead tigers kill the most hunters." Be prepared to fight until you are certain that it has stopped.

When You Stop, He Won't Stop

Anger may in time change to gladness; vexation may be succeeded by content... But a kingdom that has once been destroyed can never come again into being; nor can the dead ever be brought back to life.
— *Sun Tzu*

In my strategy, the training for killing enemies is by way of many contests, fighting for survival, discovering the meaning of life and death, learning the Way of the sword, judging the strength of attacks and understanding the Way of the "edge and ridge" of the sword.
— *Miyamoto Musashi*

When you stop, there is no guarantee that the other guy will too. You are taking a monumental risk if you roll up into a ball on the ground and assume that your submission will end the fight. This may be taken as nothing more than a green light for the other guy to stomp and kick you... a lot. In fact, you can pretty much count on it.

The only way you can stop a fight when you are losing is to escape. Run away as fast and as far as you can. Do not stop; do not look behind you, at least not right away, just run. It is really tough to capture someone who is bound and determined to get away. Use this to your advantage.

Breaking off your attack, in and of itself, is probably not going to end the fight, particularly if the other guy wants to be in control. His goal is complete and utter dominance over you, supremacy for all to see. You may agree with Musashi's missive above that killing or beating down a person unnecessarily is not honorable, not "the way." But, as Sun Tzu so aptly points out, once something has been destroyed it is over. What's done is done.

You cannot count on honor, ethics, or mercy from an adversary. If you depend on his good nature, you are bound to lose the fight in a very bad way. It is smart to show honor yourself, yet prudent to expect none from your opponent.

If you are thinking "fight" and he is thinking "combat," you are in for a world of hurt. A fight implies a rules-based event, something like a boxing match or mixed martial arts competition. In a fight you might punch, kick, and/or throw each other down, but you are not likely to kick the other guy's head in or stomp on his throat once he has fallen. Combat, on the other hand, is a no-holds-barred struggle for survival. That's where weapons come into play, eyes are gouged out, ears are bitten off, and serious, life-altering repercussions can be expected.

It's very hard to stop someone who is fully committed to combat. You must either knock him unconscious or cause enough physiological damage that he can no longer continue. Most folks, however, give up long before it gets to that point. No matter how much you are tempted to do so, don't quit. Pain alone should not stop you. Remember Sgt. Young's confrontation with Neal Beckman? His courage graphically demonstrated that if it hurts you are still alive. Deal with it and press on.

The best way to avoid getting beaten down is not to fight in the first place. If you cannot escape violence, however, you must fight with all your worth. Your goal does not necessarily need to be to win, but it must at least be to not lose. In other words, you don't need to beat the other guy to a pulp but you do need to escape successfully. That is not going to happen if you give up the struggle. If you stop, there's no guarantee that he will too.

> As the Chinese proverb states, "Dead tigers kill the most hunters." Remain vigilant during any pause in the fight. You may be facing multiple assailants, an adversary who pulls a weapon in the middle of a fight, or an opponent who just won't quit. Once you have removed yourself from the danger and are absolutely certain that you are no longer under threat you can safely begin to relax your guard.

> If you cannot escape or avoid violence, you must be prepared to fight with all your worth. Your goal does not necessarily need to be to win, but it must at least be to not lose. You cannot afford to give up. Never forget that if it hurts, you are still alive. If you stop, however, there's no guarantee that he will too. You cannot count on honor, ethics, or mercy from an adversary. Keep fighting until you can safely get away.

Six Techniques You Can Use in a Fight

If in training soldiers commands are habitually enforced, the army will be well disciplined; if not, its discipline will be bad.

— Sun Tzu

In single combat, we can confuse the enemy by attacking with varied techniques when the chance arises. Feint a thrust or cut, or make the enemy think you are going to close with him, and when he is confused you can easily win. This is the essence of fighting, and you must research it deeply.

— Miyamoto Musashi

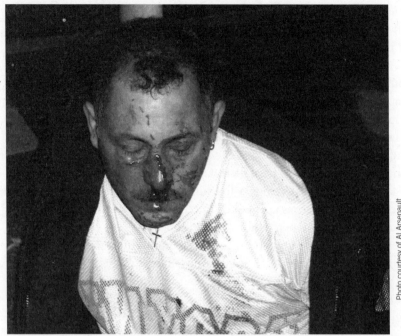

Photo courtesy of Al Arsenault

If you are thinking "fight" and the other guy is thinking "combat" you are in for a world of hurt.

You don't need to be a master martial artist, professional boxer, or seasoned combat veteran to survive a street fight. It helps, of course, but it's not a requirement. You do, however, need to have a few solid techniques you can draw upon, stuff you can pull off when you're surging with adrenaline, scared witless, and really need to stop or deflect the other guy so that you can escape to safety. So, how do you know what's going to work and what's going to fail in a real-life violent conflict? Well, you can never know for sure, since much depends upon your adversary. There are three important, yet very simple rules when it comes to self-defense that you can use as a guideline:*

1. Don't get hit
2. Stop him from continuing to attack you
3. Always have a Plan B

The first rule we've already described to you. "Don't get hit" is always sound advice. Previously we've discussed this rule from the context of awareness, avoidance, and de-

---

* The fourth rule not mentioned here is, "Don't go to jail." We've already covered judicious use of force previously so we won't rehash it again in this section.

escalation, but it's true for fighting techniques as well. If whatever you do doesn't keep you from getting hit, the rest simply doesn't matter all that much. Once you've been hurt by the other guy, it gets progressively tougher and tougher to fight back. Consequently, you need to block, deflect, or evade his attack before you can do anything else. Sometimes that's done by preemptively striking him first, though more often than not it's by some sort of defensive movement. Not ideal, just reality…

The second rule, "Stop him from continuing to attack," is just as important. You can block, deflect, or evade all you like but that won't end the fight. You need to perform a technique or combination of movements that incapacitate the other guy outright, persuade him to leave you alone and break off his attack, and/or facilitate your escape. The goal is to ensure that he can no longer hurt you. The faster you can do that the better; conversely, the longer the fight the more likely you are to get hurt.

A solid blow or two to a vital area, a part of the body that will break relatively easily, can end a fight very quickly whereas blows to non-vital areas will have minimal effect. Consequently, it's important to know where to aim. Appendix D lists the vital areas that you may want to target during a fight. Some may be struck (for example, punch or kick) while other targets must be manipulated (for example, joint lock).

Winston Churchill wrote, "No matter how enmeshed a commander becomes in his plans, it is occasionally necessary to take the enemy into consideration." In other words, no matter how crafty you are, whatever you try is not necessarily going to work. The other guy is trying his damnedest to pound your face in, pulling out every dirty trick he can think of in an effort to mess you up. It's prudent to have a Plan B, some alternative you can move to without missing a beat when things go awry. Whatever you attempt may knock him on his ass straight away, of course, but oftentimes it just doesn't work out that way. When things go wrong, there's no time to stop and think in the heat of battle.

It's intuitively obvious that if you can pummel the other guy into submission that you will win the fight, but that's not your only option in a battle. If the other guy can't get close enough to reach you in the first place, he will not be able to strike. Consequently controlling distance is important. It's very tough to fight if he can't see, so the eyes may be a viable target, at least in life-or-death encounters. If he is on the ground when you're still standing, you have a much better chance of getting away. Of course, you can always hit him… a lot. To this end, we suggest six things that you may wish to try in a fight.

- Don't let him get close enough to touch you.
- Throw debris to distract or injure him.
- Attack his eyes.
- Use neck cranks or chokes to put him down.
- Throw him to the ground with force.
- Strike with impetus.

You've probably noticed that, with the exception of controlling distance, these are offensive techniques rather than defensive ones. While it's important to be able to block or deflect the other guy's attack, it's even more important to take him out of the fight as quickly as possible. Our goal here is not to turn you into the ultimate street fighter, but rather to give you a few options that you might be able to pull off without a whole lot of practice. If you really want to get good at the physical aspects of fighting, however, you are going to need to find a martial arts school and sign up for hands-on instruction.

Don't let him get close enough to touch you

Distance is crucial in a fight. If you are too far away, he can't strike you. If you are too close, the range limits the available weapons your attacker and you can use to fight each other with. Distance plays out this way: Combat begins at about ten or more feet from you. Positioning is initiated, openings are looked for, reactions, and responses are judged. This entire process may take as little as 1/10,000 of a second, as that is how long it takes for the brain to process information. Or it could take the better part of an evening as you see with the prolonged interview process.

Letting somebody get close to you is an invitation for a fight. Think of it this way: The two of you have had a verbal altercation, and the other guy backed down, said, "Oh, okay pal, I was wrong, let's shake." No! That handshake is an opportunity for him to get close, control one of your weapons and your balance, and give you a sucker punch.

An arm around the shoulder is the same thing. Think about it, who do you let put their arm around your shoulder? You best mate, a drunken college buddy? Sure! An unknown guy who was about to kick your ass three-and-half minutes ago? Definitely not.

No matter what he asks, your answer should be "No." If he is sincere in his attitude, he will shrug it off and go about his business. If not, he will take offense and escalate the situation again. His response tells you everything you need to know about how it was going to go down so either way you are ahead.

Here is an example of distance and perception. One night Wilder left a bar late with Sgt. Rory Miller and his wife. It was a weeknight so the streets were very calm with very few people out and about. Wilder crossed the street heading for his car. As he opened his car door, a twenty-five year old(ish) man jogged up to him and said, "Hey, I need some help."

Wilder paused inside the doorjamb of his car and replied, "What's up?" He assumed from the other guy's frantic look that the problem he needed help with was something and the lines of a flat tire. Yet the unexpected response was, "I need some money for my wife and me."

"Odd," Wilder thought, suddenly realizing that he was blocked by somebody who was not who he thought they were.

Two cars down, Sgt. Miller was at the panhandler's back. He had not gotten in his car

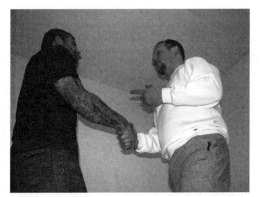

Letting a hostile person get too close to you is an invitation for a fight.

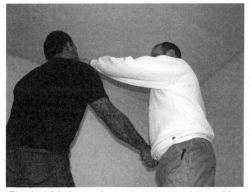

That handshake was just a ploy to get you into position for a sucker punch.

and was watching the event. He slowly closed his car door so that nothing was between the guy's back and himself.

"Okay," Wilder said. Not usually inclined to give to panhandlers, he nevertheless reached into his pocket and pulled out some loose change hoping that compliance would make the guy go away and leave him alone. "Here," he said handing over the money.

"I need more than that!," the other guy growled. "This doesn't help me one bit."

As the other guy's tone became increasingly agitated, Wilder realized that he was not dealing with a guy with a flat tire nor was he dealing with a panhandler. He had just let a mentally unbalanced person, some guy off his medications most likely, get too close to him. Miller knew it too. Watching intently, he shifted his weight a bit so that he could respond appropriately if things got violent.

"This does me crap!" the other guy shouted, throwing the coins to the ground and then reaching for Wilder.

"Don't touch me and get back!," Wilder commanded. He was blocked in, with his

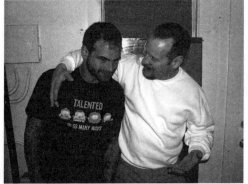

Are you really going to let the guy who was about to kick your ass three-and-half minutes ago put his arm around your shoulder to make nice?

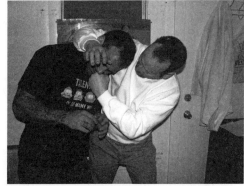

Not if you're smart.

back to the open door of his car so he had no space to maneuver in. "Get back! Get away from me, now!," he repeated.

"I need real money!" the other guy snarled. This was clearly escalating. The other guy was too close and not responding to verbal commands. Wilder knew that if the other guy had a blade he was going to get cut. His mind flashed to the fireman who was stabbed to death some ten years earlier, randomly, by a mental patient after a Mariners baseball game in Seattle… "Crap," Wilder thought.

Then, the other guy made his move. As abruptly as he had switched from a guy in trouble to a guy demanding more money, real money, he snapped, "Screw you!" He then turned and jogged back across the street and around the corner.

Wilder looked at Miller who had waited calmly the whole time. "So, see you later," he said as he got into his car.

"Yeah," Wilder replied, "See ya later."

While driving home Wilder reviewed the entire event in his mind and started criticizing himself for letting the guy get so close. Finally, he relaxed a little, thinking, "These things happen. You can't go through life all prickly at Condition Red. You assumed good will and that is not always a bad thing." He told himself, "The context was all wrong for that kind of behavior. Would it have hurt me to keep my distance coming out of bar late on a weeknight with a guy jogging toward me? No! I wasn't all prickly, or at Condition Red, but I did fail the distance test."

There are no absolutes in self-defense. Every situation will be different and unique. In England and much of Europe, for example, you are likely at risk from a head butt in a fight whereas that type of attack is rarely seen in the United States where a punch to the face is more common. Either way, your adversary must get close in order to reach you. It is critical, therefore, to maintain sufficient distance between you and a potential assailant to give yourself time to respond to whatever he tries to do.

You may be in imminent danger from an unarmed attacker within about 10 feet. For an armed attacker, this range is extended to a bare minimum of 21 feet. The bad guy can close that distance shockingly fast. A second or two is all he needs to move in and strike.

While that may seem a rather lengthy separation, several tests, including the famous Tueller Drill, have been conducted that validate this assertion. This drill, named for Sergeant Dennis Tueller of the Salt Lake City Police Department, was first described in his 1983 *S.W.A.T. Magazine* article "How Close Is Too Close."

In his drill, Tueller conducted a series of tests showing that people of various ages, weights, heights, and physical conditions could close a distance of 21 feet in an average time of 1.5 seconds, about as long at it takes a highly trained officer to draw a handgun and fire one or two aimed shots. Knowing that people who have been shot do not often fall down instantly, or otherwise stop dead in their tracks, Tueller concluded that a person armed with a blade or a blunt instrument at a range of 21 feet was a potentially lethal threat. A defensive handgun instructor whose class Kane took reiterated this point, stating that it takes a fatally wounded person between 10 and 120 seconds to drop, so you must fire and then move off-line while expecting your attacker to continue his assault even after your bullets have hit him.

In training as well as in real-life encounters, even highly trained police officers are frequently unable to draw their guns and fire a shot before being cut, sometimes fatally, by a knife-wielding opponent moving toward them from distances as great as 20 to 30 feet. It is reasonable to assert that the average civilian is somewhat less prepared for such encounters than the typical law enforcement professional.

While it's intuitively obvious with fists, distance can even keep you safe from bullets. Most gunfights take place at a distance of less than ten feet. In fact, according to FBI statistics, 95 percent of officer-involved shootings occur at less than 21 feet, with approximately 75 percent taking place at less than 10 feet and a little over half at closer than five feet. The farther away the other guy is, the tougher it is for him to hit you. Further, you have a much better chance to escape to safety or dash toward some source of cover that can protect you.

Throw Debris to Distract or Injure Him

Throwing debris is really an extension of distance. It is not a stand-alone technique, but rather a facilitator that can keep the other guy back and help you escape. You can kick dust, throw rocks, hurl trash, swing garbage cans, or otherwise chuck stuff at the other guy to distract or potentially injure him. Don't throw your weapon if you have one though. You're going to be giving up your best source of defense by throwing it away.

Here is a rough way to estimate your ability to throw an object and have a reasonable chance of hurting somebody: Wilder calls this the "baseball test." It was developed through rigorous threshold testing while he was at college. To do the test, march off about a quarter of the dormitory hallway floor, turn and face the fire door at the end of the hall. Make sure no one else is around.

Using a baseball, not a softball, hurl the ball at the fire door at the end of the hall. If you can hit the door good for you. If you can dent the door, in theory you have thrown hard enough to injure the other guy in a fight. Both accuracy and force are required. We're not actually advocating that you go out and damage someone else's property, but hurling a baseball at a door hard enough to make a dent really does indicate the kind of speed and accuracy necessary to injure someone with a thrown object. Since it's tough to actually injure, you're most likely going to use this tactic to distract.

Before you employ this tactic, however, identify your escape route. You need to know that before you do anything else. It doesn't do much good to throw things unless you can do it strategically to get away. Before you begin to run, it is very important to have a good

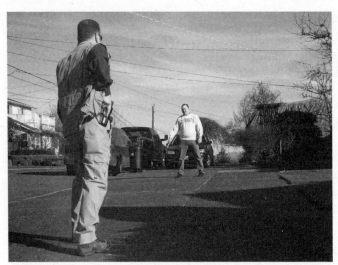

The Tueller Drill demonstrated that a person armed with a blade or a blunt instrument at a range of 21 feet can still be a lethal threat. Maintain sufficient distance between yourself and a potential assailant to give yourself time to respond to whatever he tries to do.

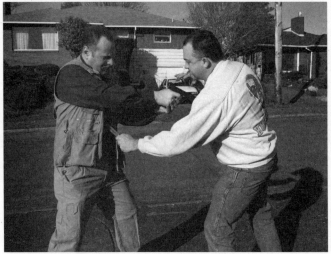

Too close. Any victory at this point would be Pyrrhic.

escape path figured out. Be sure to note the location of any improvised weapons or obstacles you will have to pass along your route. These items could be employed for countervailing force, used for cover or concealment, or simply get in your way, barring your escape. In addition to your physical location (for example, building layout, street map, terrain), pay attention to any bystanders in your proximity. They may be a source of aid, additional threat, and/or witnesses to corroborate your claim of self-defense should things get ugly.

This information can help keep you safe not only during an armed confrontation but also during a fire, earthquake, or other emergency as well. In areas you frequent, such as your workplace or school, it is imperative that you know where fire extinguishers, first aid kits, Automated External Defibrillators, and other safety resources are located. Some of these items can be used as improvised weapons during armed attacks while others are lifesaving devices for more mundane emergencies.

Pay attention to available escape paths wherever you go. On an airplane, for example, know not only where the exit doors are located but also how many seats you must pass before you get there. That way if you need to navigate in smoke, darkness, or other adverse conditions you will know what to do. Similarly, in public places such as restaurants, bars, schools, and office buildings note the locations of all available exits. If a gunman enters from one side of the building, you will want to know how to escape out the other.

So not that you've got a way out, what debris can you use to help you get there? For our purposes, if it isn't nailed down, it is debris. Look around the space you are in right now to see what is available to you. Are the chairs too heavy? What about a couch? Dresser drawers? How about a silverware drawer full of pointy objects? Pictures on the walls, stuff in your pockets, objects on your desk, or whatever is lying around that you can get to quickly that's heavy enough be some sort of threat but light enough to throw with some accuracy will do the trick.

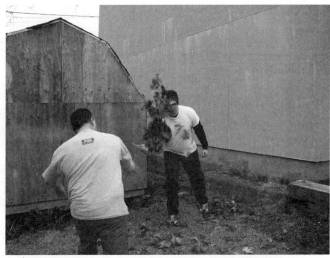

At what targets should you throw? Answer: the face. It's the most distracting and potentially damaging target. Weight and size of the debris may affect your accuracy, but it's important

Throwing debris is an extension of distance; it can distract or injure an adversary, helping you escape.

to target where you will get the most reaction. When you throw move to the escape route at the same time. The debris will only give you a second or two so you need to use it to your best advantage.

The basic way to explain this is this phrase: "Throw at the face and run away." Sophistication isn't really necessary for this technique. It's as simple as determining your escape route, chucking something at the other guy's face to make him flinch, and running away.

Attack His Eyes

It's really tough to fight if you can't see. Take a look at any kind of warfare through the course of history and you will see that blinding the opponent is one of the most significant actions taken. In fact blinding the opponent is often the first thing that is done. During WWII, pilots did their level best to have the sun at their backs during dogfights, attempting to blind the enemy with the glare. In modern warfare, one of the first things attacked is always the command, control, and communications infrastructure. It is jammed, blown up, or otherwise taken out of action so that the enemy will not know what's coming. Any attack is more likely to succeed with this advantage.

The same thing applies in hand-to-hand combat. If he can't see, it's really tough for him to fight you. That makes the other guy's eyes a very important target in a legitimate self-defense scenario. Compared to all our other senses, eyesight is dominant in its impotence. It's not only how we view the outside world but also how we acquire targets and defend ourselves against assaults.

When you have an opportunity to attack the eyes during a fight, the chance will only be there for an instant. If you're going to go for the shot, you've got to take advantage of that

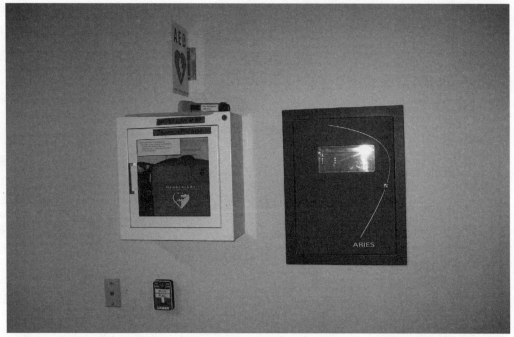

Know where fire extinguishers, first aid kits, Automated External Defibrillators, and other safety resources are located. Some of these items can be used as improvised weapons for self-defense while others are lifesaving devices for more mundane emergencies.

moment of opportunity. The thing about attacking the eyes is that it is similar to attacking the groin; there is a natural guarding reflex, even in unskilled fighters, that is difficult to get past.

Think back to the last time you were riding in a car and something hit the windshield. You instinctively flinched didn't you? When the rock hit the windshield, your eyes closed, your shoulders lifted, your head went forward and down, and your hands came up. In essence, you tucked your head in like a turtle pulling its head into its shell. This reflex action protects the neck, eyes, and face. It gets as much flesh around the eyes as it can by squinting too, making them well defended.

Knowing that the other guy is going to have this natural protection for his eyes means that there is a good chance that you won't be successful the first time you try to strike him there. You need to be fast, well-trained, and usually a little lucky to get his eyes on the first try. Assuming you are fast and/or lucky, but not highly trained, you will need to follow the shampoo rule—lather, rinse, and repeat. In other words, keep trying until it works.

Be cautious though, this is serious stuff. Not only can you cause horrific injuries with eye attacks, but also you let the other guy know that this is a very serious confrontation. If you attack his eyes and miss, you're really going to piss him off in a primal way, becoming the target of a lot more anger and violence than you might expect. Anything goes from that point on.

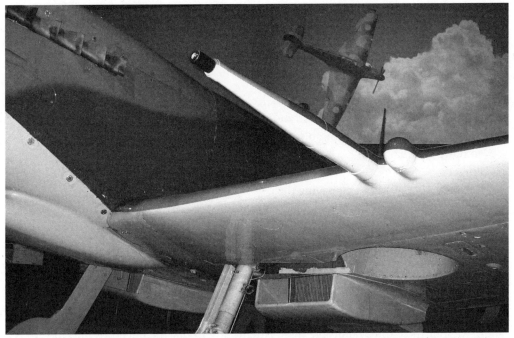

It's really tough to fight if you can't see. Until the advent of modern missile technology, pilots did their best to keep the sun at their backs during dogfights in the hopes of blinding or disorienting their enemies with the glare. This same principle can apply in hand-to-hand combat as well.

Anybody who wears glasses can relate to this action. Have your glasses knocked off by another guy, even accidentally, and it pisses you off. It is personal, it is primal, and it's instantaneous. Even in an accident, it takes a certain amount of effort to control the instinctive reaction. This gives you a glimpse of the type of response you will elicit from a person when you attack his eyes.

So, while attacking the eyes can incapacitate an adversary, it can inflame him too. Consequently you need to know how to do it right. The best techniques use either your thumbs or fingers. Here's how to attack the eyes most effectively.

Thumbs

The thumb can be used as a wedge to displace the eyeball from the eye socket. This is done by placing your thumb against the inside of the bridge of his nose and pushing into the corner of his eye socket. Typically, you'll use your fingers as a guide alongside the other guy's face. It works much better if you can support the head with your other hand or block it with a solid object such as a wall or the ground so that he cannot move his head back or twist away.

When shoved forcefully into the eye socket, your thumb works much like a wood-splitting wedge, displacing the eyeball. This ultimate result is not a full removal of the eye from the socket, which is very challenging, but rather a stretching of the optic nerve that attaches the back of the eye and shoots excruciating pain into the brain. Stretching this nerve makes the eye short out, for lack of a better phrase. It can cause blurred vision, disorientation, shock, and in some cases blindness, more than enough trauma to let you escape to safety in most cases. If you actually displace the eyeball, the disabling affect is even more severe.

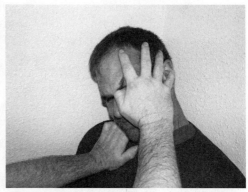

When shoved forcefully into the eye socket, your thumb can stretch the optic nerve or displace the adversary's eyeball, causing debilitating pain, shock, and disorientation.

Fingers

Raking the eyes is about damaging the cornea of the eye, the outer lens. Scratching the eye in this manner causes excessive tearing, light sensitivity, and pain. A vertical claw brought down the face from eyebrow to cheek will most likely fail. The brow above the eye and the cheek protect the eye, an imperfect and poor attack but an attack nonetheless. Moving your fingertips laterally across the eye, on the other hand, is likely to be much more successful.

Again, this attack is done powerfully, more than once, and with resolve. The chances of failure without these three points are high. Attempting to put the fingertips into the eye is a strike better left to the skilled martial artist. It is fast and effective but can hurt your hand if you do it incorrectly. Everyone else should follow this method of horizontal raking.

In this example, we will use the right hand. Palm thrust to the attacker's cheekbone. This bone will serve as an anchor and guide. Thrust the finger tips into the eye (the number or which fingers is not important) and in a twisting motion, similar to tying to take the lid off a jar of pickles, twist away from attacker's nose toward their ear. Keep trying until it works.

If you are a trained martial artist, you almost certainly know how to do an open-hand chest block (for example, *hiki uke*). After initially intercepting the opponent's blow, you can bounce off his arm in a circular clawing motion to rake the eyes. Any time your open hand crosses in front of the other guy's face, you may have the opportunity to scratch at his eyes. Even if you do not make contact, such movements can be very distracting, leaving the adversary open to a follow-on attack such as a low kick or a knee strike.

If he wears prescription glasses (or in some circumstances sunglasses) and you can flip them off, it may be very disorienting. This same finger motion can catch the edge of the frame and jerk it free. Be cognizant of this if you wear glasses and keep an extra pair in your vehicle in case they get broken. It's hard to drive when you can't see.

Inclement Weather

The old dog-fighting trick with sun can be used in hand-to-hand fighting too. If you can get the sun to your back, particularly early in the morning or late in the afternoon when it's low in the sky, you gain an additional advantage in a fight. The same thing goes

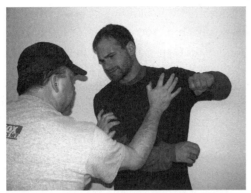

This classic chest block can be a set-up for a follow-on eye strike.

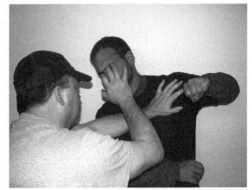

Bounce off his arm in a circular clawing motion to rake across the eyes.

for wind, hail, driving rain, and other inclement conditions. If something is blowing in the other guy's face, it's tougher for him to fight. Good footwork and body positioning can help protect against these things being used against you, though it is prudent to wear sunglasses and brimmed hats such as a baseball cap to protect your face from the weather too.

Use Neck Cranks or Chokes to Put Him Down

It's important to have both a "standing" game as well as a "ground" game, as you never know where a fight will lead. Chokes and neck cranks are very effective, particularly on the ground, but also very dangerous. Security guards generally don't use these techniques. In many cases, the techniques are categorized by law enforcement as being at the same level as lethal force on the force continuum or banned outright by policy. The reason for this is the same reason that the guillotine made such an effective means of execution during the "Reign of Terror" that followed the French Revolution in the late 1700s. These are all methods of separating the control system (brain) from the supply system (heart/lungs) of the body, because they attack the neck, the "super highway" between these two systems.

There are different ways to choke someone effectively. You must either close off his carotid arteries or compress his trachea. The carotid arteries run down both sides of the neck. By restricting the blood flow in those arteries, you can impede the oxygen flow to the brain. After a short time in an oxygen-depressed state, the brain effectively goes to sleep. When that happens, it no longer has any control of the body. Brain goes to sleep, bad guy passes out, and you win. A carotid choke is relatively safe because if you let off shortly after the other guy loses consciousness, he should revive. You can see this kind of thing happen in martial arts tournaments all the time. Medical intervention is rarely necessary. However, if you continue to compress the carotid arteries after the other guy has passed out, you can cause brain damage or death.

Compression of the trachea or the windpipe is another way of doing a choke. The trachea is on the front of the neck directly underneath the chin. You can stop or restrict the flow of air to the lungs by compressing the trachea. This causes suffocation, a condition that if left untreated will rapidly lead to unconsciousness, brain damage, and death. This is a more dangerous technique than a carotid choke because you can damage the trachea in a manner that simply releasing the choke won't often restart the flow of oxygen to the brain. Consequently, carotid chokes tend to be safer than tracheal chokes.

Architecture of the Neck. You can look at the neck as a pentagram. It has five points that are important for martial applications. The two trapezius muscles at the back of the neck form the first two points and the carotid arteries form the second two points. The carotid arteries are located along side the sternocleidomastoid and the trachea. The trachea forms the fifth point.

Choking Weapons—the Arms and Hands: We are only going to demonstrate chokes that utilize the forearms and hands in this book. While other parts of the arms, hands, and fingers can be used for choking, they require more study with a qualified instructor to pull off effectively on the street. The techniques listed here are those that we believe are the easiest to learn and apply.

- Arms: When using the arms it is helpful to think of them as propeller blades. Airplane propellers have a leading edge and a trailing edge. Look at the palm of your left hand. The edges of your arm, to the left and to the right are the leading and trailing edges that are used to perform the techniques. Those hard, bony edges give you solid leverage for performing chokes. The flat parts of your arms, directly in front of you and directly on the backside, are not used in these applications because they are softer and provide less mechanical leverage.

- Hands: The grips you use with your hands are very important. The interlacing of the fingers, as if in prayer, is never to be used. Your fingers can be crushed and/ or dislocated if you grip that way. Grabbing your own wrist can, at times, be a correct technique, but for our discussion here, it will not be used, as it is a bit more complicated to perform properly due to sweat and grime that can make a good grip go bad fast. The correct position is to clasp your hands together as if clapping, and then to grip a forefinger and thump around your opposite hand's thumb.

Subtlety. Being subtle while attempting a choke is the beginning of a path to success. Both authors, having trained with champion *judoka* Kenji Yamada, can attest to the subtlety that he used while choking. Wilder says, "The first time Yamada *Sensei* choked me, I had no real concept of what was taking place. I wasn't really able to feel his intention until he had the choke applied. I remember the technique too; it is called 'The Hell Choke.' By the time I realized what was happening it was too late." Kane has had similar

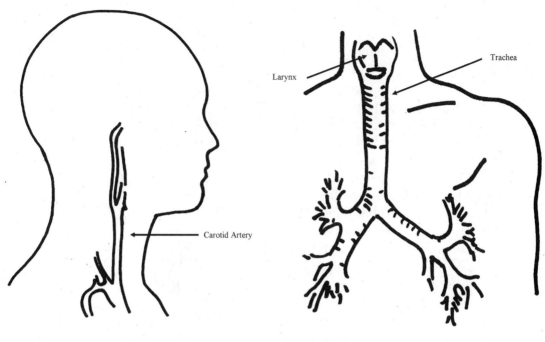

Carotid Artery

Trachea

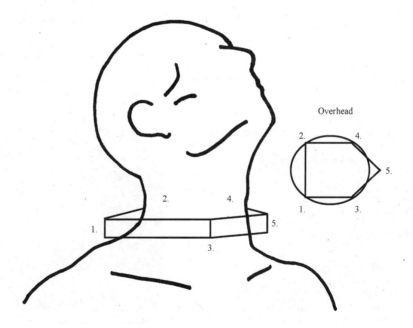

Architecture of the Neck

experiences. The first time he was choked-out in a judo tournament, he did not realize what the other guy was doing until he woke up afterward.

An attack to the neck is perceived as life threatening. While you might be choking to knock the other guy out, he is bound to think you are intent on killing him. Once he feels the choke, he is going to switch on his "fight or flight" reflex immediately and instinctively. You'll be in for a wild ride. You need to be sneaky and subtle. Not showing your intent until it is too late is the key to getting a successful choke or crank begun. Once it's on properly, an untrained opponent will very unlikely get away from your technique until you choose to release him.

An important ingredient in successful choking is control. In most cases, this means controlling your opponent's hips with your legs. If you have a solid hold, he cannot buck you off of him or find some way to squirm away and break your chokehold. In a standing choke, this might simply mean dragging him backward so that he cannot

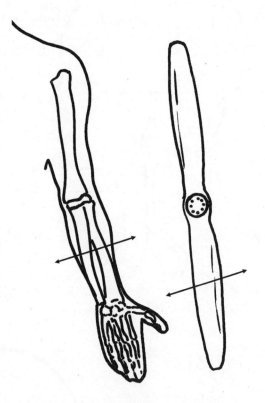

Arm—Comparison with Propeller Blades

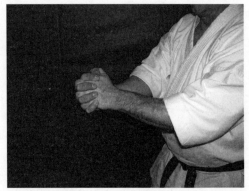

Incorrect grip: interlaced fingers can be easily crushed or dislocated as you try to apply the technique.

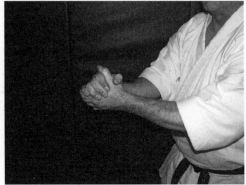

Correct grip: clasp your hands together with interlocking thumbs.

get his feet under him or achieve any leverage to take the pressure off and continue the fight. In groundwork, that typically means controlling his hips with your legs.

Four Chokes and Cranks You Can Use

The type of chokes and cranks discussed here are designed for the street. Several of them have been banned from judo competition because they are too dangerous for sport. Since they may result in life-threatening injuries to your opponent, you must only use chokes when the situation warrants a high level of countervailing force (see the section "Use Only as Much Force as the Situation Warrants" for more information). There are some fantastic neck-crank takedowns that can be executed from a standing position that we have not included here because they are far too dangerous to attempt without properly supervised instruction. Performed incorrectly, they can prove fatal. If you decide to take martial arts classes, you can learn such things there.

Attempting a choke on the street without practice is a poor choice for combat, one that is very likely to fail. Chokes require both subtlety and control. Supervised practice is essential. You will most likely learn these techniques by practicing with a uniform *gi* initially. This heavy clothing not only facilitates many chokes, but also does not tear easily. Once you get good, practice with a t-shirt too. Use an old one as it will quickly get trashed, but it is very important to be able to use these kinds of techniques in street clothes. Finally, practice against a shirtless opponent so that you will be prepared for every eventuality.

Successful chokes and neck cranks require that you control the other guy's movement until he passes out or gives up. That's easiest to do, and most commonly done, from the ground. If both you and your adversary are on the ground, you can hold him in place with your legs while choking him with your arms and/or hands. Never intentionally go to the ground in a real fight, however, unless you can do so safely. While you're working on your opponent, paying attention to getting the choke in place, his friends may intervene and put the boots to you. Be wary of bystanders if you decide to try these techniques on the street (see "Six Things to Avoid in a Fight" for more information).

Once you have successfully choked an opponent unconscious, release the pressure while maintaining the architecture of your technique. You can never know for sure if he's playing possum until you let up a little, so don't relinquish control too quickly in case he begins to fight back. Conversely, you do not want to inadvertently choke him to death either, so loosening up is a happy medium that maintains your control but provides a window of safety.

Kubi Hishigi – Neck Joint Crush

This is done from the 'mount' position. When in the mount, you need to be straddling your opponent, sitting on his lower stomach to control his hips. Your knees are on each side, riding along by his floating ribs. With both hands, not necessarily at the same time, reach behind your opponent's head and cup the back of his skull with the palms of your hands. Once both hands are behind his head, cover one with the other and place both of your elbows on his collarbones. Using the shoulder and collarbone area as a fulcrum, pull his skull forward, crushing your opponent's chin into his sternum.

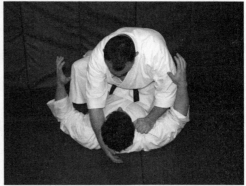

Kubi Hishigi – step 1

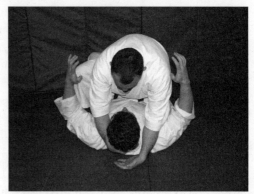

Kubi Hishigi – step 2

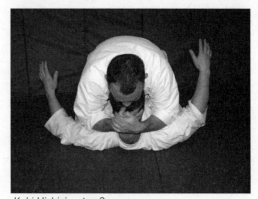

Kubi Hishigi – step 3

Gyaku Hishigi – **Opposite or Reverse Crushing (Guillotine)**

This is a reverse choke and neck crush. While the guillotine can be done from a standing position or a ground position, the ground is most common and generally the most effective. Consequently, we demonstrate how it works from the standing version. *Gyaku hishigi* often comes from an attempted tackle, or wrestler's take down by your opponent.

The opponent's head is pushed into your armpit, in this illustration the right armpit. The right arm wraps around his head placing the blade of your arm across his throat. As this arm wrap comes across the opponent's throat, you drop to the ground, opening your legs so you can wrap them around his lower abdomen and hips. This leg wrap is very important, as without it you will not be able to maintain control of your adversary and the choke will fail.

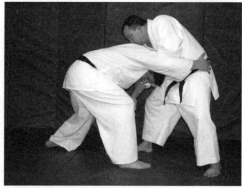

Guillotine Standing – step 1

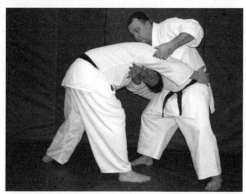

Guillotine Standing – step 2

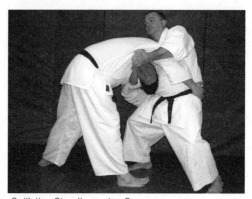

Guillotine Standing – step 3

You can grab your own hands, left to right, to apply the choke, or in this instance grab your own clothing with your right hand. This one-handed method is preferred, if possible, as it frees up the left hand for striking the opponent's kidneys. Unlike a sports competition, you will want to augment your controlling techniques with striking techniques to help subdue your adversary. With the choke set, use your legs to push the opponent's hips away from you so that you can stretch his spine. Arching your back can also create more stretch. This technique can be very fast, yet it can also work into it very slowly. Ratchet into position smoothly, getting each component in order or it is unlikely to work properly on the street.

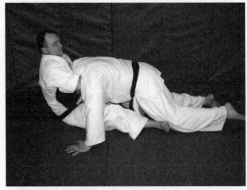

Guillotine on Ground – step 1

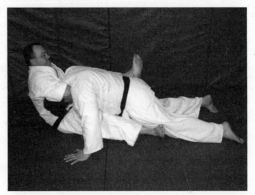

Guillotine on Ground – step 2

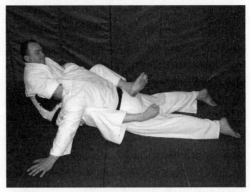

Guillotine on Ground – step 3

Hadaka Jime – Rear Naked Choke

A "naked" choke is one that does not require an opponent's heavy clothing or uniform *gi* to be effective. It only requires your arms to execute properly. When untrained individuals and practitioners who focus on sports competition are thrown or fall to the ground, they frequently give up their back, landing on all fours with their face pointing toward the ground. This is a common wrestling position as well.

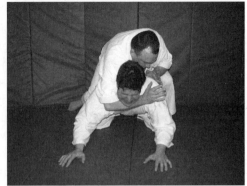

Hadaka Jime – step 1

If your opponent gives you his back, it is relatively easy to perform a rear naked choke. It is important to get his hips secured by wrapping your legs around the waist first though. This assures that you will have adequate control. You may wish to lock your feet together at the ankles for additional support.

The choke itself is done with the inside (thumb side) of the arm, placing the ulna bone against your opponent's trachea (or the carotid artery of your adversary's throat). Grip your off-hand arm in the crook of the elbow and wrap that hand across the top of your adversary's head. Cinch your arms together like a nutcracker with his neck in between them. Rotating your choking arm can change the technique dramatically, depending on the placement of your arm and hands. Cinch your grip while driving your arm bone into the other guy's throat to secure the choke.

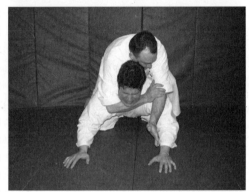

Hadaka Jime – step 2

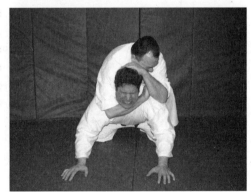

Hadaka Jime – step 3

Gyaku Juji Jime – Reverse Cross Lock and *Nami Juji Jime* – Front Cross Lock

Gyaku juji jime is a reverse cross lock choke performed from the front with your fingers inside the lapel of your opponent's jacket, shirt, or uniform *gi*, while *nami juji jime* is a front cross lock choke performed from the front with your thumb inside the lapel of your opponent's clothing. These two applications are so similar that we'll cover them together.

These techniques are very popular as they can be used from the guard (bottom) or the mount (top) when fighting on the ground. Each of these chokes requires a heavy piece of cloth (for example, coat, shirt, scarf, towel, belt) to execute successfully. The hands are placed differently in these two chokes yet they appear very similar.

Let's begin with the hand positions: *Gyaku juji jime* places the fingers inside the opponent's lapel. Your knuckles are placed across your opponent's skin, gripping the collar in the palm of your hand as you are face to face. *Nami juji jime* uses the opposite grip with your thumb inside the lapel.

Whichever grip you choose, your hands must be placed deep alongside the neck in order to be effective. Grip deeply along the collar toward the back of your opponent's neck, keep your elbows close to your ribs, and then pull downward. Yamada *Sensei* wanted us to actually touch the mat (or ground) with the knuckles of our hands to insure that the hands were deep enough around the opponent's neck; this is a good rule to follow.

The legs are used once again to hold the opponent in check by immobilizing his hips as in the previous techniques. Not only can you control the hips, but you can also use your legs to once again stretch your opponent from head to hip. Often when the opponent has paused and has stopped fighting momentarily, you know that you have sunk the choke into their neck well. This may be followed by a sudden burst of frantic thrashing as he attempts to break free before his oxygen supply is cut off.

Throw Him to the Ground with Force

Unless you're a very competent martial artist, the ground can hit a lot harder than your fists, particularly when you hurl the other guy onto it with force. The challenge is that many throws are commonly taught for sporting applications rather than for street combat, so the setups require you to turn your back on your foe or otherwise leave yourself open to a counterattack. Consequently, it's good to know a few ways of dumping him on his butt without eating a fist while you do it. When executed properly these techniques can do much damage and facilitate your escape. When done poorly, however, throws can get you hurt so you need to choose the right distance and timing to pull them off.

Let's pretend for a moment that the distance between you and your attacker has closed, closed fast and not by your choice. At very close range, your options become limited. You can shorten your weapon, for example, moving from using the fist up the arm to striking with the elbow. Similarly, you might be able to strike with your knee or forehead. Or, perhaps, you can turn your palm over and strike with an uppercut.

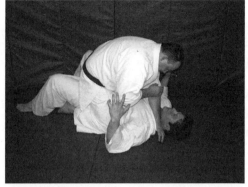

Gyaku Juji Jime 1

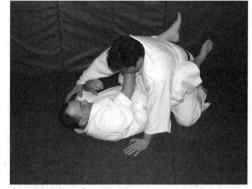

Nami Juji Jime 1

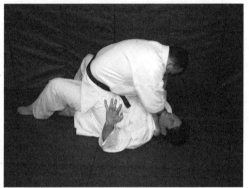

Gyaku Juji Jime 2

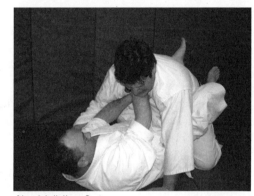

Nami Juji Jime 2

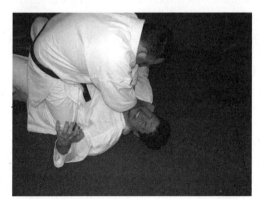

Gyaku Juji Jime 3

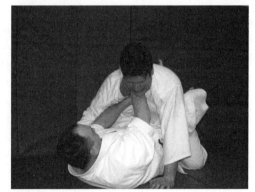

Nami Juji Jime 3

Another viable option at very close range, however, is a throw. If executed correctly, it can come out of your natural reflex response. When someone closes distance fast and aggressively, your natural tendency will be to lift up your hands in a warding-off motion. This reflex action can be turned into the opening you need to make a throw, using your closing attacker's force against him.

To throw a person effectively, you need to not only be able to touch him but rather to seize him, grab hard, and control him with both of your hands. Some very skilled practitioners can throw with one hand, but in all likelihood, you can't. The bottom line about throwing is that is takes practice, lots of it, to become good. If you throw a person and you use poor technique, you will either be counter-thrown or dragged to the ground. Not exactly your goal and most definitely a bad place to be.

The goal of your throw is to knock him down hard so that you can run away fast. Becoming entangled with your attacker is not a good thing. In close quarters combat, a throw can help you gain a superior position yet it should not be your primary technique useless you have years, and we mean yeeeaaaarrs of experience in the throwing arts like judo, *jujitsu*, *Hapkido*, *Samozashchita Baez Oruzhiya* (*Sambo*), western wresting, or *shuai-jan* (Chinese wrestling), to name a few. When you have years of experience, then the art becomes your primary form and you go with what you know.

If you have opportunity to train in a throwing art, it is suggested that you take advantage of it. You need not look for the best or the most expensive to gain an introduction to the throwing arts, just get on the mat, and go at it. You will soon learn just how over-matched you are when you come up to a skilled and experienced thrower because he will throw when and where he chooses to and you will be unable to stop him. Even when you think you are good enough to counter or block his chosen technique, you will discover he has more technique and more skill than you do. He will be slick, deceptive, tricky, and powerful when he wants to be and you will feel nothing but the mat as you hit it.

It works on the mat and it works in real life too. For example, 20-year-old Tyrone Jermain Hogan tried to carjack the wrong people when he went after the Florida International University judo club's van. The *judoka* were in Los Angeles to teach a self-defense class when they had an opportunity to put their skills to the test on the street. They quickly threw him to the ground and held him there until police could arrive and make an arrest. Hogan pled guilty on February 7, 2003 and was sentenced to 11 years in prison for kidnapping, robbery, and carjacking.

Here are five throws that you can practice that don't require a high level of skill to pull off. Further, only one requires you to turn your back on your adversary in order to throw him, a somewhat dangerous movement unless you have excellent timing. They are all judo throws, hence named in Japanese, yet you can find similar, if not identical, throws in other arts. If you choose to get some formal training as we recommend you will not necessarily learn these throws, nor learn them in this order, yet they are a good place to start. While we may show any given movement to one side (for example, right), it can just as easily be reversed to the other side (for example, left).

Osoto gari – Major Outer Reaping Throw

Basic throw:

Pull the attacker's right arm with your left to make the attacker plant his right foot as he is pulled forward or stiffen his leg to maintain his balance. Either way this motion temporarily immobilizes the adversary.

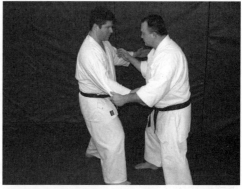

Osoto gari – Step 1

Step forward with your left leg so that it is next to the attacker's right foot. At the same time, you must swiftly place your right leg behind his right leg. Note: you are touching your attacker with your entire body from the leg up to your head. There must be virtually no space between you and your attacker to make this move successful.

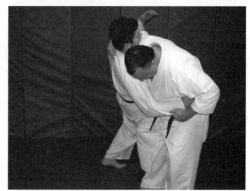

Osoto gari – Step 2

Sweep your right leg backward in a cutting motion while driving your right shoulder downward to the ground. Pull with your left arm and push with your right simultaneously. If he resists strongly you can rotate your hips to the left a bit to facilitate the throw.

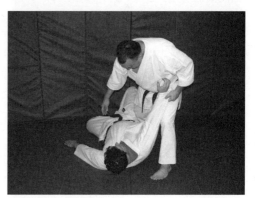

Osoto gari – Step 3

Street application:

During Step #1: Use the right fingers to the eyes.

During Step #2: Punch the attacker in the neck or jaw.

During Step #3: Stomp on the knee instead of sweeping with your leg.

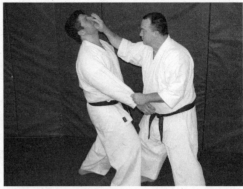

Osoto gari – Fingers to Eyes

Sasae tsurikomi ashi – Lifting/Pulling Ankle Block Throw

Sasae tsurikomi ashi requires precise timing to be effective. You must execute Steps 2 and 3 in precise sequence to bring your adversary up onto his toes at the same time you sweep his leg.

Basic throw:

Close distance and grab the adversary.

Lift upward to shift his center of balance upward and bring him onto his toes.

Twist your hands, as if turning the steering wheel of the car, left hand down and right hand up, while simultaneously sweeping the attacker's right leg.

When *Sasae tsurikomi ashi* is done traditionally and well by a skilled practitioner, it is beautiful and appears effortless. In the hands of an unskilled practitioner, it appears ugly and sloppy, yet it is still an effective throw nevertheless.

Street Application:

During #1: Grab flesh, not clothing.

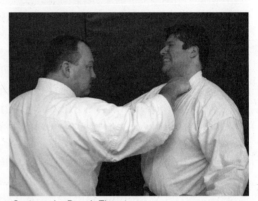

Osoto gari – Punch Throat

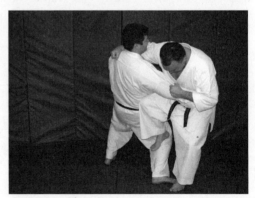

Osoto gari – Stomp Knee

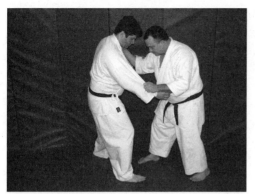

Sasae tsurikomi ashi – Step 1

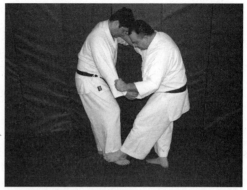

Sasae tsurikomi ashi – Step 2

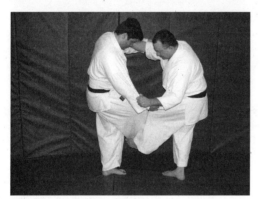

Sasae tsurikomi ashi – Step 3

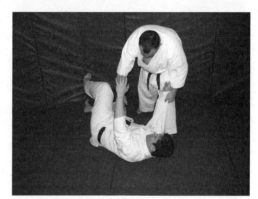

Sasae tsurikomi ashi – Step 4

Osoto gake – **Major Outer Hook Throw**

Basic throw:

Thrusting off of the right foot, drive your body into the attacker's body while hooking behind the attacker's right leg with your right leg. It is critical to pull downward on the attacker's right shoulder/sleeve to shift his weight momentarily and pin his right foot to the ground so that he cannot step away.

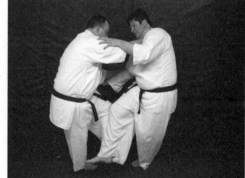

Sasae tsurikomi ashi – Grab Flesh not Clothing

Driving forward with your upper body, look over your attacker's shoulder to the ground. You must pull with you left hand and push with your right as you do this.

Drive the attacker over your right leg onto the ground.

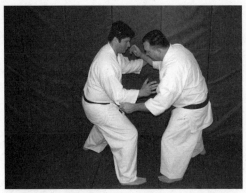

Osoto gake – Step 1

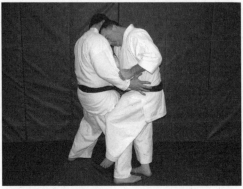

Osoto gake – Head Butt

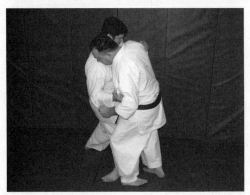

Osoto gake – Step 2

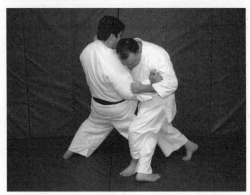

Osoto gake – Tear Knee]

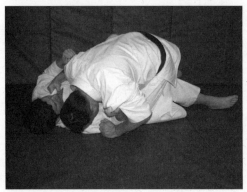

Osoto gake – Step 3

Street application:

During #1: Head butt the attacker.

During #2: Spin your upper body away (while driving downward) tearing the attacker's right knee with your entangling leg.

Koshi guruma – Hip Wheel Throw

Basic throw:

Grab the attacker's right bicep with your left hand while reaching behind the attacker's neck with your right. The deeper and further you reach around the neck with your right arm the better.

Turn your hips into the attacker. You must turn completely 180 degrees to your attacker

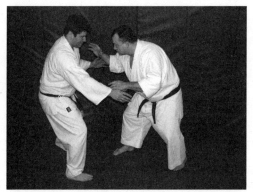

Koshi guruma – Step 1

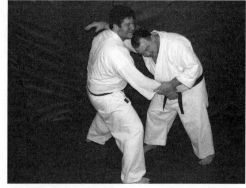

Koshi guruma – Head Butt

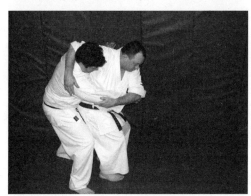

Koshi guruma – Step 2

with bent knees. As you do this, your hips must be below your attacker's hips such that you are below his center of gravity.

Lift your attacker by extending your knees while simultaneously pulling leftward with both hands.

Street application:

During #1: Head butt the attacker.

During #3: Drive your right knee into the attacker's groin as he lands on his back.

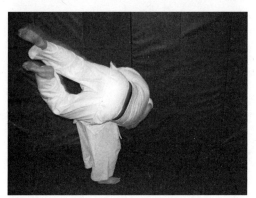

Koshi guruma – Step 3

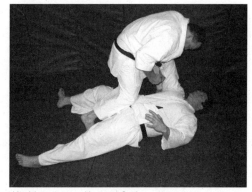

Koshi guruma – Knee to Groin

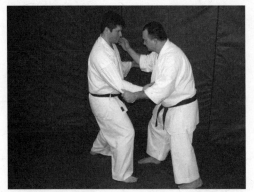

Kosoto gake – Step 1

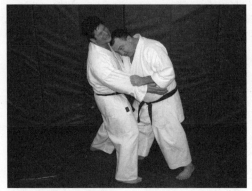

Kosoto gake – Head Butt

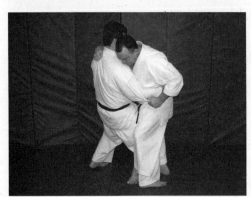

Kosoto gake – Step 2

Kosoto gake – **Minor Outside Hook Throw**

Basic throw:

Charge the attacker by stepping forward with your right foot.

Hook your left leg around the attacker's right leg and drive your chest into the attacker's chest, while simultaneously pulling the attacker's right elbow downward.

Look downward and behind your attacker's shoulder while driving backward and down.

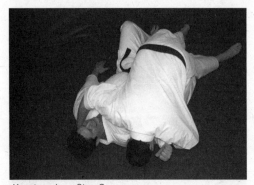

Kosoto gake – Step 3

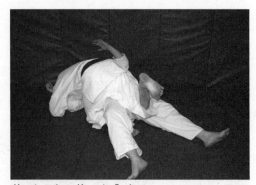

Kosoto gake – Knee to Groin

Street Application:

During #2: Head butt the attacker.

During #3: Drive your right knee into the attackers groin as he lands on his back.

Try all five throws. Find the one that is easiest for you and train with that one throw, forgetting the rest. You are not trying to become good at these throws, but rather to develop apprentice-level skill with the one throw you can use in an extreme stress situation. Here are a few tips that will make your training safer and more effective.

Training tips

Find a good instructor. Martial arts are dangerous and should not be attempted without competent instruction and oversight.

1. Have padded mats or use a mat room. Practicing without them is a sure path to injury.
2. Have plenty of space available to work in. Uncontrolled falls are just that, uncontrolled. Without an ample amount of room, a wall or other solid object can become very dangerous.
3. Go slow. As odd as it sounds if you go slowly, you will progress faster. This is because slow work forces you to develop solid body mechanics, good muscle control, and excellent balance.
4. Relax. If you relax, the technique will emerge. Using too much strength masks the working of the technique so it won't work on larger, stronger foes.
5. Repeat the movement over and over again. Don't throw your partner, but move in and set the technique, and then reset it. Your first fifty repetitions mean that you are just getting started. And we mean just getting started for that day and training session.

Strike With Impetus

Sometimes hitting the other guy is your best tactic in a street fight. If you're a skilled martial artist, for example, there are dozens of hand striking techniques that you might attempt including fore-fist punches, standing-fist punches, sword-hand strikes, palm-heel strikes, hammer fist blows, back fist strikes, wrist strikes, swing strikes, uppercuts, and single knuckle strikes, to name a few. Unless you have substantial skills, however, it is dangerous to hit a solid target with your closed fist. If your alignment is off, you will break your hand and/or damage your wrist. Wilder has broken his hand three times; it's not all that hard to do in a fight.

If you want to become a skilled fighter, you will need to study a martial art. Despite what we will cover here, there's really no substitute for hands-on experience. Since striking can be an excellent tactic, albeit one that takes a fair amount of skill to avoid hurting yourself while attempting to do it, we'll cover a small number of strikes that are relatively safe to perform yet powerful enough to end a fight if you do them correctly.

Before we begin, however, it is important to cover a few overarching principles surrounding striking in general. No matter how skilled you are (or are not), strikes work best when you catch your opponent by surprise, control distance and direction of your blow, relax until the moment of contact, and strike ferociously and repeatedly until the conflict is over.

- **Surprise**. As with any fighting application, if the other guy doesn't see it coming you're much more likely to be successful. Be careful not to telegraph your blows; you give your adversary a huge advantage whenever you do. Each punch should suddenly explode from wherever your starting point is into your target as fast as possible with no warning. Avoid cocking your arm back, taking a sudden breath, tensing your neck, shoulders, or arms, widening your eyes, grinning, grimacing, or making any other inappropriate or unnecessary movement before each blow. The same thing applies to elbow strikes, kicks, and knee strikes as well. If you train in martial arts, practice in front of a mirror can help eliminate these tells. Videotaping training sessions can also be a great way to objectively evaluate your performance and look for areas for improvement.

- **Distance**. Ensure that you are close enough to strike before you throw a blow. That's often closer than you'd naturally think. If you have to roll your shoulder or lean forward, you are too far away. Whenever you have to stretch to reach the other guy, your alignment will be off, your blow will be slower, and your power will be significantly reduced. Worse still, it will be easy for your adversary to disrupt your balance and drive you into the ground. Furthermore, if you lock your elbow to get a few extra inches of reach, you can damage the joint as well. Once you are in range, strike directly at the target covering the shortest distance possible. Keep your elbow pointed downward and your arm as close to your side as possible. Hook punches, haymakers, and other wide-swinging blows take

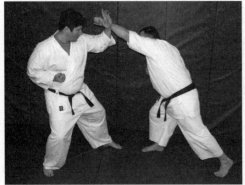

Punch from incorrect range: overextending your reach dramatically reduces your power and leaves you vulnerable to counterattack.

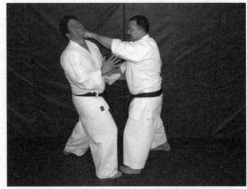

Punch from correct range: proper body alignment focuses all of your strength and power.

longer to reach your target than straight punches. They are much easier to spot, hence easier to block or avoid as well. The same thing applies for kicks. Unless you are skilled enough to disguise your intent, roundhouse and hook kicks are easier to block than more direct applications such as front kicks or joint kicks.

- **Relaxation.** Controlling the mind is the difference between being good and being great. In Major League Baseball, a pitcher can have a ten million dollar arm, but paired with a $10 head he is worthless. It's the same in fighting. If you are tense, letting your amped-up mind control your body, you will be slow and easy to block. It might sound counterintuitive, but it's not. Try it for yourself. Make a tight fist, lock all your muscles down hard, and try to throw a fast punch. Now, try it again with an open hand. Flick your hand forward as fast as you can as if you're trying to touch or poke someone. Which is faster? When you are relaxed, you can move much more swiftly. Experienced martial artists know that relaxation does not require you to sacrifice power. The trick is tensing at the moment of impact, not before. Here's how it works: *Fa jing* means explosive or vibrating power. It is sort of like a sneeze, a sudden unexpected movement that is very difficult to anticipate or block, followed by an instant of tension at the moment of impact. Both speed and relaxation are necessary to achieve *fa jing*. All strikes should be performed in this fashion. If you are relaxed until the moment of impact your speed and power will be greatly increased. And, importantly, you will make it much harder for the other guy to defend himself from your blows.

- **Ferocity.** All things equal, the guy who attacks with the most ferocity wins. Even if the other guy is a bit stronger or more skilled than you are, he's likely to disengage if he realizes he's bitten off more than he can chew. If you have no other choice but to fight, do so wholeheartedly. Your adversary should feel like he's run across a rabid wolverine wielding an industrial buzz saw. Strike fast, hard, and repeatedly until it's over and you can escape to safety. Throwing a single blow or short combination and dancing aside to see if it had any effect may work well in the tournament ring, but it's woefully inadequate on the street. Give it everything you're worth and don't stop until it's over.

Now that the principles are out of the way, let's talk about some common striking techniques that lesser skilled individuals can usually pull off successfully. These include hand strikes, forearm strikes, elbow strikes, knee strikes, foot strikes, and head butts.

Hand Strikes. The hand is a great weapon in a fight. We've already mentioned that you don't want to hit a solid object with your knuckles unless you are very skillful, yet you don't need to make a fist to hurt the other guy. Palm-heel strikes, for example, can be very powerful yet relatively safe if you contact something hard like the other guy's jaw. You can thrust straight out with your open palm (for example, to the face) or slap sideways, for example, to the ear. When we teach children how to break boards for the first time, we have them strike with an open palm because they can generate much power with relative safety.

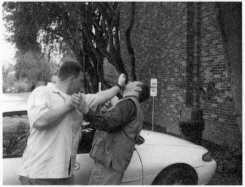
Palm Heel Strike

Rotate your hand upward and pull your fingers back so that you won't tangle them on anything. Aim so that you will hit with the meaty heel of your palm at the bottom. You can improve your power if you can get your bodyweight behind the blow too. The easiest way to do that is to step forward as you strike. Begin with the hand movement and then follow with the step. Your opponent will undoubtedly see the blow coming if you step first and then strike. The goal, however, is to land the blow at the same time you complete your step, adding impetus to the strike.

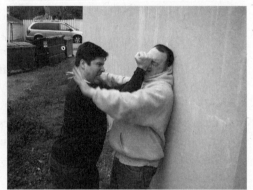
Hammerfist Blow

Another way to strike with reduced chances of injury to your hand is with a hammer fist blow. While this is done using a closed fist, you hit with the bottom of your hand rather than with your knuckles. This softer striking surface protects the hand yet can deliver solid power in your blows. You can strike downward (for example, to the face or nose) or sideways (for example, to the side of the head or temple). The hammer fist is a smashing type of blow not a penetrating blow.

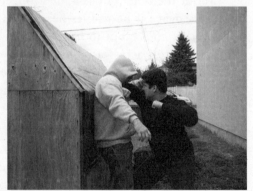
Forearm Smash

There are dozens of other effective hand strikes yet they require a fair amount of training to execute successfully and safely so we won't go into detail here. If you do choose to punch with a closed fist, however, it's critical that you straighten your wrist and strike primarily with your first and second knuckles so that the line of power passes directly through the knuckles, traveling up your arm and into your body. If you connect with something solid like the other guy's jaw with a bent wrist or with your third and fourth knuckles you can hurt yourself severely.

Forearm Strikes. A forearm smash can be extraordinarily powerful, though you need to be relatively close to an opponent to make it work. It looks like a basic head block, if you have trained in a striking art such as karate, yet is designed to be offensive rather than primarily defensive in nature. Forearm blows work best when you rotate the hard ulna bone along the outside edge of your arm into the other guy, using the torque from your twisting movement to augment your upward force. Adding a forward step to magnify the blow with your bodyweight can be beneficial as well. Forearm strikes can also be executed sideways like a hammer fist blow, though that's usually intended as a defensive technique to block or deflect an opponent's punch.

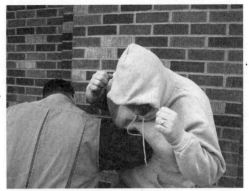

Horizontal Elbow Strike

Elbow Strikes. The elbow is a pretty hard bone, one of the hardest structures in the human body. Nature knows that you are very likely to land on your elbows in a fall, so the bone is very resilient. The elbow also serves as an excellent short-range weapon when you are too close to generate good power with your palm heel strike or punch. You can create enormously powerful blows at very short distances using your elbows, one of the reasons this type of strike is favored in martial arts such as *muay Thai*.

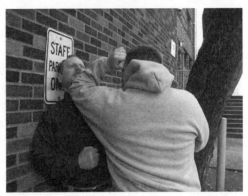

Vertical Elbow Strike

You can strike upward (for example, to the solar plexus), downward (for example to the head or neck if the other guy is bent over), or sideways (for example, to the ribs or head)

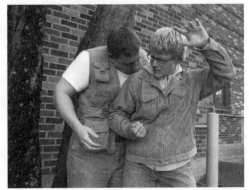

Reverse Elbow Strike

with your elbow. You can strike directly behind you too (for example, forcefully pulling your fist into a traditional karate chamber at your side). It is a very versatile weapon. It is also important to note that only the most skilled practitioners have the forethought and

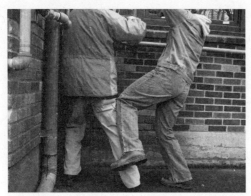

Knee Strike to Thigh

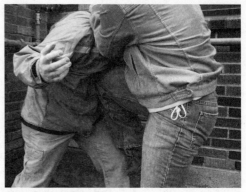

Knee Strike to Solar Plexus

skill to use their elbows as weapons in most cases. The majority of people default to their closed fists in a fight, even when the distance is better suited to a shorter-range weapon such as the elbow. Consequently, elbow strikes can have an additional element of surprise when you use them on the street.

Knee Strike. Your knee is much like your elbow. If you know how to joint-lock an arm, you know how to joint-lock a leg. If you know how to strike with your elbows, you also know how to use your knees. Once again, short range is key for knee strikes. If you are too far away, they do not work effectively. Obviously, the groin is a default target, one that is often taught in women's self-defense classes (notice the authors yawning here). The challenge is that men are inherently good at protecting their genitals. Further, groin strikes do not always end a fight right away. Fortunately, there are alternatives you might choose.

There is an easily accessible nerve bundle along the side of your thigh, about where your fingers touch if your hands are hanging down at your sides. That's a great place to hit with a knee strike if you've tangled up with a standing opponent. You can also knee-strike his chest or solar plexus if you are a skilled grappler or can find a way to off-balance or bend him over first. For example, you can hook the back of his head with your hand, or cross your arms behind him to strike the back of his neck, and then pull him downward into your blow. Trying to use this technique without training can be dangerous, however, as it is fairly easy to become unbalanced when you strike that high with your knee.

If your adversary is on the ground, your knee can be used to strike to his ribs too. This type of knee strike is often a precursor to grappling as it is intensely painful and can flip your opponent onto his back or side. You can also strike to the head if he's down, of course, but that's very dangerous and challenging to justify in court unless he's armed with some type of weapon. The knee can generate extraordinary power so be cautious that you don't overdo things if you strike with it.

Foot Strikes. While most martial artists train barefoot, in today's world the foot is

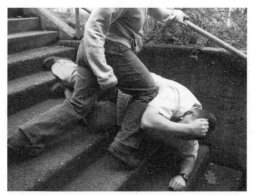

Knee Strike to Ribs of Downed Opponent

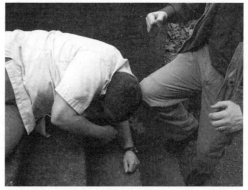

Knee Strike to Head of Downed Opponent

rarely bare in combat. That means your boot or shoe can become a weapon in its own right. Not only do certain types of footwear make great striking surfaces (for example, steel-toed boot), but they also protect your foot as well. Furthermore, proper foot positioning is not as critical when you're wearing shoes as it is when you are barefoot. For example, a front kick should hit with the ball of the foot. If you don't pull your toes back, you are likely to jam them when barefoot yet sturdy shoes can let you do this technique incorrectly without hurting yourself. The similarity between the boxing glove and the shoe should not be lost. The shoe protects the foot in the same way the boxing glove protects the hand. Similarly, it often cushions and softens the blow too such as running shoes would.

The top of the foot can be used to strike as well as the toe and the heel. The top of the foot is used anywhere on the opponent's body. You will see the top of the foot and/or toe used on the face, usually when the opponent is down. If you are the person on the ground, be prepared to have incoming blows aimed at your face. The heel, or stomp

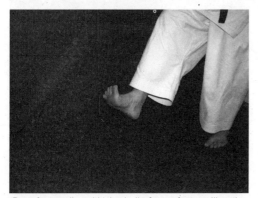

Bare foot: strike with the ball of your foot, pulling the toes back so that they are not jammed by contact with the opponent.

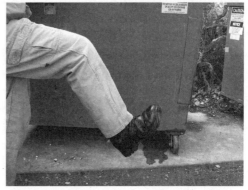

Shod foot: when wearing boots or sturdy shoes the position of the toes doesn't really matter all that much.

kick, is frequently used when the opponent is on the ground as well. It's simply a matter of downward vs. sideways motion. Once again, be aware of the legal ramifications of utilizing such techniques.

If you are going to kick the other guy in a fight, the safest place to aim is below his waist. Low kicks are faster, more direct, and harder to block than high ones. They also help you retain your balance. Front kicks, stomps, and sidekicks are generally the easiest kicks for beginners to learn. All of these kicks begin by forcefully lifting your knee as quickly as you can. The higher you lift your knee, within reason, the better. To do a front kick, swing your foot up and snap it forward. For a stomp kick, drive it back downward leading with your heel. To do a sidekick, rotate your hip and snap the kick out to the side. Good targets include the side of the knee, the middle of the thigh, the ankle, and the foot. You can also target the groin, though that's often challenging.

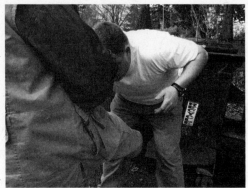
Front kick to groin

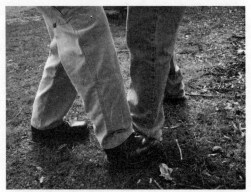
Stomp kick to foot

Head Butts. Head butts are oddly a cultural artifact. While they are very common throughout most of Europe, they are rarely seen in America. Perhaps this has something to do with the popularity of soccer, yet it really doesn't matter all that much why. What matters is that it works. Head butts can used in very close quarters combat. The goal of the head butt is simple, forcefully striking one of the stronger bone architectures of your body onto a weaker area of your opponent's skull. This is usually done by driving your forehead into the occipital bone surrounding the other guy's eye, into his temple, or into his nose.

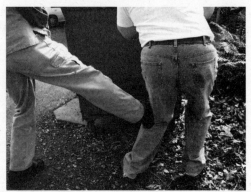
Joint kick to knee

While the forehead is the most common striking surface for head butts, you can attack with all four sides of your head, connecting with the area covered by your sweatband.

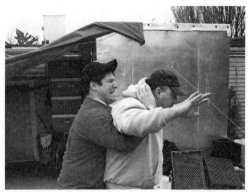
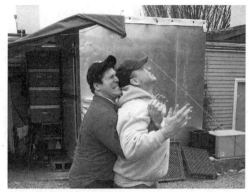

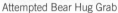
Attempted Bear Hug Grab   Reverse Head Butt to Face

Avoid hitting with "softer" areas such as your face, ear, or temple. It is imperative to note that the head butt is a body move not a head move, especially when butting with the back of the head. If you strike solely with your head/neck, like nodding, you are quite likely to injure yourself, particularly if you miss. Use your whole body. Loren Christensen likes to call it "bowing with prejudice," an apt analogy.

Distance and surprise are critical for a successful head butt. Additionally, it's also important to note that you are momentarily blind when you perform the technique. Like trying to keep your eyes open during a sneeze, it's nearly impossible not to close your eyes on contact.

There are many ways to secure the other guy's hands and arms to keep him from interfering with your head butt but that is not always necessary, particularly when you have the element of surprise on your side. An infamous example of this was when French soccer star Zinedine Zidane head-butted Italian Marco Materazzi during the 2006 World Cup Final. The two players reportedly exchanged heated words before Zidane began to walk away. Materazzi said, "I prefer the whore that is your sister," to Zidane, who turned around, made a run-up and head-butted Materazzi in the chest, knocking him to the ground. He was subsequently ejected from the game.

Combinations

While all of these techniques can be used in isolation, they are more effective when combined together. The best combinations move along the body going high-low-high or low-high-low to create openings by disrupting the opponent. They work because your adversary's head and hands will follow the pain when you strike him. His attention should shift to where he has been struck, particularly if he is not a trained fighter who has become desensitized against pain. Further, there is a natural physiological reaction that draws a person's hands toward the body part that hurts. This gives you a momentary advantage to strike an unguarded area, providing that your combinations flow smoothly and quickly in concert with each other.

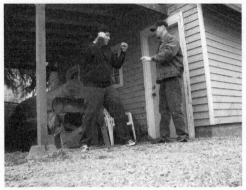

Combination, step 1

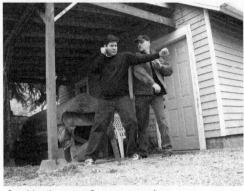

Combination, step 2

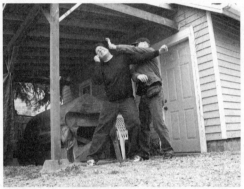

Combination, step 3

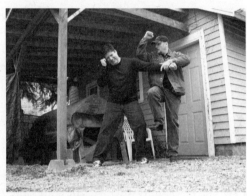

Combination, step 4

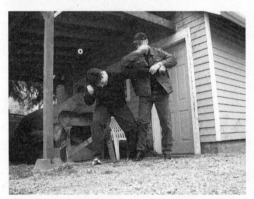

Combination, step 5

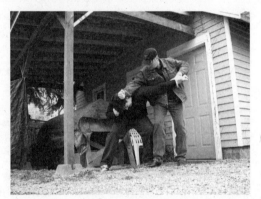

Combination, step 6

For example, let's say that your adversary opens the fight with a punch to your mid-section. One way to respond is by twisting to the side, evading, or shoulder blocking his punch and then immediately riposting with a palm-heel strike to his face. As he reels back from your hand strike, you can fairly easily stomp on his foot or ankle (or throw a low kick to his knee, depending on the angle of the opening). As his attention is drawn to the damaged limb, you can finish him off with a hammer fist blow to the face.

If Something Works, Keep Using It Until It Stops Working

He who knows these things, and in fighting puts his knowledge into practice, will win his battles. He who knows them not, nor practices them, will surely be defeated.

— Sun Tzu

Chase him towards awkward places, and try to keep him with his back to awkward places. When the enemy gets into an inconvenient position, do not let him look around, but conscientiously chase him around and pin him down.
— Miyamoto Musashi

If something works, keep using it until it stops working. This idea can be said many different ways. Examples would include the old farmer's axiom, "If it ain't broke, don't fix it," or the business phrase, "Go with what you know."

Have you ever loaded a supposedly "new and improved" program onto your computer only to find that it crashed everything else you had installed? Maybe you had intra-program conflicts, ran out of disk space, or your processor chip was just too slow? Or you quickly discovered that you wanted to print out a short report and couldn't even do that. Or you were forced to upgrade to a new operating system only to find that you needed a whole new computer as well.

The same thing happens in a fight. If you just hit the other guy with your hand, don't try a jumping, back-spinning, split kick to follow it up. If it ain't broke, don't fix it. Go with what just worked. Do it again and again and again until it doesn't work anymore. Then go to plan B.

Standardization and simplicity are the hallmarks of a good fighter. Oh sure, there are the professionals who can do these wild techniques and make them work, but frankly that is not you. And for the most part it's not us either. If you watch these guys, professional cage fighters, boxers, wrestlers, judo, or *jujitsu* players, they all have strong basic and non-complicated techniques. They go with what is simple and effective. They are professionals that stay with something that works until it doesn't.

Street fighters, gang members, bouncers, bikers, law enforcement officers, and anybody else who settles things with violence has a set of favorite techniques that they will use over and over again. Why? Because they work. The cost of failure is far too high to attempt things that might not work.

Do not get fancy in any fight, but especially not against an armed assailant. On the street, there are no points for executing a technique with perfect form. Do whatever it takes to win no matter how messy or sloppy it becomes.

Once the fight begins, adrenaline will affect your fine motor skills so you have to keep things simple if you wish them to be effective. Use well-directed, efficient techniques— things you know you are good at and can rely on under extreme stress. There are techniques you know, techniques you can do, techniques you practice, and techniques you would be willing to bet your life on. Apply only the latter in a real fight. Use your favorite one again and again until it no longer works and then pull another one out of your bag of tricks.

Any mistake you make in a street fight could be your last, so stick with what you know. Hick's* law states that response times increase in proportion to the logarithm of the number of potential stimulus-response alternatives. That is a fancy way of saying that the more choices you have to make, the longer it takes to make a decision. While you may know and even practice hundreds of techniques in your martial arts training, assuming you practice such things, a limited subset is required in self-defense situations. Choose your favorite and keep using it until it stops working.

Six Mistakes to Avoid in a Fight

If equally matched, we can offer battle; if slightly inferior in numbers, we can avoid the enemy; if quite unequal in every way, we can flee from him... Hence, though an obstinate fight may be made by a small force, in the end it must be captured by the larger force.

— Sun Tzu

In single combat, we can confuse the enemy by attacking with varied techniques when the chance arises. Feint a thrust or cut, or make the enemy think you are going to close with him, and when he is confused you can easily win.

— Miyamoto Musashi

Real fighting on the street is nothing like practice in the *dojo* due to the fear factor, among other things. When it's real, the consequences are real too. Your body knows this even if your mind does not. Adrenaline surges through your system, making you faster, tougher, and more resilient. It helps you survive, yet robs you of fine motor control and higher thought processes at the same time. Your animal brain (amygdala) rears up and takes control, making it hard to respond, plan, or think your actions through. Consequently, you need to keep things simple and straightforward in order to be effective.

You must employ techniques that do not require fine motor coordination or complicated thought. These applications must also cause serious damage if you want to stop

---
* British psychologist William Edmund Hick (1912–1974) conducted reaction-time research to develop this model.

a determined aggressor who, like yourself, is also hopped up on adrenaline. Last, but not least, the techniques you choose cannot take very long to execute. John Wayne-style roundhouse punches, high kicks, and the like take a circuitous route, hence don't connect very quickly, at least not when compared to other techniques.

Because it is hard not to telegraph these types of big movements, they are easier for the other guy to see, hence easier for him to counter or block. This is not only bad because it doesn't work very well, but also because the longer the fight lasts, the better the chances that you will get hurt in the process. It is much better to use low kicks, straight punches, and other applications that hit hard, fast, and immediately.

To this end, we suggest six things you should remember in a fight.

- Don't kick above the waist.
- Don't play "tank."
- Don't hit with a closed fist… unless you've got skills.
- Don't forget to use your mouth too.
- Don't play the other guy's game.
- Don't use the wrong technique for the situation.

> Street fighters, gang members, bikers, bouncers, law enforcement officers, and anybody else who settles things with violence has a set of favorite techniques that they will use over and over again. Standardization and simplicity are the hallmarks of a good fighter. These guys use simple, straightforward applications and uncomplicated techniques because they work well under extreme stress. When it works, keep on using it until it is no longer effective. The cost of failure is far too high to attempt complicated things that might not be effective.

Don't Kick Above the Waist

Funny things happen when you work stadium security. Way back when Kane was a green belt in karate, he had occasion to attempt to throw a patron out of the stadium for rowdy behavior. That sort of thing happened incessantly, yet this particular occasion was somewhat unique. Kane didn't know it at the time, but the other guy wasn't just disruptive and annoying; he was also a black belt in *taekwondo*.

As they approached the gate, the rowdy suddenly wrapped his brain around what was happening and made up his mind that he wasn't going to leave quietly. Without warning, he suddenly spun and launched a lightening-fast roundhouse kick at Kane's head.

Sensing movement, Kane shifted slightly, instinctively scoop blocking the kick. It's not that he was better or faster than the other guy; he most certainly was not, yet the movement was so broad and telegraphed, and took so long to connect that he was able to intercept the kick successfully. We're talking fractions of seconds here, yet it was enough, particularly since Kane had been practicing that technique over and over for a couple months prior to the incident while working on advancement requirements toward his next belt test. Since it was ingrained into his muscle memory, his body reacted without much conscious thought.

Once he had captured the other guy's leg, it was no effort at all to clamp it down onto his shoulder with both hands, holding it in place. He then started walking backwards, dragging the other guy over to a police officer who was stationed at the gate nearby. The officer calmly watched Kane dragging the fan towards him, the former rowdy wincing in pain as his leg and groin were stretched, and hopping along in an attempt to keep up without falling over. As the pair approached, the officer sardonically stated, "Hey, I can come back in a while if you'd like to hurt him some more." While Kane laughed, the other guy went a little pale.

The guy was underage, but he was not drunk so he was off the hook for that one, but worse things were yet to come. The officer examined the rowdy's identification. Since he'd seen the kick and knew that most folks couldn't pull something like that off without practice, it was a logical question to ask about his training. The other guy solemnly answered and that's where things got ugly.

Given the guy's black belt, he'd just committed aggravated assault. A kick to the head from a trained martial artist is reasonably likely to cause death or serious physical injury so he was in just as much trouble as he would have been had he pulled a knife or a gun. Fortunately, for everyone involved, the kick hadn't connected with its intended target. The fan, suddenly contrite, was given a choice: He could tell the officer who his *sifu* (instructor) was so that his unseemly behavior could be reported to his instructor, or he could be arrested for the assault. Interestingly enough, he selected jail as the safer choice. That says something about the character of his instructor.

Let's face it, high kicks look really cool. That's why they are often seen in tournament competitions and movie choreography. Unfortunately, these techniques are simply not practical in most real-world self-defense situations. Unless you are vastly more skilled or a lot faster than your adversary is, high kicks are not going to work.

Self-defense entanglements typically happen fast, furious, and at very close range. Balance and unimpaired movement are paramount when you tie up with an opponent. If you are knocked to the ground, you could easily be injured from the fall. Further, you can get stomped, maimed, or squashed like a bug while lying there momentarily defenseless.

From very close range, you can often strike with your knee as *muay Thai* practitioners like to do, yet there is not even enough room for a full-on leg strike or kick much of the time. On the other hand, if you land a good shot from your knee and your opponent bends over from the impact you can easily follow through with a kick from the foot, but that is a secondary movement.

Even if there is enough room for a traditional high kick, you still should not attempt to perform it in a street fight. Whenever you raise your foot high into the air, you take more time to strike your opponent, weaken your balance, and very likely open yourself to counterattack. Low kicks to vital or painful areas such as the feet, ankles, or knees on the other hand, are much more effective. They are harder to see and avoid, hence more likely to connect. Further, they do not disrupt your balance very much and can easily be performed in most regular street clothing.

No matter how fast you are, it takes way too long to cover the distance required to execute such maneuvers efficiently. They are relatively easy to anticipate, block, and counter. And they leave you off balance far too long. Kicking below the waist, on the other hand, covers a lot less ground and is, therefore, much faster for you to use. In addition to the benefits of more speed and less distance, low kicks are considerably better at helping you maintain your balance when you throw them. Whenever your foot leaves the ground, you become vulnerable and temporarily rooted to the spot where your support foot rests.

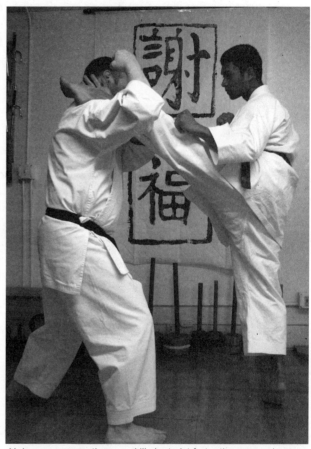

Never try to kick a weapon. That's another thing that looks great in the movies but that can cost you dearly in the real world. For example, if he's got a knife it takes only a quick flick of the wrist and you impale yourself on his blade. Unless you're some kind of super-evolved mutant life form, his hands are faster than your feet.

A great kicking tactic in such encounters is to chop away at your opponent's knees, shins, ankles, and/or feet. Such attacks are quick and vicious. They are difficult to see, even harder to avoid, and cause significant physiological damage with minimal effort. Kane, who has had arthroscopic surgery to repair cartilage tears in both knees, will be among the first to tell you that damage to a knee is debilitating.

Unless you are vastly more skilled or a lot faster than your adversary is, high kicks are not going to work. Don't kick above the waist in a real fight.

Once you have entangled an opponent's feet with your low kicks, you will have a much better chance of landing upper body blows with your hand strikes. If you really want to kick him in the head, wait until you've knocked him to the ground first, and then do it. Watch your back legally though; such actions might have adverse repercussions.

When was the last time you had time to stretch out before a real fight? We certainly never have. No matter how flexible you are, it is fairly difficult to execute a high kick at full speed and power with cold muscles. Even if you can snap off a few high kicks, you'll almost certainly pay for them later with strained muscles.

Further, you are not necessarily going to be wearing loose-fitting clothing such as a karate *gi* the next time you find yourself in a real-world life or death encounter. The constrictive street clothes that most people wear are simply not conducive to the extreme leg movements necessary to kick above someone's waist. While that may be pretty obvious with dresses or long skirts, it often holds true for jeans and slacks as well.

Don't kick about the waist in a street fight. It's foolish, ineffectual, and tactically unsound.

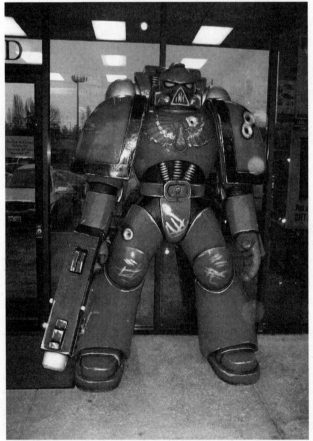

Standing toe-to-toe with your adversary is just plain dumb, particularly if he's big, highly skilled, or armed with some type of weapon. You're not a tank, so don't try to fight like one; keep moving, control the distance and the angles between yourself and the other guy, and you'll have a good shot at taking him down.

Don't Play "Tank"

Sadly, inexperienced fighters tend to stand in place while whaling away at each other without regard to evasive movement, stances, or mobility. You're not a heavily armored tank. It hurts to get hit. Consequently, standing toe-to-toe and duking it out with your adversary is just plain dumb, particularly if he's big, highly skilled, or armed with some type of weapon. Don't forget that he's attacking you for a reason, thinking he can win, so chances are good that he's going to be big, nasty, and mean.

The only time Kane has ever been sucker-punched was at a college fraternity party in 1985. The guy who hit him was a 22-year-old, 310-pound Samoan football player, a guy twice his weight and strong as an ox. Although the football player's blow caught him along the side of his jaw, knocking him to the ground, he was back on his feet doing his best Bruce Lee imitation seconds later.

The two flailed at each other for what seemed like several minutes trading blows, though it was probably much shorter than it seemed. While neither combatant

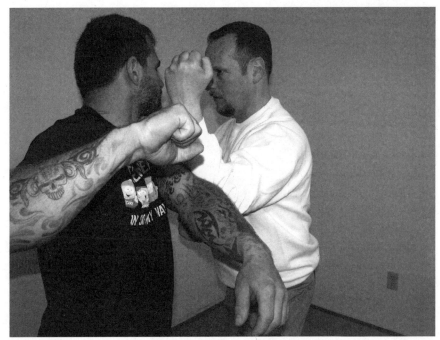

Closing is done by moving to the outside while blocking across the opponent's body to tie up his limbs, forcing him to reposition before successfully counterattacking.

realized it at that time, despite the Samoan's strength and Kane's agility neither of them could throw a decent punch. They didn't move too well either. While Kane ultimately lost, he received only a sore jaw and a bloody nose. His opponent, who barely flinched under his best shot, wasn't seriously injured either.

In retrospect, the thought of the two of them thumping on each other to no effect was pretty funny. By the time it was over, they held a grudging respect for each other's ability to take a punch and even became friends after a fashion later on, yet not all fist-fights end so sociably. Going toe-to-toe with a big Samoan was just plain dumb. Standing in place only exacerbated the stupidity.

If you don't want to get hurt in a fight, you will need to move away from the strength of the other guy's attack. It is imperative to not only get off line, but also keep your attacker from being able to reorient immediately at the same time. In a typical martial arts example, we often call this "closing."

Closing is done by moving to the outside while blocking across the opponent's body to tie up his limbs, forcing him to reposition before successfully counterattacking. Fighting down the centerline is advanced martial arts, very difficult to perfect, whereas moving off-line and closing is taught to beginners because it is relatively easy to learn. And it works pretty well too. It is even better if you can manage to get behind the other guy.

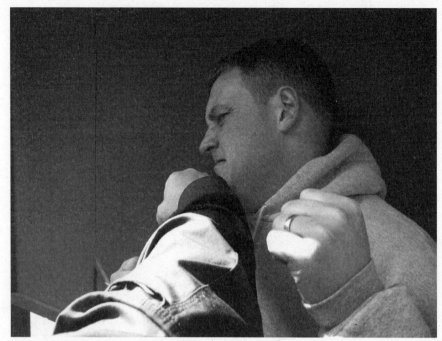

Punching his jaw with your closed fist is probably going to hurt you as much, if not more, than him. Strike hard to soft and soft to hard for best effect.

Use movement and distraction to imbalance and overcome. Stay balanced, upright, and mobile, keeping your weight centered over your feet. Body positioning and mobility not only keep you out of harm's way but also afford opportunities to counterstrike, knock your adversary down, and escape. Good balance is also needed if you are to generate powerful, effective techniques.

Don't let yourself get boxed in. Use mobility to control the distance and the angles between yourself and the other guy. While this is paramount for armed assaults, it is very important for unarmed ones too. You're not a tank so don't fight like one.

Don't Hit With a Closed Fist... Unless You've Got Skills

Unless you are an experienced martial artist, don't punch using a closed fist in a street fight. The odds are good that you'll damage yourself at least as much as you will hurt your adversary. Even former heavyweight champion Mike Tyson, a guy who clearly knows how to hit, broke his hand in a street brawl when he hit fellow boxer Mitch Green incorrectly. The incident took place in Harlem during August 1988. Furthermore, striking with a closed fist looks bad for potential witnesses, as it is clearly an offensive movement.

Go ahead and test it for yourself, it is easy enough to do. Find a brick or cement wall, make a good fist, and give it a light tap with your knuckles. Now, slap it good and hard with your open hand. Which one hurts more? The closed fist, of course. If you really insist on hitting with a closed fist, avoid targeting the other guy's face. Body shots are much less likely to damage your hand, though you can still mess up your wrists if you do it incorrectly. Incidentally, that's why boxers tape their hands and wrists.

Look at any teenage boy who has his hand in a cast, especially his right hand. If you see the two smallest fingers curled up in the cast, he's got what's called a "boxer's fracture." That means that he threw a looping right to the head and broke his metacarpal bones at the ring and/or pinky finger knuckles.

This brings us to the concept of contouring, a very important component of fighting. It is also an aspect that is commonly overlooked since it becomes pretty much irrelevant in tournament competitions where safety gear and heavy gloves dramatically change the dynamics of the situation. Contouring helps you identify the best target for any given technique. In general, hard parts strike soft targets and vice versa.

Here's how it works: If you have ever punched someone in the jaw with your closed fist you undoubtedly know how painful that can be for both parties. Hard fist to hard jaw is simply no good. We have seen quite a few broken knuckles resulting from such mistakes. A palm-heel strike to the jaw, on the other hand, can be quite effective. Soft palm to hard jaw is a good equation. It not only meets the contouring rule but it is far more painful for the other guy.

If you take a close look at all of your striking surfaces, your feet, hands, knees, and elbows, you can see how targeting

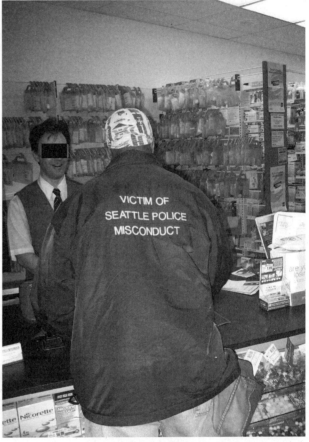

Law enforcement officers are highly trained, yet they are frequently accused of overreacting and abusing the criminals they arrest. How much more likely is the average civilian, who has no policy or procedure to follow, to be similarly accused of wrongdoing in a fight?

works at a more granular level. For example, the blade edge of your foot aligns best with the other guy's joints (for example, the knee), while the ball of your foot makes a good fit with his groin or midsection, particularly if you use an upward arc when you strike. As you can see, different types of kicks are best for different targets.

The same thing applies to punches too. A single knuckle or finger strike fits the solar plexus better than the whole fist, even when you make it properly by connecting solely with the first two knuckles. A hammer fist aligns much better with the temple or the forehead than it does with the base of the jaw or stomach where an uppercut or palm-up straight punch might better apply.

If you have to defend yourself on the street and don't have much training, you are best off trying to knock his attack aside so that you can get away. Open hand slaps are great defensively, deflecting incoming blows with relative ease. If you are going to strike back, we recommend that you connect with you open hands, elbows, or knees in a fight. Stay away from most closed-fisted techniques, save for the hammer fist where you strike with the bottom of your hand rather than hitting with your knuckles.

Don't hit with a closed fist unless you have sufficient training to do so without hurting yourself in the process. If you really want to strike with a closed fist, plan where you strike carefully, aiming for soft areas of the opponent's body such as his kidneys or solar plexus.

Don't Forget to Use Your Mouth Too

If you have ever watched football, basketball, or other college or professional sports, you have, no doubt, seen instances where one player fouls another who subsequently retaliates. In the majority of those cases, it is the second player that the referee observes committing the infraction. His eye is drawn toward the initial motion, yet he only notices the retaliatory strike. Consequently, it is often the victim who is penalized rather than the guy who started the confrontation.

Unfortunately, it works that way on the street as well. Witnesses frequently see the reaction of the victim and think that his defense is the first blow. Consequently, the person who initiates a fight is perceived as the good guy. If witnesses misinterpret what actually occurred, that could be highly problematic for you when the police arrive or things get to court.

We recently did an online news search of the key words "police brutality," which resulted in 918 stories reported within 30 days of our query. Law enforcement officers are highly trained, following specific policies and procedures as they conduct their business, yet they are frequently accused of overreacting and abusing the criminals they arrest regardless of whether or not they stay within procedural specifications. How much more likely is the average civilian, who has no policy or procedure to follow, to be similarly accused of wrongdoing?

If you really want to protect yourself, you need to make sure that everyone around you knows that you are the good guy when it comes to a fight. So, how can you create a witness who is likely to interpret your just actions favorably? You create witnesses by using your mouth as a weapon. It can be just as potent as your fists or feet in a fight and is often even more important in the long run.

Start by acting afraid—you probably are anyway— by verbally calling for help. There is an off chance that you can ward off your assailant or convince someone to intervene on your behalf simply by shouting for help. Even if you can't, you might still convince others around that you are the good guy. Shouting something along the lines of, "Oh my God, don't kill me with that knife!" is a pretty good indicator of peril. It clearly differentiates you from the other guy and should help justify your use of force in court if it gets that far.

"I don't want to fight you," "Please don't hurt me," "Put down the weapon," and "Help, he's got a gun" all put you in a much better light than "Go ahead, make my day!" or "I'm gonna kill you sucker!" Think about various scenarios ahead of time so that you will have a better chance of articulating strategically. It is pretty easy to shout something during a fight. The real challenge is finding words that put you in the best possible light and your assailant in the worst. In other words, it is easy to shout but hard to verbalize so you need to practice this. Many martial arts classes do role-playing and scenario drills that give you the opportunity to exercise your verbal skills while fighting.

What you say before, during, and after a confrontation holds much weight in convincing witnesses that you are the good guy in the fight. What you do has significant impact as well. Once you have evaded the initial attack and disarmed, disabled, or escaped your assailant, be wary of reengaging the enemy. It is not only dangerous physically but also puts you on dangerous ground perceptually as well.

If, for example, you knock your attacker to the ground then proceed to kick or pummel him, you will be seen as overreacting even in many cases where you are on sound tactical ground. A far better tactic in this example would be to precede any further action with verbal commands such as, "stay down," "stop fighting me," "drop the weapon," or "don't make me hurt you."

Your mouth is an important weapon. Don't forget to use it. There is a long list of phrases in Appendix B that you might choose to use.

Don't Play the Other Guy's Game

Darrell, a burly 200-pound logger friend of Wilder's, had a very near miss. His chainsaw tangled on a log, bucked up, and bounced toward his throat. The good news was that he saved his life by blocking the running saw blade with his hand, but the bad news was that it ripped open his palm and tore him up pretty good.

A week or so later, long before the injury had healed very much, he decided to go drinking with some friends, trying to unwind. Unfortunately, he ran afoul of another guy who was spoiling for a fight. The bully saw Darrell's injury and hoped to take advantage of his weakness. This other guy was big, maybe even a bit bigger than Darrell, yet he wasn't used to getting up at the crack of dawn, climbing up and down hills through the woods, and wrestling logs for a living. He came on strong, but the fight was short. Using his left, uninjured hand, Darrell picked the other guy up, carried him flailing in the air for half a dozen steps, and tossed him out the door down a flight of stairs.

As the bully found out, it doesn't pay to play the other guy's game. The bully was used to being the stronger guy, throwing his weight around to his best advantage. Unfortunately, he ran across a guy who was not only stronger, but sore, tired, and irritable as well. When you're going to fight a big guy, it doesn't make in sense to face him toe-to-toe. Moving off line, striking at his knees, or otherwise cutting him down to size is not only safer, but far more likely to succeed too.

Jeff, a *nidan* (2nd degree black belt) in karate was a big guy, about 6 feet 3 inches and built like a tank. He was not only skilled and strong, but in extremely good shape too. One day he got into a fender bender on the highway. Both he and the other guy got out of their cars to take a look at the damage. This dude was big too, a lineman who played a starting role on a nationally ranked college football team. Unfortunately, what could have been a civilized exchange was not. Tempers flared and things got physical.

As a karate expert, Jeff thought he could hold his own; after all, he was nearly the same size as the other guy. Much to his surprise, the football player simply grabbed him by the throat and slammed him into the side of the car. And there was nothing that he could do about it. The fight was over almost as soon as it began. What went wrong? Well, the lineman was used to using his weight and his hands to move big, strong, highly skilled guys on the field. Pac-10 college football is a pretty elite group, and this guy could play with the best. Gross physicality was his game, and Jeff stumbled right into it and lost big time.

No matter how big you are, there's always somebody bigger. No matter how strong, there's always somebody stronger. If you're used to playing the big guy game and that's all you've got, you're in for a nasty surprise when you find yourself the smaller or weaker man. If you're going to train to fight, you need to understand both the big guy's and the little guy's role. There are different strategies for each and knowing how to fight in either role is key. While you cannot fight him down the middle if you're overmatched, you can still break him down from the outside. If he's big, fight like a small guy, and vice versa.

The size differential is but one aspect of disparity in a fight. The other has to do with your training and natural tendencies. Here's how it works: Let's say for the sake of argument that you're a striker. Maybe you study karate. While the art of karate encompasses grappling, throwing, pressure points, and submission applications, it's primarily a striking style, attacking with fists, elbows, and open-hand techniques. Maybe you've practiced boxing or are just plain good with your hands. If that's your strength, use it. Karate and boxing are both very solid in-fighting styles. Get close, throw a lot of punches and maybe a short kick or two, and pound the other guy into submission so that you can escape to safety.

Taekwondo practitioners, on the other hand, are very good with their feet. If you're a

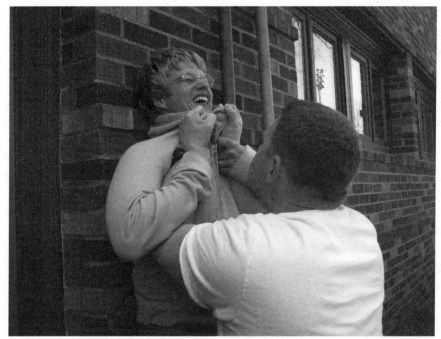

No matter how big you are, there's always somebody bigger. No matter how strong, there's always somebody stronger. Play your game, not the other guy's.

hand striker, tangling up in kicking range would be a recipe for disaster. That's playing to the other guy's strength. You'd need to get in close to take away his range advantage in order to do the most damage with your hand techniques. Similarly, *judoka* and *jujitsu* practitioners will want to go "ground and pound," knocking you down and busting up your joints or choking you into submission. That's their game, not yours. It's very hard to throw an effective punch when you're lying flat on your back with the wind knocked out of you. Watch just about any MMA match and you'll see good examples of that.

It's foolhardy to think that you can overcome an adversary by doing what he's best at. Play your game, not the other guy's.

Don't Use the Wrong Technique for the Situation

When Kane first began training in karate, he was frequently matched up with another practitioner named Mike. They took their training very seriously, often practicing late after class and/or on weekends. Working toward their green belt tests, they repeatedly performed a prearranged tandem sparring drill using techniques from one of the *kata* (forms) that they were supposed to know on the test. One of these sequences called for a front kick toward the groin from one partner, while the other guy turned his body to pull his family jewels off of the line of attack while simultaneously sweeping aside and deflecting the kick with his arm.

Kane and Mike worked this drill for several weeks, quickly reaching a point where they could perform it swiftly and well, or so they thought. One day in class, they had the opportunity to perform this drill with Scott, a visiting black belt. Kane went first. The first time Scott threw the front kick, Kane took a solid strike to the groin, a severely painful and thoroughly embarrassing incident.

He realized that during their friendly practice sessions, he and Mike had subconsciously aimed their kicks away from each other, eliminating the need to seriously block the techniques. Turning their bodies a little was all it took to avoid getting hit by these un-aimed strikes. Since the deflections were relatively unnecessary, they had not been training realistically even though they thought that they had been. The first properly aimed, full-speed blow clearly pointed out that shortcoming. Thankfully, it happened on the practice floor rather than in actual combat on the street.

Kane found out the hard way that there is a big difference between "honoring" your partner's technique and simply letting him do what he wants to unhindered. You don't want to squash your training partners yet if you are too nice you do just as great a disservice. Many martial artists, particularly newer ones, fall into this same trap of thinking that they are training realistically when they are not. Sadly, many discover their shortcomings for the first time when they try something out on the street—clearly not a good idea.

If you expect to do well in a fight, you must examine what you are doing through the lens of an opponent rather than a training partner. The other guy is going to be doing his damnedest to sabotage whatever it is that you want to do. And he wants to hurt you in the process.

Let's say for a moment that you want to restrain him. You cannot just walk up to the other guy and apply a lock or a hold. Well, perhaps you can if he goes along with you, but certainly not if he is an unwilling adversary, so that's the perspective you must take. Grappling techniques require very close proximity and a good set up. No matter how skilled you are, the other guy will smack you upside the head before you can get close enough to try your technique if you don't have a good set-up first.

Throws work the same way. You must maneuver him into a position from which you can imbalance him and then apply the technique. Frequently that's done by striking him to cause pain and disorientation. We oftentimes call this set-up the "blow before the throw," borrowing from internationally renowned martial arts instructor Iain Abernethy who coined the term. This concept of striking to disrupt is critical to street-effective techniques. In fact, the goal ought to be to drop him with your initial blow, applying a lock or hold only when further control is required such as restraining the other guy until the police arrive.

Striking to disrupt and disrupting to strike is a very effective way of breaking through the other guy's defenses in general, not just for facilitating control techniques. If you try to punch him in the face, for example, odds are pretty good that he will block it. Even untrained individuals are instinctively good at protecting their heads; it's in the nature of the human beast. We cover up our "soft bits" instinctually. Stomping on his foot or kicking his ankle first, however, causes his head and hands to follow the pain. He involuntarily looks down and flinches inward. This usually opens up the head shot. So, you strike his foot, disrupting his stance and concentration, and then you use the disruption to gain the opportunity to attack his head.

In this fashion, you can work the other guy's body—striking to disrupt, and then using the temporary disruption for an even better strike. Attacks to the feet, knees, or ankles; slaps to the ears; and assaults to the hands, wrists or elbows are all disruptive strikes that are much easier to achieve than starting off with the core where all his vital areas are. It's really tough to get there directly. With a good disruption, you can follow up with shots to his eyes, throat, solar plexus, groin, and other painful, vital targets.

Notice that these are all striking techniques, the kind of stuff that boxers, *taekwondo* practitioners, and *karateka* like to employ. Hitting someone in a street fight is a good way to retain your mobility. When you are moving and striking, you are much safer than slugging it out in place or rolling around grappling. Although many locks and holds can be applied standing up if you have sufficient training, the majority are most effective when applied to an adversary on the ground. It is simply easier to control the guy's movement or immobilize him that way. The problem is that if you go to the ground in a self-defense situation and your opponent has any friends around, you have put yourself in an extremely vulnerable position.

This means that locks, holds, and throws have limited utility in most street fights. They can certainly be used in the right situations, but by no means universally. Be very sure that the tactical situation warrants such applications before attempting them outside the tournament hall. It's not just going to the ground or constricting your ability to move and escape that you need to worry about. If you have competed in tournaments, you undoubtedly know that many opponents will yield to submission techniques, tapping out before the lock damages their joint or the choke knocks them unconscious. Unfortunately, it rarely works that way on the street. Unlike the competitor who knows he's going to be immediately revived if you choke him out, for example, the other guy will think that his life is on the line and fight for everything he's worth. Consequently, if you attempt a strangulation technique on the street you need very good form and solid control. Expect a wild ride before he collapses or submits.

A black belt in judo, Wilder once tried to subdue a knife-wielding attacker using the classical *hadaka jime* technique from his sport. A so-called "naked" choke because it does not use the other guy's uniform *gi* to strangle him with, this application can readily be applied on the street. While he was able to take the knife away from the bad guy, he simply couldn't knock him out. As a black belt in karate too, he certainly could have pounded the guy yet he was trying to capture and hold him until the police could arrive.

Nevertheless, the bad guy fought like hell and was eventually able to wiggle free and get away. His determination to escape was probably fueled, in part, by an incident that occurred about a week earlier where a would-be car thief named Edward Zanassi was accidentally choked to death by the owner of the vehicle he was trying to steal when the good guy tried to restrain him. The guy Wilder fought may very well have had heard about Zanassi's demise, since it was extensively covered in newspaper and television broadcasts. The news undoubtedly motivated him to fight even harder to break free.

Adrenaline robs you of fine motor coordination in a fight, so you have to keep things simple and direct. Finger locks, for example, are great parlor tricks. Imminently painful, you can latch onto a victim and really make him dance with one, yet they are virtually impossible to pull off in a real fight, particularly when sweat, blood, pepper spray, or other slippery substances are thrown into the mix. While precise grabbing movements are extraordinarily tough, even imprecise ones like grabbing a wrist or hooking a leg can be problematic unless you're highly trained. If you try to get too fancy or precise, you will dramatically hurt your chances for success.

However, gross motor movements, especially those that target vital areas of the adversary's body, work pretty well. Applications on the street just don't work the same as they do in the training hall, in part because you are fighting an adversary who's doing his all-out best to defeat you. It's tough enough to get in a few solid blows without getting thumped yourself; don't compound the mistake by trying the wrong thing.

Avoid Going to the Ground

Now an army is exposed to six several calamities, not arising from natural causes, but from faults for which the general is responsible. These are: …(3) collapse…
– Sun Tzu

When the fight comes, always endeavor to chase the enemy around to your left side. Chase him towards awkward places and try to keep him with his back to awkward places. When the enemy gets into an inconvenient position, do not let him look around, but conscientiously chase him around and pin him down.
– Miyamoto Musashi

Avoid going to the ground in a fight. The ground is where you can easily get stomped, kicked, and maimed, if not outright killed. If you land on the ground, get up as fast as you can. Grapplers will tell you that submission techniques, or "ground and pound," are great means to end a fight. They are absolutely correct, in the tournament ring. On the street however, they are flat-out wrong.

Going to the ground in a real fight puts you in a position where your adversary can easily

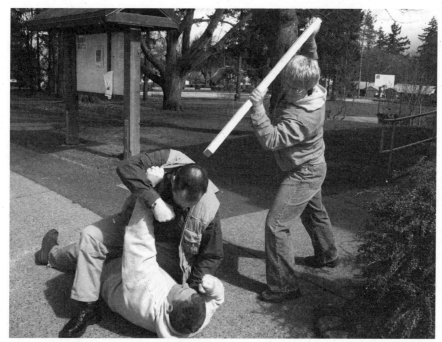

Going to the ground in a real fight puts you in a position where your adversary and/or his friends can stomp a mud-hole in you. It's a very precarious place to be.

stomp a mud-hole in you. Even if he chooses not to do so or drops down with you to grapple, his buddies will most likely put the boots to you. Or his girlfriend will. Either way, you are in dire straits; the ground is a very bad place to be.

Sitting in a bar one day Wilder watched a conversation between two men at an adjoining table grow in intensity. As they argued, these men sat side by side, turned slightly toward each other. One of them was wearing a white t-shirt. Without any telegraphing of his intensions, white t-shirt guy suddenly reached up behind the other man's head and grabbed a wad of hair. Grip secured, he stood up and jerked the other guy down to the floor.

In the one deft motion, the other guy went down hard. Mr. T-shirt spread both hands out, supporting his weight between two tables, and swiftly kicked the other guy six or seven times in the face. Before anyone could react, he launched himself forward and ran from the bar.

The elapsed time for the entire fight was, perhaps, four or five seconds. By the time it was over, the other guy probably needed serious dental work and definitely needed stitches. This is a good example of the how going to the ground will get you stomped.

And if you think you want to be doing the stomping, like white t-shirt guy, listen up. One of our students came into the *dojo* one night and told us the story of a fight at his high

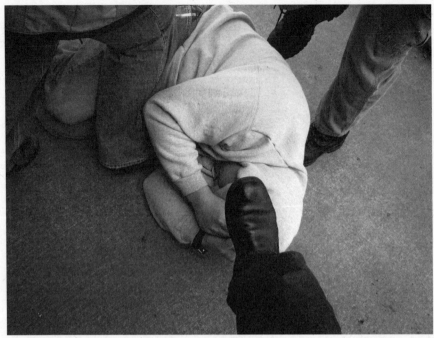

The only people who can safely go to the ground in a real fight are police officers, security personnel, and other people who work in highly trained, well-coordinated teams. For most civilians, it's an invitation to a boot party with you as the guest of honor.

school. When one student hit the ground, the other guy managed to remain standing. He used this advantage to kick his fallen opponent viciously several times in the head hard enough to dislocate the other kid's eye. His kicks actually crushed the bone in the side of the other kid's head, collapsed the eye socket, and popped out the eyeball.

The kid who did the kicking, oh, he had been in trouble before, in and out of juvenile detention several times in his young life. This particular fight happened just after his eighteenth birthday, however, so his reality shifted a bit. Suddenly he faced aggravated assault charges; cooling his heels with other incarcerated adults until his trial. He enjoyed Thanksgiving, Christmas, and New Years in jail. He not only missed his high school graduation but also faced a five- to seven-year prison term. Try to get a decent job with no high school diploma, or rent an apartment after you have checked the yes box that is on every apartment rental application where it asks, "Have you ever been convicted of a felony?"

Working stadium security, Kane has helped break up hundreds of fights. In his experience, combatants tend to go to the ground about 30 percent of the time, not counting situations where one person falls and the other stands over him while continuing to attack like white t-shirt guy or felony student have done. The most severe injuries he has seen occurred when two guys became enjoined in a wrestling contest and then one or the other's friends weighed into the battle. Kicks to the head are brutal. They are vicious, bloody, and extremely dangerous. You really do not want to be the recipient of one.

Ever seen the victim of a Berkeley stomp? That's when a guy, usually someone who pops off verbally to the wrong person, is shoved up against a curb with his mouth wrapped around the cement. He is then kicked in the head, fracturing the jaw and knocking out his teeth. It's ugly. Perhaps not quite as bad as having your eyeball popped out from the force of a blow, but ugly enough that it is clearly something you will want to avoid.

The only people who can safely go to the ground in a real fight are police officers, security personnel, and other people who work in highly trained, well coordinated teams. As one or more officers take down, control, and restrain the subject, the rest secure the perimeter so that they will not be overly vulnerable during the process. Unless you are a skilled professional working with an experienced team, the ground is a dangerous place to be, one best avoided if at all possible.

> Submission grappling works great in the ring, but not so well on the street. If you are on the ground, you are vulnerable. You can easily get stomped, kicked, and seriously messed up by your adversary. If you become tied up while wrestling, your opponent's friends might put the boots to you as well. Unless you are a skilled professional working with an experienced team, the ground is a dangerous place to be, one best avoided if at all possible.

Don't Let the Other Guy Get Behind You

When you leave your own country behind, and take your army across neighborhood territory, you find yourself on critical ground. When there are means of communication on all four sides, the ground is one of intersecting highways.

— *Sun Tzu*

Stand in the sun; that is, take up an attitude with the sun behind you. If the situation does not allow this, you must try to keep the sun on your right side. In buildings, you must stand with the entrance behind you or to your right. Make sure that your rear is unobstructed, and that there is free space on your left, your right side being occupied with your sword attitude.

— *Miyamoto Musashi*

It was going to be a great night. Motorhead was in town and Wilder and his buddy James were going to the show. Of course, nobody expects a kindergarten game of hopscotch at a heavy metal concert, but this was going to be different. You see the club that was hosting the band opened the bar at 7:00 P.M., yet Motorhead wouldn't take the stage until about 11:00. You do the math; that's a lot of drinking time. Oh, and to add to it, several bars were just across the street and down the block.

By the time the band started to play, the booze-fueled crowd was ready. There was slam dancing, puking, and so many ejections from the show that Wilder lost count. A flicked cigarette landed on Lemmy's (the bass player and singer) set list and it caught on fire, the equipment was not sounding right, and the band left the stage until everything could be fixed. As you might expect, this interruption in the middle of the show added the proverbial fuel to the fire. By the time things got going again, the crowd was in a very rowdy mood.

The bartenders handed out Ziploc baggies of ice to bruised patrons. Down front against the rail was sheer combat, as Wilder quickly found out. The guy behind him suddenly decided that Wilder had his space and was ready to fight to get it back. Wilder, in turn, was not keen on giving up the spot. Nudges turned to pushes, to shoves, to blows. Wilder was sober, heavier, and had some martial arts skills. The other guy was drunk, stupid, and felt no pain. Sort of an even match in an odd way... Ultimately, however, Wilder was able to put enough hurt on the other guy to make him back down. He didn't crush him because he wanted to watch the show rather than go to jail, yet he did make the other guy stop trying to fight and disappear back into the crowd.

At the end of the show, Wilder was confident that the pushy guy would be back, however, most likely with friends. Moving through the crowd at the end of the show would place him at risk, since he didn't know what the other guy's friends looked like. He didn't like the idea of being exposed on all sides, so Wilder turned and put his back to the stage, leaning against the rail. He now only had to sweep 180 degrees to spot any potential danger, not try to look across a full 360.

As the crowd dwindled, a young guy broke from the throng and started toward Wilder. Wilder watched him warily and adjusted his stance. The younger guy stopped, held up his hands, and said, "Thanks man, that guy was an asshole. He was hitting everybody."

"Oh, okay," Wilder replied, "You seen him around?"

"No I think he left," the kid said.

Assuming that would be a good time to leave, Wilder moved deliberately and swiftly through the residual crowd, heading for the door, up the stairs, and out to the street. Two separate fights were going on when he got outside. These altercations attracted a lot of attention as the bouncers dragged combatants apart and told them to get off their sidewalk.

Moving away from the fights, Wilder placed his back against the brick building near the band's tour bus and waited for his buddy James to show up. The bus screened him from the street while the wall protected his back. Luckily, the pushy guy never showed up. Either he'd forgotten all about the confrontation, was scared off by Wilder's preparedness, or lost track of his intended victim. Consequently, instead of having to fight as Wilder had feared, he got to meet Phil Campbell, the band's guitarist instead. Campbell had to take his arm down from around one of the blonde groupies in order to shake Wilder's hand, but that's not really the point.

The point is that nothing bad happened as a result of the altercation because Wilder protected his back. Don't let anybody get behind you if you can help it. That's not entirely possible in a crowd, however, so in such settings you need to keep your awareness level high.

One of the best tactics you can use during a fight is to get behind your adversary. Humans are really good at perceiving and responding to danger that is in front of them. With a bit of training, we can become pretty good at defending against attacks from either side, yet we are really lousy at dealing with dangers coming from directly behind. If you are behind the other guy or tucked a bit to the side in behind his shoulder, it's very hard for him to reach you, yet you can strike with impunity, delivering one or two solid blows before he can reposition himself to respond effectively.

In part, this is because humans cannot see directly behind themselves without adjusting to face the threat. It's nearly impossible to block an attack from behind you either. Dodging is often the best option. Further, there are only a limited number of counterattacks that you can launch to the rear, stuff like back kicks, and reverse elbow strikes, and reverse head butts. It's even tougher if someone manages to tuck himself behind your shoulder where your only option is an elbow strike.

Consequently, if you're behind the other guy you're very well positioned to strike and/or escape. Conversely, if he's behind you, you're in a lot of trouble. Don't let the other guy get behind you in a fight. It's a losing proposition.

Fighting is Not a Democratic Process

All warfare is based on deception.
> *– Sun Tzu*

Always chase the enemy into bad footholds, obstacles at the side, and so on, using the virtues of the place to establish predominant positions from which to fight. You must research and train diligently in this.
> *– Miyamoto Musashi*

Fighting is not a democratic process. There is no exchange of ideas here, no 'I'm going to hit you first and then let you think about it a bit before it becomes your turn to hit me.' Hopefully, there is no exchanging of strikes at all. Street fighting is about physically beating your opponent down as rapidly as possible and escaping the scene. No hanging out, no going back.

Modern warfare works pretty much that way too. When it comes to one-on-one aircraft dogfights, for example, they simply don't exist in the modern world. The entangled maneuvering from World War I and II flying aces, or the tricky choreography from movies like *Top Gun* really don't happen anymore. This is because the pilot that can identify an enemy first, from the farthest distance possible, is at the greatest advantage. Because modern technologies let pilots identify potential targets from miles away, there is no longer a need to spot an enemy up close or fight in visual range.

The modern strategy is to spot the enemy before he sees you, strike first, and kill him before he even knows you are there. It really is more of an assassination than a fight. There is no sizing each other up, maneuvering for position, and exchanging blows. In fact, it is a lot like the bad karate school in the movie *The Karate Kid*. They would yell their motto, "Strike first, strike hard, and show no mercy." That pretty much sums up a real fight. Combatants gain advantage, use their lead, and unrelentingly attack until it's over. Not very democratic at all.

> Humans are really good at perceiving and responding to dangers in front of them and to a lesser degree from either side. Unfortunately, we are really lousy at dealing with dangers coming from directly behind. Consequently, if the other guy gets behind you he can strike with impunity, delivering at least one or two solid blows before you can reposition yourself to respond effectively.

Here's a real life example: A high school football game went badly for Wilder's team. The game started poorly and tempers escalated throughout the competition. The officiating was poor, the coaches got mad, and the fans in the stands were irate. By the end of the game, most everyone was furious.

Players began pushing and shoving each other. Name-calling escalated the tension to the point where the two teams stopped in the parking lot on the way back to their respective locker rooms. A fight was clearly about to begin. Before we describe what happened, it's important to point out that if you have ever played football you know that taking your helmet off on the field is a foolish thing to do. With all the pads you wear (for example, shoulder, forearm, hip, knee), exposing your head by taking off your helmet is much like asking to get hit in the face. It's the easiest unprotected area to strike.

You'd think the same rule would apply in the parking lot, but not so. Darren, Wilder's team's defensive captain, took off his helmet, held it by the facemask, and swung it right into the temple of another guy's helmet. That blow buckled the other guy's knees, sending him reeling. Suddenly the rest of the fight was on.

After a few minutes, the fight was broken up, ending everything but the name-calling, but Wilder learned an important lesson in the process. While everybody "knew" that taking your helmet off was an invitation to get hit, Darren saw his helmet as a weapon. He broke the rules as everyone else understood them. He came up with an unconventional approach, struck first, and did not allow a response from the other guy.

Most fights work this same way. When the other guy attacks, he will employ surprise and cheat to win, perhaps utilizing a weapon. He will bend the rules as much as possible to gain advantage. No, fighting is not a democratic process.

Don't Self Destruct

Now the general who wins a battle makes many calculations in his temple ere the battle is fought. The general who loses a battle makes but few calculations.

beforehand. Thus do many calculations lead to victory and few calculations to defeat: how much more no calculation at all! It is by attention to this point that I can foresee who is likely to win or lose.
                                                            — *Sun Tzu*

Some of the world's strategists are concerned only with sword fencing, and limit their training to flourishing the long sword and carriage of the body. But is dexterity alone sufficient to win? This is not the essence of the Way.
                                                  — *Miyamoto Musashi*

Wilder's judo instructor, a two-time national grand champion back in the 1950s, had a simple mantra when it came to fighting. Kenji's principle was, "If you have a position that is not the best or not the one you want, stay with it anyway until your opponent gives you something better. Don't go looking for a better position. Wait until he gives you one."

Keeping what you've got until something better comes along is sound advice not only for sport, but for street fighting as well. If, for example, you grasp the other guy's arm, keep it. Use it to control him until he gives up something better, say, his head. Neck cranks are much better for takedowns and control techniques than arm locks or throws, yet they are also much harder to get without the other guy doing something stupid first. Sure, you can trick him, of course, but don't force things you can't naturally get.

Forcing techniques is dangerous. Your opponent will be doing his damnedest to beat you down, so do your best not to let him win. Keep things simple and straightforward and you won't self-destruct. Don't get stupid. Don't get too smart for your own good, trying fancy or flashy techniques.

> If you meet a jet fighter pilot today and ask him if he has ever been in a dogfight like the movie *Top Gun*, the answer is most likely going to be "No." With today's technology, the real fight is about spotting and destroying the enemy before he even knows that you are there. Acquire the enemy first, strike first, and never let him know what hit him. It really is more of an assassination than a fight. Not a very democratic exchange of blows, now, is it? Well, aerial combat is not democratic and neither is street fighting.

This is important whenever you practice martial arts. What gets trained gets done, so if you practice for a fight, you need to do so realistically. Sadly, many folks, even veteran police officers, fail to do so. In his outstanding book *On Combat*, Loren Christensen described what can happen when you bake in bad habits through repeated, unrealistic practice.

> *One police officer gave another example of learning to do the wrong thing. He took it upon himself to practice disarming an attacker. At every opportunity, he would have his wife, a friend, or a partner hold a pistol on him so he could practice snatching it away. He would snatch the gun, hand it back, and repeat several more times. One day he and his partner responded to an unwanted man in a convenience store. He went down one aisle, while his partner went down*

another. At the end of the first aisle, he was taken by surprise when the suspect stepped around the corner and pointed a revolver at him. In the blink of an eye, the officer snatched the gun away, shocking the gunman with his speed and finesse. No doubt this criminal was surprised and confused even more when the officer handed the gun right back to him, just as he had practiced hundreds of times before. Fortunately for this officer, his partner came around the corner and shot the subject.

Whatever is drilled in during training comes out the other end in combat. In one West Coast city, officers training in defensive tactics used to practice an exercise in such a manner that it could have eventually been disastrous in a real life-and-death situation. The trainee playing the arresting officer would simulate a gun by pointing his finger at the trainee playing the suspect, and give him verbal commands to turn around, place his hands on top of his head, and so on. This came to a screeching halt when officers began reporting to the training unit that they had pointed with their fingers in real arrest situations. They must have pantomimed their firearms with convincing authority because every suspect had obeyed their commands. Not wanting to push their luck, the training unit immediately ceased having officers simulate weapons with their fingers and ordered red-handled dummy guns to be used in training.

As you can see by these examples, it's very easy to train yourself physically or mentally to self destruct. Visualization exercises can be an important aspect of your training. As with hands-on practice, you need to conduct your mental exercises realistically and with solid forethought. Plan to succeed and don't hinder yourself with destructive practice.

If you use visualization exercises, be sure to only see perfection in your mind's eye. If necessary, elongate the component movements of your techniques as you think about them, breaking things down into small enough pieces to imagine doing each one flawlessly, even it takes significantly longer than a real-life performance. It is okay to imagine doing things in slow motion until you feel comfortable that you have captured all the important nuances properly. Once you are confident that you have covered everything important, increase the speed at which you see yourself performing in your mind.

> The other guy will be doing everything he can to win in a fight. Don't make his job any easier. Don't get too smart for your own good, trying fancy or flashy techniques. Keep things simple and direct so that you won't self-destruct.

The other guy will be doing everything he can to win. Don't make his job easier. Keep things simple and direct, using techniques you are good at and comfortable with. Practice realistically, both mentally and physically. Don't self destruct!

You Will Get Hurt

What the ancients called a clever fighter is one who not only wins, but excels in winning with ease.

— Sun Tzu

You should not speak of strong and weak long swords. If you just wield the long sword in a strong spirit your cutting will become coarse, and if you use the sword coarsely you will have difficulty in winning.

– Miyamoto Musashi

Wilder and his friend Kim had gone down the hill toward the river to visit with a bum who had been camping out in the area. Wilder remembers standing there wide-eyed in wonderment as the old bum and intermittent jailbird explained how to put a sharpened screwdriver or toothbrush into an unsuspecting fellow inmate. "You stick 'em in the butt, right about here," he said. "That way the leg doesn't work so well and he can't run from you."

You may be thinking fistfight but that doesn't necessarily mean that the other guy is too. Knives, guns, bludgeons, beer bottles, and a host of other nasty tools may be in your adversary's arsenal. Think about that old jailbird's advice. It's chilling to think that he was counseling eleven-year-olds how to ambush someone in a fashion that ensured that the victim couldn't escape until they'd be able to kill him. Sadly, that attitude isn't really all that uncommon.

Whenever you fight, you are almost certainly going to get hurt, even if you don't run up against a psychotic foe. It's unavoidable if the battle lasts more than a few seconds. The real question is how bad you will get hurt. If he's armed and you're not, the damage will almost certainly be severe. If he's bigger, faster, or stronger than you are, or he's got friends that join in, it's all bad. Remember, if he's attacking, he thinks he can win and is probably cheating in some way in order to do so.

Take this example: most young men carry pocketknives these days. Many are willing to use them on you, either because they don't fully appreciate the consequences of their actions or, in some cases, because they are too furious to care. Then again, they may just be a sociopath like that old jailbird.

Knives are great tools, yet they automatically bump the encounter up from simple assault to aggravated assault or possibly even murder. Use one on another human being without just cause and you'll undoubtedly spend a whole lot of quality time in prison, yet your average street punk isn't thinking that far ahead. He's reacting to the emotions of the situation, paying attention solely to the encounter he's in, right here, right now. In other words, all he cares about is defeating you, no matter how he has to go about doing it.

The vast majority of people who carry a knife have never used it as anything other than a tool for slicing fruit, opening envelopes, cutting down boxes, or similar routine endeavors. They have never hurt another human being with their blade. They have never seen what the smallest amount of blood can do, how the smallest amount of blood can make them lose their grip on the knife, slip on the floor, or lose their lunch down the

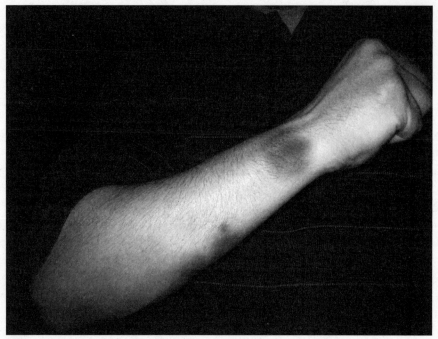

If all you got was a few bruises on your arms after the fight, you did just fine. Unfortunately, most street fights don't end quite so pleasantly, even for the victor.

drain. Unfortunately, they don't need any experience, special skills, or extraordinary intelligence to hurt someone bad with that knife. Heck, most any sharp object will do.

Think for a moment about the type of person it takes to truly want to stick you with his knife, the guy who looks forward to ambushing you with a blade. Premeditated attacks are even worse than unhampered rage. Here's why: knives are very intimate weapons. That means that if you're facing the pointy end, the guy holding it either hates you with a white-hot passion or is totally out of his mind with fury and/or terror.

There is no reasoning with someone who is fully prepared to become drenched in your blood and viscera, to smell your bowels as they release, and to hear your cries for help as they fade to whimpers of pain and finally to the rattling gurgle of your last breath. If you are facing someone like this, he is ready, willing, and able to cut you as many times as it takes, to stab you as deep and as often as necessary to finish the job he has in mind. That kind of guy is real damn scary, be he a big brawny biker or skinny little computer geek. The blade makes them both deadly.

Fighting should be avoided whenever possible because you simply cannot predict the chaos and mayhem that comes along with it. If a knife or other weapon enters the fight, experience says that you are not very likely to see it before you have already been hurt. You will get hurt and you may get hurt very, very badly.

It's hard for many people to visualize dying in a fight. Because of this, the threat of death isn't really much of a deterrent for most young men. Visualize instead spending the rest of your life maimed, crippled, or grossly disfigured, confined to a bed or a wheelchair. Think about all the things you'll never do and the places you'll never see in such a condition.

Although all violence is bad, armed assaults are far more dangerous to the victim than unarmed ones. Sadly, ordinary citizens are victimized an average of 1,773,000 times per year by weapon-wielding thugs in the United States alone. While crimes of non-lethal violence committed with or without weapons were about equally likely to result in victim injury, armed assaults are three-and-a-half times as likely as unarmed encounters to result in serious damage to the victim, such as broken bones, internal injuries, loss of consciousness, or similar trauma resulting in extended hospitalization. Worse still, 96 percent of all homicides involve some type of weapon.

Because you are going to get hurt, it is prudent to end the fight as quickly as possible to minimize the damage. This means that if you cannot avoid fighting altogether, your initial response needs to place you in control of the momentum. You need to keep from getting hit, stop the other guy from continuing to strike, and do it in as few moves as possible. Once you have dealt with the immediate threat, your next move needs to cross him up, destroy his balance, or knock him on his ass. If he's got a weapon, your response should be, if not fatal, at least severely disabling.

> When you fight, you are almost certainly going to get hurt. It's unavoidable if the battle lasts more than a few seconds. The real question is how bad it will be. If he's armed and you're not, the damage will be quite severe. It's in your enlightened self-interest, therefore, to avoid fighting when possible and when it's not, end confrontations as quickly as possible. Your initial response needs to place you in control of the momentum. If he's got a weapon, it should be severely disabling if not fatal.

Recognize Your Own Limitations

He will win who, prepared himself, waits to take the enemy unprepared.
— *Sun Tzu*

It is difficult to know yourself if you do not know others.
— *Miyamoto Musashi*

There was an amusing scene on *The Drew Carey Show* where the star was challenged to a fight in a bar. Always the comedian, Carey responded, "Okay I'll fight you, but I am going to have to kill you quick since I'm out of shape." That's an entertaining response, yet it has some bearing in real life. It's important to recognize your limitations and account for them as you strategize the way in which you will fight.

Limitation comes in two flavors: inherent and manufactured. Inherent limitations are then broken into two more categories: mental and physical. Physical limitations are a hard wall to hit. You can work out in the gym to become stronger, practice speed drills to become faster, or perform aerobic exercise to build your endurance, yet you cannot get around your natural genetic limitations. Some people, for example, are blessed with an abundance of fast-twitch muscles. If you are not that lucky, you will never be as fast as someone who is, yet you can train yourself to become as fast as your body is capable of being. Some people are tall while others are short. You cannot change how you are born; you can only make the most of what you've got.

The more you are involved in a physical activity, the more in touch you are going to be with your body. Physical activities like aerobics, weightlifting, yoga, or martial arts, or tough jobs like logging or construction give you a contact with your body that is beneficial. It helps you understand what you're physically capable of.

Following the completion of the physical aptitude test battery, Coach Garner stated firmly, "The

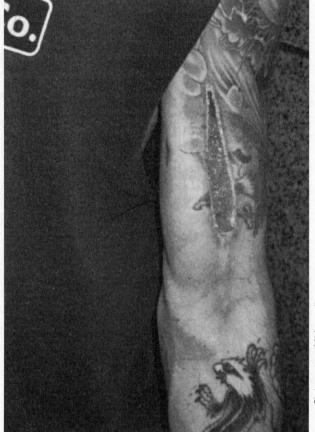

Photo courtesy of Al Arsenault

The presence of a weapon changes everything. There is no reasoning with someone who is fully prepared to become drenched in your blood and viscera, to smell your bowels as they release, and to hear your cries for help as they fade to whimpers of pain and finally to the rattling gurgle of your last breath.

vertical jump is the one single best test of athletic ability." He looked at his clipboard, "Wilder, you better wrestle. Don't even think about basketball." That direct, blunt, and very honest comment set Wilder on the path of wresting, judo, and football, and has held his martial arts training in good stead. He simply doesn't have the right body type to excel at certain other sports like basketball.

In some ways, the mental game is even tougher than the physical. There is a saying that goes "Fatigue makes cowards of us all." There are moments in all these sports where you want to say, "Get me off the mat." You can choose to win or lose at that point, whatever it takes to get it over with. Then the limitation turns to mental.

Have you ever been hit so hard that you lost control of your body? Have you ever had to run away from something as fast as you could for as long as you could? Such things transcend the mere physical to become significant mental challenges. Surviving a fight is often more of a mental issue than a physical one.

Look at members of the military, especially specialists in their field. These guys are well-conditioned athletes yet they are not bodybuilders. They may not be exceptionally big or strong yet they simply do not quit. Quitting isn't even in their vocabulary. It turns into a mental attitude of "I will never quit." As an example of this attitude, here are some United States military groups and their mottos:

- The 2nd Battalion 7th Marines: *Ready For All, Yielding To None*
- The 1st Marine Division, USMC: *Mors De Contactus (Death on Contact)*
- The 1st Recon Battalion: *Celer – Silens – Mortali (Swift-Silent-Deadly)*

Wilder sat across from a former Army Supply Officer Joe one day. Joe told him how he had deep respect for the specialists in the military. Wilder asked, "They must be physical monsters, super soldiers, and weightlifters. Real tough, right?" "No," Joe said. "They are not defined by that. They are defined by the fact that they don't quit... ever. They *never* quit." He went on to talk about a friend of his that really wanted to be in this special elite military group, but during the training session he fractured his leg, not badly, but enough to have him wash out. He was going to have to wait until next year to attempt to qualify again, or so the manual read. Joe's friend was stopped trying to leave the medical center with his fractured leg. His intent was to rejoin the training session; he was not going to quit.

If you'd like to get a deeper appreciation of what elite force training is truly like, we suggest you pick up a copy of *Lone Survivor: The Eyewitness Account of Operation Redwing and the Lost Heroes of SEAL Team 10* by Marcus Lutrell (and Patrick Robinson). While much of the book focuses on a failed attempt to capture or kill a notorious al Qaeda leader in 2005, it also delves into the rigorous training that helped Lutrell forge the mental and physical fortitude necessary to survive being blasted unconscious by a rocket-propelled grenade, blown over a cliff, and left for dead. He had to fight off a group of Taliban assassins who were sent to finish him and then crawl seven miles through sheer mountains with a broken back before he was taken in by Pashtun tribesmen who risked their lives to protect him from the encircling killers. It's a true story and a thrilling read that gives you great appreciation for the kind of mental conditioning elite forces develop and what that makes them capable of enduring.

Many people are aware of their physical limitation, at least to some degree, yet few are truly aware of what they are mentally capable of until put to the test in a life-threatening struggle. We hope you will not have to take that test, yet a "never quit" attitude can pull you through nearly anything you are physically capable of handling.

For example, during a routine hike in 2003, Aaron Ralston suddenly found himself in dire straights when an 800-pound boulder shifted unexpectedly and pinned his wrist to a canyon wall in a remote area of Canyonlands National Park in Utah. After six days of captivity, he realized that desperate measures were needed for survival. Using a cheap, dull pocketknife, he managed to amputate his own arm, rappel one-handed down a hill, and then hike six miles through the wilderness before someone found and rescued him. This extraordinary tale of survival shows what a sufficiently motivated person is capable of doing.

Manufactured limitations are important too. It is good to know what you are wearing on your feet for example. Cowboy boots are not the same as a pair of running shoes when it comes to footing; poor traction limits you in a fight. Tight fitting jeans restrict your range of movement in ways that cargo pants do not. A heavy meal recently consumed can adversely affect your performance as can a steady diet of hamburgers, fries, and other unhealthy foods.

> Limitations can be mental or physical, inherent or manufactured. Knowing your limitations helps you find creative means for achieving your goals. Surviving a fight is often more of a mental issue than a physical one. Seek out your limits and know them.

Knowing your physical limitations helps you find creative ways achieving your goals. Knowing your physical strengths gives you ways to resolve situations. Seek out your limits, and know them. Ask your closest friends to speak to you about your weaknesses and limitations, your boss, you family, just as Wilder's high school coach did for him, and then audit yourself. Find the one thing you'd like to improve and work on it; drill it just as you would drill it in the weight room. Once you have progressed sufficiently, set it aside and work on another. Improvement is a continuous process.

You May Think, "My Enemy's Enemy is My Friend," But It's Not True

To secure ourselves against defeat lies in our own hands.
— Sun Tzu

When it is difficult to cut an enemy down either one hand, you must use both hands.

— Miyamoto Musashi

The idea that someone else is going to join you in a fight out of the goodness of his heart or because he simply doesn't like the other guy too is about as dumb an idea as they come. Even in a clear-cut case of self-defense, an honest-to-God crisis that can affect everyone around you, you simply cannot count on others to get involved. People tend to act in their own self-interest. Why help you if they might get hurt, jailed, or killed too? Some people will, yet most won't.

For example, there was a fairly dramatic incident on US Airways flight 78 from Phoenix to Seattle during the final approach in June 2007. An unruly passenger fought with flight attendants and tried to open an over-wing escape hatch, something that would have depressurized and crashed the plane had he been successful. At first, no one came forward to intervene. Then, despite pleas from his girlfriend not to, off-duty Benton County Sheriff's Deputy Doug Stanley decided he needed to step into the situation. After trying unsuccessfully to calm the man down, Stanley then physically subdued and restrained him until the aircraft landed safely. By way of thanks, the airline awarded him two free tickets to anywhere he wanted to travel and a model airplane featuring an inscription that reads, "Our Hero."

Let's say for a moment that you get into a confrontation with some other guy at your favorite drinking hole, a far less significant incident than the one on the airplane. If a fight ensues, are you really going to trust someone else that you have never met before, some guy whose name you don't even know to guard your back? You can't and you shouldn't.

Plan on being on your own if things get physical. If you're not positive that you can handle the situation yourself, you had better look it over again. The idea of being on your own should make you think twice about fighting. Don't trust others to help; don't depend on them even if they are your longtime friends. Most people intuitively know that fighting has consequences. Some guys will join in so long as there is strength in numbers where others will bail out at the first sign of conflict.

Good Samaritans who may be drawn to your aid could just as easily be frightened away over concern for their own personal safety. You simply cannot count on receiving any help unless they are people whose job it is to act, such as emergency services personnel and law enforcement officers like Deputy Stanley. In fact, the presence of bystanders can be good, bad, or neutral. They may be inclined to help you but could just as easily ignore your plight.

For example, on September 23, 2002 at least ten people allegedly saw 18-year-old Rachel Burkheimer bound and gagged, lying on the floor of an Everett (Washington) garage shortly before she was taken out into the woods and murdered. None of them stopped to help. None of them even called the police. Legally, none of them had to. Many people simply will not get involved, even in cases of life or death.

Interestingly enough, the more bystanders present, the more likely it is that people will assume that someone else has called for help or that someone else will intervene. And the larger number of bystanders, the less obligated each is likely to feel that he has an imperative to do so. A person by himself cannot assume that someone else is responsible for taking action and do nothing.

> Plan on being on your own if things get physical. If you're not positive that you can handle the situation yourself, you had better look it over again. The idea of being on your own should make you think twice about fighting. Don't trust others to help; don't depend on them. People tend to act in their own self-interest. Why help you if they might get hurt, jailed, or killed in the process? Some people will, yet most won't.

Anyone who did not see an incident from the beginning may also be unsure about what is going on. Who is the bad guy and who is the victim? To the extent that we are unsure about what is going on or the situation is ambiguous, we are more likely to look

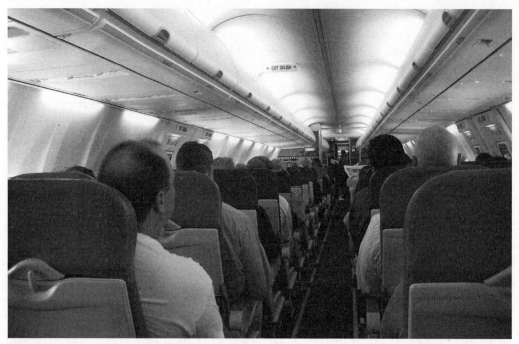

An unruly passenger fought with flight attendants and tried to open an over-wing escape hatch to depressurize the plane. At first, no one came forward to intervene. Then, despite pleas from his girlfriend not to, off-duty Sheriff's Deputy Doug Stanley decided he needed to step in to control the situation. You cannot expect others to help you in a fight, even where it makes sense that they should.

to others for help in defining whether intervention is appropriate or necessary. If others do not get involved, we may decide that whatever is happening does not require our assistance. That is one reason why first aid/CPR students are taught to look a specific person in the eye, describe the emergency, and tell that person to dial 9-1-1 for assistance.

Many people try to avoid showing outward signs of worry or concern until they see that others are alarmed as well. After all it would be quite embarrassing to be worked up about something everyone considers a non-event. This sort of caution encourages bystanders to appear nonchalant about a potential emergency, inhibiting everyone's urge to help. The larger the number of people who appear unconcerned about a situation, the stronger that inhibiting influence will be on everyone else, a cycle that feeds upon itself.

The converse of this is also true. The more people who appear alarmed the more likely that someone would decide to intervene. We saw that on United Airlines Flight 93 when passengers and crew banded together to fight back against the terrorist hijackers on September 11, 2001.

Bystanders may help, yet they may even be inclined to hurt you, especially if they are friends of your assailant. You cannot count on anyone else to help you out in a fight.

As Stress Goes Up Intelligence Goes Down

Amid confusion and chaos, your array may be without head or tail, yet it will be proof against defeat.

— *Sun Tzu*

As the enemy attacks, attack more strongly, taking advantage of the resulting disorder in his timing to win.

— *Miyamoto Musashi*

When adrenaline hits your system, your ability to think rationally gets reduced, you lose peripheral vision, and your ability to hear is reduced as well. You become tougher and more resilient, yet the downside is that you become a one-task, knuckle-dragging troglodyte.

When Kane took a defensive handgun course several years ago, he was taught to train for handling the survival stress reaction commonly associated with actual combat. To simulate this reaction, students had to do as many pushups as they could as fast as they could for one minute. Immediately after completing the pushups, they sprinted to the parking lot and raced around the building four times, as fast as they could go, covering close to a mile in the process. They then sprinted back into the building and attempted to accurately fire down range under the watchful eye of the instructors.

While Kane could normally hit the bulls-eye of a static paper target much of the time at 25 feet during shooting competitions and always put every shot in the black, the first time he attempted to do so after this "stress test" he missed the paper completely. It was an illuminating experience. Fortunately, he discovered this in training rather than on the street.

The New York Police department did a comprehensive analysis of police-involved shooting incidents, evaluating some 6,000 violent altercations that took place during the 1970s. They found that officers hit their targets roughly a quarter of the time while criminal assailants made about eleven percent of their shots. This study dramatically demonstrated the effects of adrenaline. To look at it another way, highly trained professionals who near universally hit their targets in practice missed 75 percent of their shots during live fire situations. Criminals who presumably had far less experience handling firearms missed 89 percent of the time. Ninety percent of those shootings took place at distances of less than 15 feet.

Not all hits were fatal, of course. During the period of 1970 through 1979, law enforcement officers inflicted ten casualties for every one suffered at the hands of their criminal assailants. In all of the cases investigated, the size, shape, configuration, composition, caliber, and velocity of the bullet was not the preeminent factor in determining who lived or died. Shot placement accuracy was the overarching cause of death (or an injury that was serious enough to end the confrontation), which is clear evidence that adrenal stress must be overcome to survive a street fight.

The more stressed you are through exertion, fear, or desperation, the harder it is to perform. In a violent encounter, your heart rate can jump from 60 or 70 beats per minute (BPM) to well over 200 BPM in less than half a second. Here is how accelerated heart rates can affect you.

> When adrenaline hits your system, your ability to think rationally is greatly reduced. You will suffer degraded motor skills, experience tunnel vision, and may even suffer temporary memory loss too. In essence, you become a one-task, knuckle-dragging troglodyte. Combat breathing techniques can alleviate some, but not all of these symptoms. As stress goes up intelligence goes down.

- For people whose resting heart rate is around 60 to 70 BPM, at around 115 BPM many begin to lose fine motor skills such as finger dexterity, making it difficult to successfully dial a phone, open a lock, or aim a weapon.

- Around 145 BPM most people begin to lose their complex motor skills such as hand-eye coordination, precise tracking movements, or exact timing, making complicated techniques very challenging if not impossible.

- Around 175 BPM most people begin to lose depth perception, experience tunnel vision, and sometimes even suffer temporary memory loss.

- Around 185–220 BPM, many people experience hyper-vigilance, loss of rational thought, and inability to consciously move or react. Without prior training, the vast majority of people cannot function at this stress level.

Breath control techniques can help you recover from the effects of adrenaline to a large degree, though it takes much practice to control your breathing in an actual fight. The preferred breathing method is similar to *ibuki* breathing found in martial arts. Here's how it works: Breathe in through your nose, let the air swirl around in your belly, and then breathe out through your mouth. Break the breath into three components, clearly inhaling, holding, and exhaling with a 4-count pause in between each step. In other words, each cycle of combat breathing includes:

- Inhale for a 4-count.
- Hold for a 4-count.
- Exhale for a 4-count.

This process helps you oxygenate your blood while psychologically calming you during extreme stress. Nevertheless, it's important not to take unnecessary risks. Since it's really tough to focus on more than one thing, escape should be your primary goal. As stress goes up, intelligence goes down.

Beware of Crowds

The host thus forming a single united body is it impossible either for the brave to advance alone, or for the cowardly to retreat alone. This is the art of handling large masses of men.

— *Sun Tzu*

It is better to use two swords rather than one when you are fighting a crowd and especially if you want to take a prisoner.

— *Miyamoto Musashi*

While most violence you need to worry about takes place one-on-one or among small groups, larger clashes can occur. Military engagements and conflicts between nations are beyond the scope of this discourse, yet you may find yourself caught up in a riot or tangling with members of a crowd some day, so we'll briefly discuss how those sorts of things play out.

Mobs are dangerous. Highly emotional, unthinking, unreasonable, and quite likely to erupt into violence, you really don't want to get caught up in one. Crowds can turn into mobs if members become indifferent to laws, choose to disregard authority, or take advantage of the perceived anonymity that a large group can provide and follow instigators into unlawful, disruptive, or violent acts such as a riot. Most riots explode out of an event, things like perceived racial incidents, jury verdicts, rallies, or protests, particularly if agitators stir things up, though they can certainly arise from other causes such as out-of-control celebrations, or even develop spontaneously as well.

Riots don't happen every day though. While it is easy to plan a demonstration, it is somewhat harder to instigate a riot. Nevertheless, anarchists try to do so all the time. Even when they don't, irrational exuberance can turn darn near any large gathering into a riotous mob too, leading to situations where people overturn cars, set fire to buildings, damage property, and harm people. Alcohol and other intoxicants play a critical role as well.

For example, on June 20, 2007 an angry crowd beat a 40-year-old man to death over a slow-speed accident in Austin, Texas. According to police reports, a driver inadvertently bumped a three- or four-year-old girl while driving through a car park near the site of the annual Juneteenth festival, a celebration that commemorates the freeing of American slaves. The driver stopped his car to check on her well-being, discovering that she was scared but not seriously injured.

The passenger, David Rivas Morales, also got out of the car but he was almost

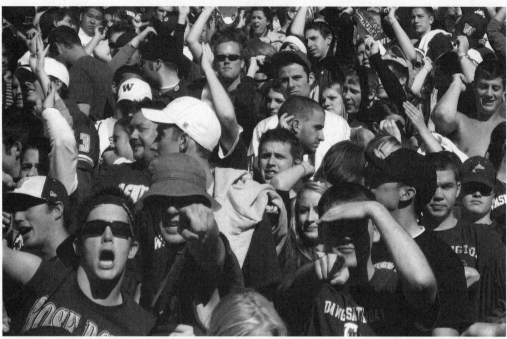

Crowds can turn into mobs if members become indifferent to laws, choose to disregard authority, or take advantage of the perceived anonymity that a large group can provide and follow instigators into unlawful, disruptive, or violent acts such as a riot.

immediately set upon by a group of about 20 people and beaten severely. He collapsed to the ground and was subsequently pronounced dead from blunt force trauma upon arriving at the hospital shortly thereafter. While the girl was shaken up a bit, the man died.

The crowd mindset of being one face among hundreds can be a very dangerous thing. It's quite easy to get caught up in the fray, not truly thinking about what is going on. It can even be fun for those involved, particularly when they don't consider the consequences, an adrenaline rush that rivals any amusement park ride. Consequently, things can get out of hand pretty quickly. When they do, they are very difficult to stop, even once law enforcement officers arrive to take control.

According to Loren Christensen, there are five psychological influences that affect rioters, their targets, and the police who try to break things up. These include (1) impersonality, (2) anonymity, (3) suggestion/imitation, (4) emotional contagion, and (5) discharge of repressed emotions. Here's a brief summary of how these factors play out.

1. Impersonality – So-called "groupthink" is an impersonalizing factor that makes it easier for people to lash out. Rioters do not see their victims as individuals with families, hopes and dreams, but rather as objects on which to vent their

rage. Impersonality makes it easier to attack victims because of their race, ethnicity, gender, sexual orientation, religion or any other factors that set them apart from the mob.

2. Anonymity – The large mass and short life of a mob tends to make many of its members feel anonymous and faceless. Participants can more easily convince themselves to act without conscience, believing that the moral responsibility for their behavior belongs to the entire group. Consequently, in their own minds they are not responsible for their actions.

3. Suggestion/imitation – The massiveness of a mob discourages many of its members to act as individuals, making them more susceptible to follow others like a bunch of lemmings diving over a cliff. There is a powerful instinct to follow the crowd. Only those with deeply ingrained convictions are strong enough to repulse this urge.

4. Emotional contagion – The size of the mob and its activities generates a building emotion that can be felt by each member of the mob. It is a powerful influence. Often called "collective emotion," even bystanders can be caught up in this wave and soon find themselves involved with the mob.

5. Discharge of repressed emotions – As a result of the other four influences listed above, certain individuals feel a sense of freedom to discharge any repressed emotions they harbor. They are free to release pent-up rage, hate, revenge, or a need to destroy, acting out accordingly.

> Mobs are dangerous. Highly emotional and unthinking, they often erupt into violence. Crowds can turn into mobs if members become indifferent to laws, choose to disregard authority, or take advantage of the perceived anonymity that a large group can provide and follow instigators into unlawful, disruptive, or violent acts. Five psychological influences—impersonality, anonymity, suggestion/imitation, emotional contagion, and discharge of repressed emotions—affect rioters, their targets, and the police who try to break things up. If you stumble across a violent crowd, your goal should be to escape to safety, remaining anonymous, and avoiding as much of the conflict as possible in the process.

The good news is that these psychological influences don't impact everyone. The bad news is that the minority of those who are influenced can cause serious confusion, destruction, and injury for everyone else. Because riots can be hard to predict and even harder to stop, it is prudent to pay careful attention to what is going on around you whenever you are part of a large crowd. Even if you sense the mood change, catch a glimpse of the opening acts, and see what's coming, it can be very hard to force your way through the press of bodies and escape to safety.

A panicked crowd is just a dangerous, if not more so, than a riotous mob. When someone believes that there is imminent danger and flees in panic, his actions can spark fear in others who act accordingly. This fear can be initiated by actions from others, such as setting off a bomb or discharging a firearm, and may be exacerbated by environmental factors, such as flooding, smoke, fire, or tear gas. It gets even worse if there are limited escape routes, blocked exits, or other factors that lead to desperation where people begin fighting each other to clear a path so that they can get away. Think about all the people who have been crushed to death at nightclubs, concerts, or sporting events when crowds got out of control.

In general, there are two divergent goals when it comes to dealing with riotous mobs. If you are a civilian concerned about self-defense, your goal will be to escape to safety, remaining anonymous, and avoiding as much of the conflict as possible in the process. You will move away from the danger. If you are a law enforcement officer or security professional, however, your goal will be to minimize injuries and prevent property damage by managing the crowd to the extent possible. Your job requires that you move toward the danger. Since this book is primarily aimed at civilians, we'll address self-protection and tactics rather than crowd control techniques here. The following guidelines can help keep you safe in a crowd.

- Recognize that riots can materialize unexpectedly – Almost any incident involving people and emotion can trigger a violent disturbance, particularly when alcohol or other intoxicants are thrown into the mix. The situation may ignite suddenly with very little warning. Maintain a higher than normal level of situational awareness when navigating crowds, identifying and evading potential sources of trouble to the extent practicable. Diligent observation can protect you not only from violence but also from more mundane threats like pickpockets. Be constantly aware of cover, concealment, and potential escape routes as you move about in case you are forced to flee with little warning.

- Monitor warning signs – Like a rock thrown into a pond, you may not spot the initial impact, but you can readily detect the ripple effect that flows outward from the point of contact. Pay attention to the body language of people around you. They may be reacting to something important they noticed that you have missed. Any sudden change in the demeanor of the crowd, gathering of onlookers, agitators urging a confrontation, or people rapidly moving into your space may be warning signs of impending violence. Look and listen to what is going on around you; shouting, screaming, or other loud commotions also constitute danger signals.

- Watch everyone – Be especially alert for the presence of weapons. If a weapon is fired, the situation immediately escalates into a very serious tactical affair. You may be assaulted directly, caught in the crossfire as law enforcement officers move to restore order, or trampled by terrified bystanders who are trying to get out of the way. Everyone can become a threat, even the good guys. In addition to monitoring the crowd, pay attention to unattended vehicles parked where they shouldn't be, packages left in high traffic areas, abandoned luggage, or anything

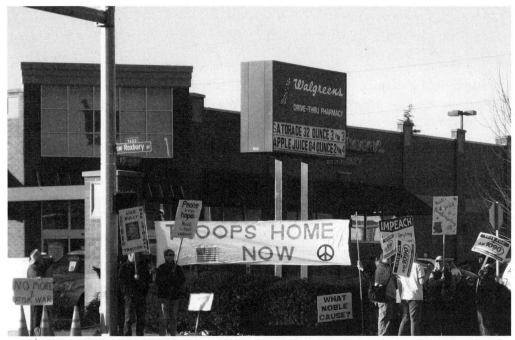

Riots typically explode from specific events, things like jury verdicts, perceived racial injustices, rallies, or political protests, particularly if agitators actively stir things up.

else that appears suspicious. The sooner you spot potential dangers the better your chances of reacting appropriately.

- Evaluate your options before you act – Sometimes it is best to flee right away, but occasionally it may be more sensible to hunker down behind something and defend in place. Take a moment to evaluate your options and make a reasoned choice before embarking on any course of action. If you are inside a building look for alternate exits, particularly in a panicked crowd scenario where the main exit will almost certainly be blocked. In nightclubs, for example, windows are often blacked-out so they are easy to miss if you are not actively looking for them.

- Don't enter an agitated crowd if other alternatives exist – There is a huge difference between a highly spirited crowd of shoppers, a restless throng teetering on the edge of violence, and a riotous mob, one that most anyone actively paying attention can sense. As things begin to turn ugly, don't hang around to watch no matter how fascinating it might be. Leave as quickly and quietly as possible. Plan your exit route to minimize contact with others, even if it means taking the "long way" around the scene. Slip through gaps between others rather than shoving people out of your way to the extent practicable.

- Don't fight unless you have no alternative – If you are forced to fight, you may attract undue attention and quickly find yourself facing multiple opponents who want to beat you down or law enforcement officers who don't realize that you are the good guy. If you are knocked to the ground or stumble and fall, you may very well be trampled. If you have to fight, you will lose valuable time and there is no guarantee that you will survive the encounter, so rather than engaging opponents directly, attempt to deflect or redirect anyone who tries to slow your escape using open-hand techniques.

Crowds can also attract adverse criminal attention, such when pickpockets find a large pool of distracted victims that they can separate from their wealth. Worse yet, terrorists bombers may find the crowd a compelling target since they try to time attacks to inflict maximum casualties.

No matter how tough you are, you cannot knock bullets out of the air or deflect bombs with your "fists of death." That only happens in the movies. As always, your best defense is awareness, spotting and avoiding dangerous situations before it is too late. In addition to monitoring the mood of the crowd, pay attention to unattended vehicles parked where they shouldn't be, packages left in high traffic areas, abandoned luggage, or anything else that appears suspicious.

Summary

The following is a brief recap of the content you have read in this section.

- Never start a fight. If you can walk away from a confrontation, you can avoid all the serious repercussions that come with violence. A preemptive strike as you sense an imminent threat, however, can be a legitimate and street-worthy defensive technique when used properly. Preemptive initiative cuts off an attack before it is fully in play, looking an awful lot like a first strike yet is still a defensive movement.

- Sometimes you truly do need to fight in order to protect yourself and/or your loved ones from an immediate and unavoidable threat. Before you throw the first blow, however, it is critical to know that you have a good case for doing so. If the four criteria of ability, opportunity, jeopardy, and preclusion (AOJP) are all met, you have a pretty good legal case for countervailing force. If one or more of these conditions are absent, however, you are on shaky legal ground should you decide to tie up with the other guy.

- It is important to exercise a judicious level of force sufficient to control the other guy in a fight without overreacting. Force options you might select from include

(1) presence, (2) voice, (3) empty-hand restraint, (4) non-lethal force, and, ultimately, (5) lethal force. The first two levels can prevent violence before it begins, the third may be used proactively as an opponent prepares to strike, and the last two take place after you have already been attacked.

- Alcohol can be a violence magnet. If you are sober and the other guy is not, you will have a significant advantage in a fight. Hitting a drunk really doesn't work all that well most of the time, however. A better strategy is to either dodge his blows in order to let him overbalance himself and facilitate your escape or spin him to cause disorientation and make him fall. Once he's down, you can more readily control him or move to safety.

- Reasonable force in legal terms is generally considered only that force reasonably necessary to repel an attacker's force. You cannot overreact and expect to stay out of jail. While women can be just as dangerous as men, the courts don't often see it that way, focusing on size, gender, and strength differences. Consequently, it is challenging to prove that you did not use excessive force if you wind up hitting a girl unless she's armed with some type of weapon.

- The classic rule is that self-defense begins when deadly danger begins, ends when the danger ends, and revives again if the danger returns. Neither a killing nor a beating that takes place after a crime has already been committed, nor a proactive violent defense before an attack has taken place is a legitimate act of self-defense in the eyes of the law. Once the immediate threat has been dealt with, you can escape to safety. When he stops fighting, you need to stop too.

- Remain vigilant during any pause in the fight. You may be facing multiple assailants or an adversary who pulls a weapon in the middle of a fight or who just won't quit. Once you have removed yourself from the danger and are absolutely certain that you are no longer under threat you can safely begin to relax your guard.

- If you cannot escape or avoid violence, you must be prepared to fight with all your worth. You cannot count on honor, ethics, or mercy from an adversary. Keep fighting until you can safely get away. If you stop, there's no guarantee that he will too.

- There are six things that you may wish to try in a fight, (1) maintaining distance, (2) throwing debris, (3) attacking the eyes, (4) using chokes or neck cranks, (5) throwing him to the ground, and (6) striking with impetus. People who are good at settling things with violence develop a set of favorite techniques that they will use over and over again. Standardization and simplicity are the hallmarks of a good fighter. If it works, keep on using it until it is no longer effective.

• There are six things you should not try in a fight: (1) kicking above the waist, (2) playing "tank," (3) hitting with a closed fist, (4) forgetting to use your mouth as a weapon, (5) playing the other guy's game, and (6) using the wrong technique for the situation. If you let a fight go to the ground, you become vulnerable. You can easily get stomped, kicked, and seriously messed up by your adversary and/or his friends. Similarly, if the other guy gets behind you, he can strike with impunity. The other guy will be doing everything he can to win in a fight. Don't make his job any easier. Keep things simple and direct so that you won't self-destruct.

• When you fight, you are almost certainly going to get hurt. It's unavoidable if the battle lasts more than a few seconds. The real question is how badly it will be. If you must fight, it is critical to end the confrontation as quickly as possible to minimize your injuries. Plan on being on your own if things get physical. You cannot trust or depend on others for help. You may think that your enemy's enemy is your friend, but more often than not, it's simply not true.

• When adrenaline hits your system, your ability to think rationally is greatly reduced. You will suffer degraded motor skills, experience tunnel vision, and may even suffer temporary memory loss too. In essence, you become a one-task, knuckle-dragging troglodyte. Combat breathing techniques can alleviate some, but not all of these symptoms. As stress goes up intelligence goes down.

• Mobs are dangerous. Highly emotional and unthinking, they often erupt into violence. Five psychological influences—(1) impersonality, (2) anonymity, (3) suggestion/imitation, (4) emotional contagion, and (5) discharge of repressed emotions—affect rioters, their targets, and the police who try to break things up. If you stumble across a violent crowd, your goal should be to escape to safety, remaining as anonymous as possible and avoiding as much of the conflict as possible in the process.

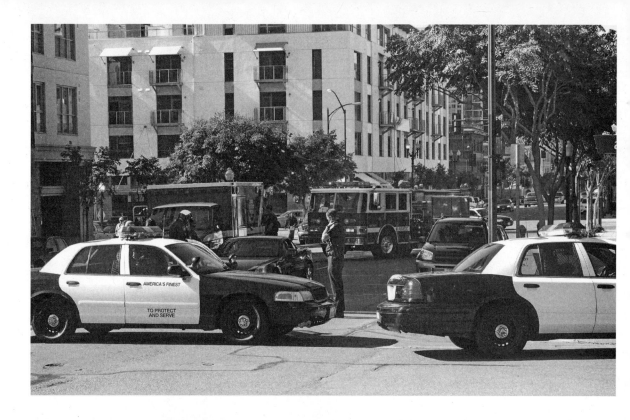

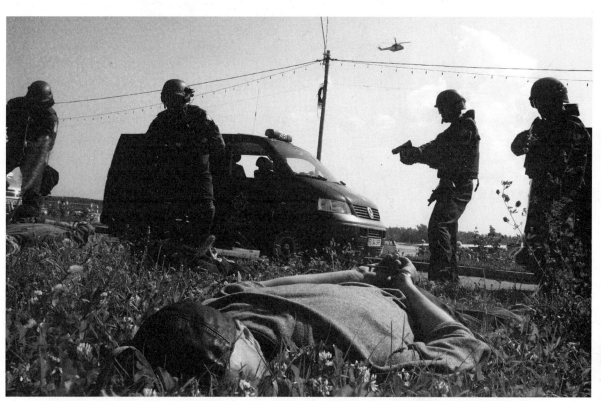

Photos on this page courtesy of BigStockPhoto.com

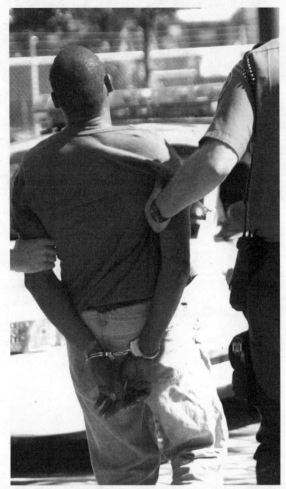

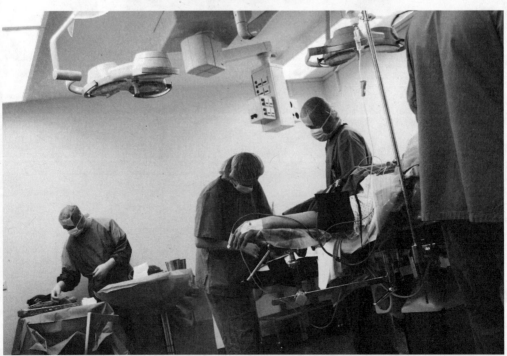

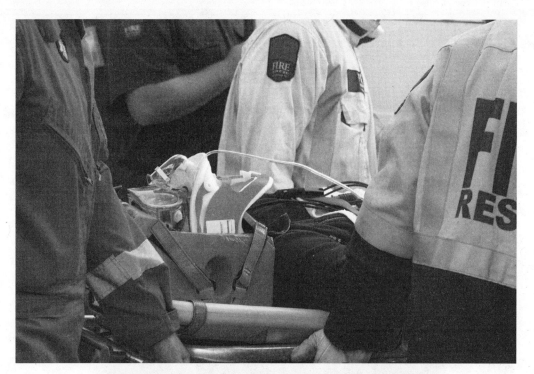

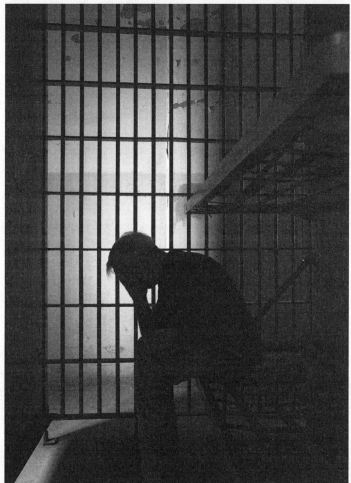

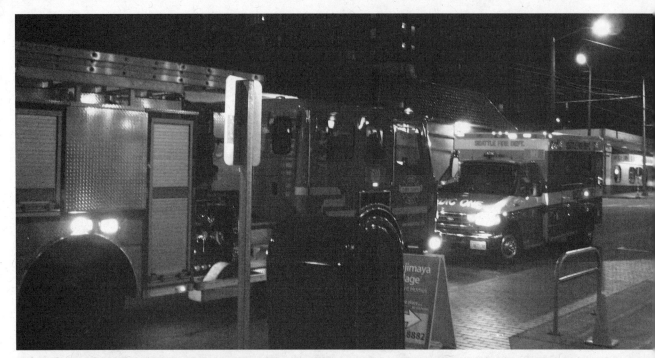

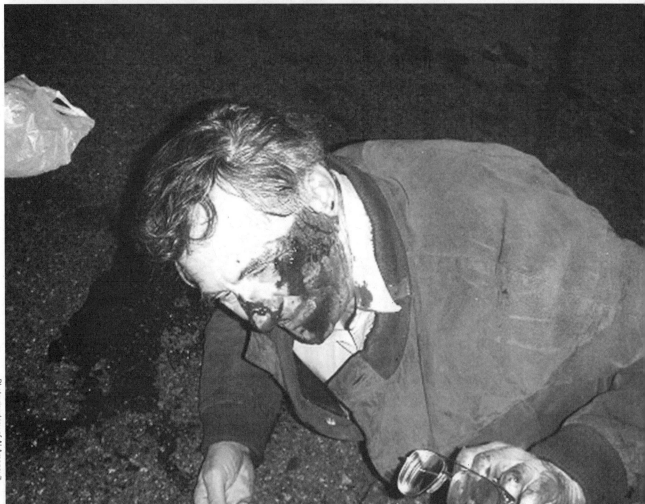

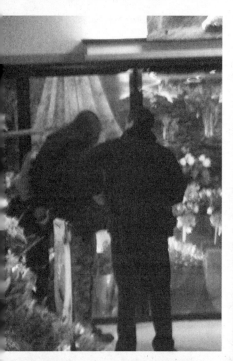
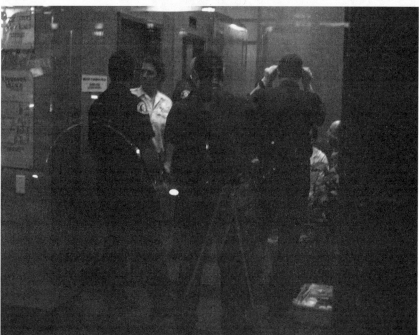
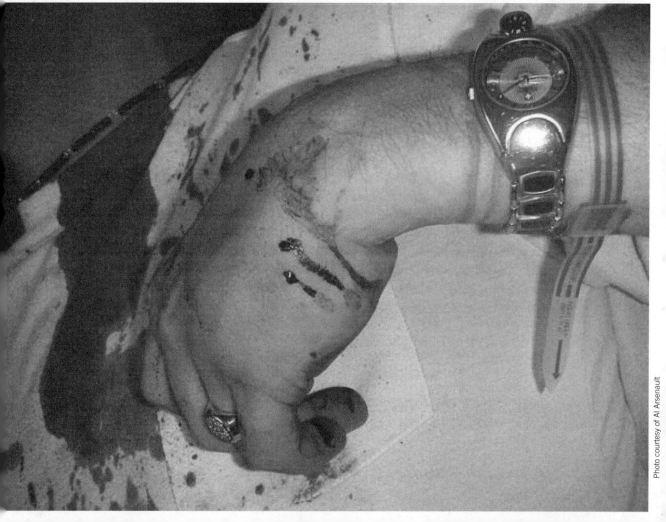

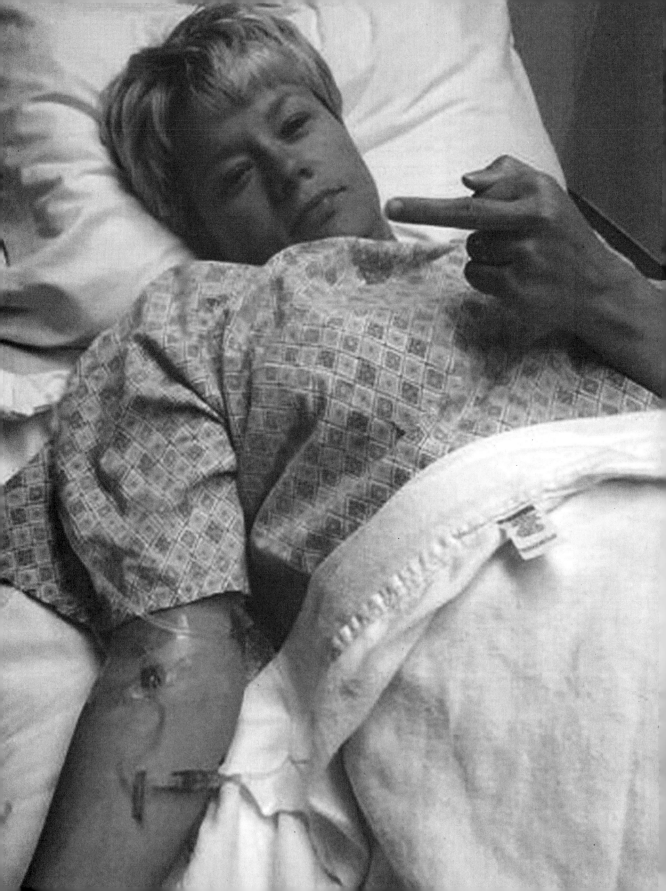

SECTION THREE

Aftermath of Violence

Man is Buddha—
the day and I
grow dark as one.
           – Ryushi (1684–1764) [7]

This section covers the aftermath of violence, showing that it's almost never over when it's over. We're going to assume, for the sake of argument, that once the dust has settled you are still alive. Otherwise, there won't be much aftermath for you to deal with; that'll be left for the authorities and your mourners to hash out. So, under our scenario, the good news is that you've survived. The bad news is that living through the fight is just the beginning. There are a host of other consequences to address, including first aid, legal issues, managing witnesses, finding a good attorney, dealing with the press, interacting with law enforcement, and dealing with psychological trauma.

If you were unexpectedly attacked, ambushed with a weapon, or suddenly discovered that what you thought would be a simple fistfight had escalated in to something far more serious, you will need to get your head in the right place after it's over. You may be gravely wounded and/or facing serious short- and long-term repercussions. Your first order of business must be to know your priorities and act accordingly.

Once It's Over, Know Your Priorities

The rules of the military are five: measurement, assessment, calculation, comparison, and victory. The ground gives rise to measurements, measurements give rise to assessments, assessments give rise to calculations, calculations give rise to comparisons, and comparisons give rise to victories.
           – Sun Tzu

All things entail rising and falling timing. You must be able to discern this. In strategy, there are various timing considerations. From the outset, you must know the applicable timing and the inapplicable timing, and from among the large and small things and the fast and slow timings find the relevant timing, first seeing the distance timing and the background timing. This is the main thing

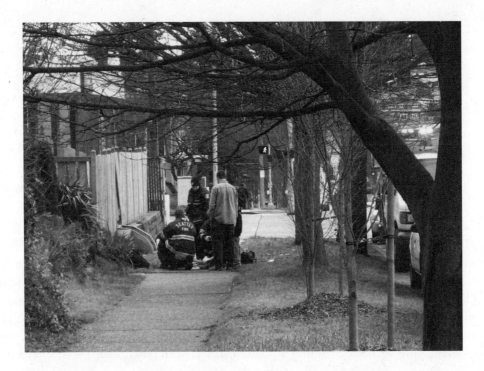

in strategy. It is especially important to know the background timing; otherwise, your strategy will become uncertain.

— *Miyamoto Musashi*

Once you survive a violent conflict, there are hosts of other consequences to address. Your first order of business, however, must be survival. If you have been injured during a fight, you may have to take care of yourself until professional help can arrive. First, you need to make a mental commitment to live. Your attitude plays a large part in your ability to survive. It's also important to know how to treat your own injuries as you may be on your own for a long time until paramedics or other assistance can arrive.

Once you have taken care of any life-threatening injuries, you will want to turn your attention to notifying the authorities, calling your attorney, contacting your wife, girlfriend, or appropriate family member, and identifying any witnesses who may be able to testify about your actions and those of your adversary. It is extraordinarily important to act in a manner that demonstrates to any who observe a violent encounter that you are the victim rather than the instigator of the attack. Always act as if you are on video camera, even if no one else is around. Assume anything you do will be interpreted in the most derogatory manner possible and likely used against you in a court of law. Calculate your verbal response and physical actions to put yourself in the best possible light.

It's tough to remember to do this if you are in pain or shock from a traumatic

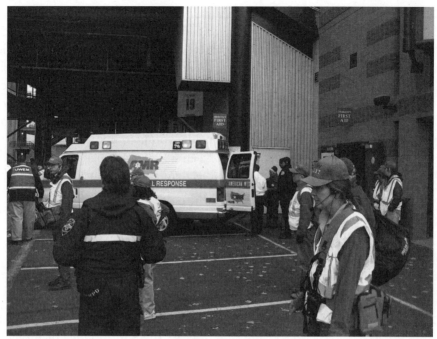

Win or lose, there's always a cost to engaging in violence.

experience but your fight on the street is only the first of several fights you may endure. While you may or may not have to fight to work through and recover from injuries and/ or emotional scars, you almost certainly will have to fight for your freedom and livelihood in court. Your defense begins before the altercation gets physical and often doesn't end for months or years to come. While the opening salvo is playing to any witnesses who might see the fight or video equipment that might record what happened, one of the most important skirmishes will be your first contact with the police.

When the authorities arrive, approach the responding officers calmly and politely. A confrontational attitude will do you no good. Follow the officers' instructions without hesitation. Expect to be arrested. It may or may not happen, but if you are arrested do not resist for any reason. Similarly, do not interfere with an attempt to arrest anyone who is with you at the time.

Do not, under any circumstances, make any incriminating statements that may be used against you at a later time. Despite Miranda[8] requirements, your fundamental rights and responsibilities may not always be clearly spelled out by the responding officers, especially in any conversations that precede an arrest. Remember that you have a Fifth Amendment right against self-incrimination and that it is often prudent to have an attorney present during any questioning. Your priority should be to alleviate or minimize any potential charges against you, so be enormously cautious about what you say and do.

The legal process is arduous, complicated, and expensive. It generally begins with an arrest followed by a booking, arraignment, evidentiary hearing, and trial. At times, an appeal will be necessary as well. Because your freedom, family, livelihood, and reputation are on the line, it is essential to have a highly skilled and experienced attorney to help you navigate the process. You should always carry the phone number of an attorney you can trust and of a person who can contact a lawyer for you if yours is not immediately available. That means, of course, that you will need to be proactive and find an attorney before you need one. More on that later...

> Win or lose, there's always a cost to engaging in violence. Once you survive a violent conflict, there are a host of other consequences to address, including first aid, legal issues, managing witnesses, dealing with the press, interacting with law enforcement, and dealing with psychological trauma. The fight itself is only the beginning. Your first priority afterward must be to ensure your survival. Once you have taken care of any life-threatening injuries, you can begin to deal with everything else.

Killing or crippling another human being is traumatic, even when it's absolutely the right thing to do in order to preserve your own life and well-being. The other guy might be a total scumbag while he's attacking you, but he's still a person, someone with a family, friends, and loved ones who will miss him when he's gone. For example, serial killer Ted Bundy's mother's last words to him were, "You will always be my precious son." She said that right before he was executed by the State of Florida for his crimes.*

If you put someone down on his street, there is no legal process, proceedings, or appeal. There is no judge or jury, only an executioner. You fight. You win. He dies. Sure, lesser outcomes are certainly possible, but it's important to prepare yourself mentally for that ultimate eventuality. It all takes place in the blink of an eye, yet you'll undoubtedly remember it for the rest of your life if it goes that far. That sort of thing is not trivial stuff. It can be very tough to deal with, a great argument for avoiding violent confrontations in the first place, as well as a great argument for seeking psychological counseling to put your head in the right place afterward. Win or lose, there's always a cost to engaging in violence.

We'll go through these things in more detail shortly. At the overview level, however, your most important priority is staying alive and dealing with injuries. Next comes managing witnesses and interacting with law enforcement. We hope you won't need to do so, but you must be prepared to navigate the legal system next. Finally, you'll have to deal with any psychological trauma you've sustained from the encounter.

It Only Takes a Microsecond... And Then You're in Survival Mode

Hence, the skillful fighter puts himself into a position that makes defeat impossible, and does not miss the moment.

– Sun Tzu

---

* Theodore Robert Bundy (1946–1989) was one of the most infamous serial killers in U.S. history. While Bundy confessed to raping and murdering some thirty women before his execution, his total number of victims remains unknown.

Speed implies that things seem fast or slow, according to whether or not they are in rhythm. Whatever the Way, the master of strategy does not appear fast.
— *Miyamoto Musashi*

Real fights occur at closer ranges and with much greater speed and intensity than any sparring match. When bad things happen on the street, life-threatening injuries can take place in the blink of an eye. Mentally shifting into survival mode, while critical for your continued existence, can be a significant challenge if you are unprepared. While this is often necessary in a fight, it can happen in other venues as well.

The following story is a real-life example of dealing with a serious injury. While it didn't happen in a fight, there was a stabbing involved.

Kane's big project over a three-day Memorial Day weekend was building a knife and fork carving set for some friends as a present for their 50th wedding anniversary. Although he had not yet sharpened the blade, he had already finished the metalwork and was in the process of attaching the handle materials when things went awry. First, he got the blade and handle all glued up, but instead of setting it back on the shelf to dry as

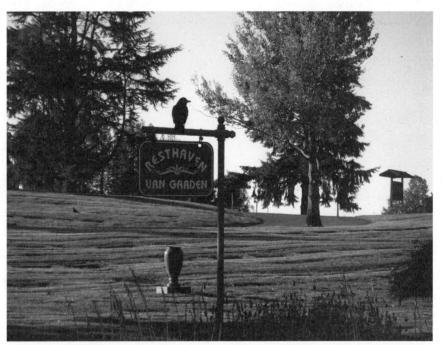

Killing another human being is traumatic, even when it's absolutely the right thing to do in order to preserve your own life. The other guy might be a total scumbag while he's attacking you, but he's still a person, someone with a family, friends, and loved ones who will miss him when he's gone.

he usually did, he left it on a low bench to put up once he got the fork done too. After he finished clamping up the fork, he turned around, took a step toward the bench, and managed to stab himself in the thigh with the knife.

Guess what, it was a lot sharper than he had realized. In a microsecond, he got a three-quarter-inch wide, one-and-a-half-inch deep hole in his leg... Thankfully, it missed all the major arteries, but it was a very serious wound nevertheless. At first, it didn't hurt much; most knife cuts don't, but the considerable pool of blood collecting in his sock demonstrated that it was not something to be taken lightly. While this particular incident stemmed from an accident, it plays out much the same way in a fight. Most stabbing victims do not realize that they've been cut until after the fight. As he peeled the pant leg away to examine the wound, it began to hurt like hell.

Kane is, sadly, quite familiar with pain. He has been stabbed, sliced, abraded, bruised, contused, and concussed, and suffered a wide range of injuries from martial arts training, physical confrontations, a hunting accident, and a few run-ins with wayward power tools. He has been a bit of a klutz at times too, yet he knows how to ascertain the seriousness of an injury and what to do about triaging it. Good skills to have if you're in the martial arts business.

He immediately went limping into the house covered in blood, hobbled over to the first aid kit, and patched things up as best he could. Unfortunately, he also found that

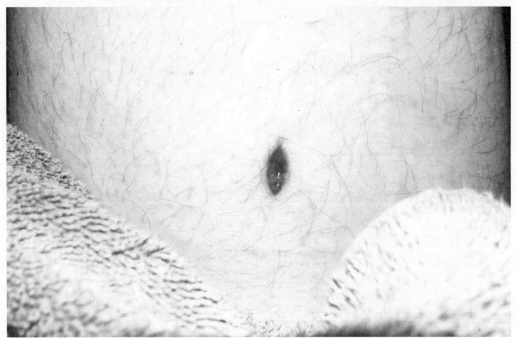

While knife slashes tend to cause more bleeding, stab wounds are oftentimes more serious. This partially healed injury was photographed about two weeks after the incident.

he had used up the last of the necessary supplies. Given the holiday, he was not sure how long stores would be open, so without taking time to change is bloody clothes he drove down to the local Target department store to buy more.

Picture this: he's got two days beard-growth, he's dusty and grimy from the shop, and he's got a massive blotch of fresh blood (not dried yet) surrounding a hole in his pant leg. He's also got blood all over his shoes and socks. And he's limping slightly.

So he went in through the parking lot, past the security guy at the front of the store, and then limped past close to a hundred customers to the back corner where the first aid supplies were kept. He packed a handcart with bandages, gauze, tape, antibiotic ointment, hydrogen peroxide, and the like, and then hobbled back up to the front of the store where the cashiers were located. He must have passed another hundred customers on the return trip.

Sensing nothing wrong, the cashier asked him how he was doing. "I'm fine," he lied. She then asked him, "Did you find everything you were looking for?" to which he replied, "Yes." She proceeded to try to sell him a Red Card (Target's store brand Visa credit card), which he politely declined, yet she still had not noticed anything amiss even though she was looking right at him while they talked.

With the transaction now completed, she told him to have a nice day and he mumbled something along the lines of "You, too." He then hobbled past the security guard at the entrance, back out into the parking lot, past a roving police patrol car, and over to his truck. He climbed in and drove home. During all that time, no one had noticed anything wrong.

While it wasn't terribly funny at the time, he found this incident highly amusing in retrospect. That was by far the worst situational awareness he had ever experienced—both on his part for walking into the darn blade in the first place and everyone else's for not noticing the "stupid bleeding guy" wandering around in the parking lot or the store.

Kane went to the doctor when his office opened a couple of days later after the holiday and got some antibiotics and a tetanus shot. Although he also got yelled at for not going to the emergency room in the first place, the wound fully healed several months later, leaving nothing worse than a small scar.

There are two important lessons here.

> Awareness is important at all times. Pay extra attention whenever you are around anything or anyone dangerous. Staying calm in a crisis is paramount. Sooner or later, you're going to get hurt doing something stupid. You may do it to yourself or the other guy may do it to you, but either way it takes only a microsecond to get severely injured. How you act after it happens can make all the difference.

- Awareness is important at all times. We've already beaten you upside the head with this concept, but seriously pay, extra attention whenever you are around anything or anyone dangerous. It doesn't matter how you get hurt; it's the wound you have got to deal with.

- Staying calm in a crisis is paramount. Sooner or later, you're going to get hurt doing something stupid. Maybe the pain will come from some other guy's fist yet it just as easily could come from your vehicle, a power tool, or a kitchen knife. How you act after it happens can make all the difference.

It takes only a microsecond to get hurt badly, whether in a fight or in an accident. How you act after it happens makes all the difference. Interestingly, it's much tougher to work through an identical injury if it came from another person. For example, a broken leg suffered in a fall on the ski slopes is much less psychologically traumatic than an identical injury caused by some street thug with a baseball bat. Regardless, you must remain calm and focus on the task at hand. Resolute determination can help you achieve what you need to do.

This is what the Japanese call *fudoshin* or indomitable spirit. Miyamoto Musashi, arguably the greatest swordsman who ever lived, demonstrated the ultimate evolution of such spirit. In his writings, he related that many opponents fell before his sword simply because they believed that they would, not necessarily, because he was the better warrior.

When your life is on the line, fight not only for yourself but also about those who care about and depend upon you—your family, your wife or girlfriend, your kids, and your friends. In the heat of battle, you will not have time to think of anything beyond the immediate but it is wise to consider beforehand what will happen to your loved ones if you do not make it. Sometimes the impact to others can be even more motivating than the impact to yourself. You must make a wholehearted commitment to survive. This same indomitable spirit is necessary throughout the entire encounter—from first contact with an adversary to the closing gavel in the courtroom (if it gets that far).

Staying calm in a crisis is paramount. Sooner or later, you're going to get hurt doing something stupid. You may do it to yourself or the other guy may do it to you, but either way it takes only a microsecond to get severely injured. How you act after it happens can make all the difference.

Know How to Perform First Aid

Triage and battlefield medicine are not addressed by either Sun Tzu or Miyamoto Musashi. While ancient warriors certainly learned these vital skills, they were beyond the scope of books on strategy at that time.

Even if you don't expect to get into a fight, it's a good idea to know what to do if you or a loved one becomes injured. The Red Cross and Red Crescent provide relatively inexpensive, comprehensive first aid and CPR classes throughout the world so access to quality training is rarely a problem. Once you have received training, it is important to keep emergency supplies in your home and carry a first aid kit in your vehicle. After all, it's pretty tough to patch yourself up if you don't have the proper equipment available. Be sure to include rubber gloves to protect yourself from blood-borne pathogens (such as hepatitis B, hepatitis C, or HIV/AIDS) if you have to treat others as well.

If you or another person with you has been injured in a fight, controlling bleeding must be your first priority. The Red Cross suggests a (1) check, (2) call, (3) care approach, performed in that order. First, discern the safety of the scene and the condition of the victim before doing anything else. Make sure that the fight is truly over and that it's safe to lower your guard. Next, call 9-1-1 (or the local emergency number) to notify authorities about what happened, asking them to dispatch an ambulance with professional help. The faster the paramedics get there, the better the victim's chances of survival. Only after these first two steps have been completed do you begin to care for the injured victim yourself.

Once you have taken care of your own life-threatening injuries, you will also want to treat your opponent. Remember that your goal in applying countervailing force is to keep yourself safe from harm. If your adversary is disabled and no longer a threat, it is both prudent and humane to try to keep him from dying from his wounds. It may play well in court too. Whenever possible, wash your hands before and after dealing with another person's injuries, even when you wear disposable gloves.

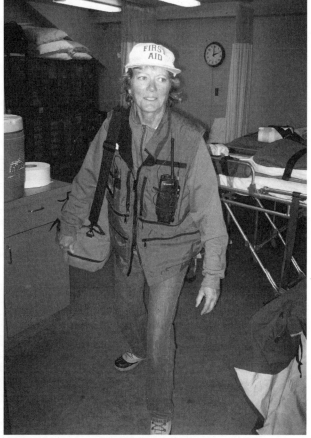

Even if you don't expect to get into a fight, it's a good idea to know what to do if you or a loved one becomes injured.

There are far too many potential wounds that victims might receive to cover them all, but we've included details about how to deal with some of the most common ones below. This information is only an introduction and should never take the place of professional, hands-on instruction.

Control Bleeding. Heavy bleeding is often the most serious, life-threatening injury victims will receive in a fight. For example, Washington Redskin's standout free safety Sean Taylor was shot in the leg during a home invasion robbery on November 26, 2007.

The bullet damaged his femoral artery, causing him to bleed rapidly to death despite the fact that he was a well-conditioned, 236-pound professional athlete.

Fire fighters, military, law enforcement, and emergency medical professionals (for example, paramedic, EMT) often use special blood-clotting sponges, or hemostatic agents as they are called in the business, to treat severe bleeding from gunshots, stabbings, shrapnel, and similarly critical wounds. One brand that is available to the general public is called QuikClot. Made by Z-Medica Corporation, this agent accelerates the body's natural clotting process by increasing the concentration of platelets and clotting factors at the wound site. Combined with a pressure bandage, this treatment can often be lifesaving even in cases as severe as Taylor's if it is applied fast enough. The challenge is that uncontrolled hemorrhaging, particularly from weapon wounds, can cause a person to bleed to death very quickly, sometimes in seconds, often in minutes.

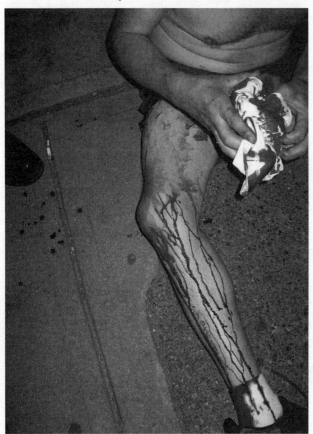

Discern the safety of the scene and the condition of the victim, and then call for help before you begin administering first aid. Once you are sure it is safe to proceed, controlling bleeding must be your first priority.

If you don't have a special hemostatic agent such as QuikClot sponges or CELOX coagulant granules available, heavy bleeding is controlled first through direct, firm pressure on the injury site, preferably through a gauze pad or sterile dressing. If it is a limb that has been damaged, it will bleed less if it is elevated so that the wound is above the heart. If hemorrhage persists, use pressure points. Only in the worst cases when emergency services will not be available for an extended period of time should you consider use of a tourniquet, which if improperly used could cause gangrene or death. The Red Cross has dropped tourniquet techniques from its civilian training curriculum, as they are rarely needed and dangerous to apply.

If you are the one who is injured and think that you might pass out, especially if you are bleeding heavily or it is very cold, you have to get help immediately. If you do not, it will most likely prove fatal. Take a moment to gather your wits and locate the nearest cell phone, payphone, or source of friendly human beings. If you are alone and

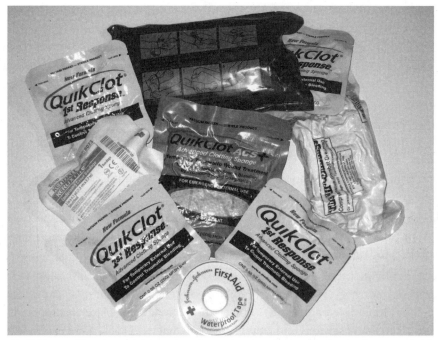

Firefighters, military, law enforcement, and emergency medical professionals often use special blood-clotting sponges, or hemostatic agents such as QuikClot, to treat severe bleeding from gunshots, stabbings, shrapnel, and similarly critical wounds. This stuff is very expensive to keep in your first aid kit but it saves lives.

bleeding badly and there is no phone readily available, you will need to decide whether to stay or attempt to go for help. Physical activity will make your heart race faster, increasing blood loss. You are likely to get dizzy and collapse, thereby losing your pressure hold on the wound, and causing even more blood loss.

If there is a reasonable chance that a rescuer will happen along soon, you may be better off dressing your wounds to the extent you can than putting yourself in "shock position" to wait for assistance. This is done by lying on your back with your legs elevated on something or with your legs bent sharply and your toes locked against a wall or similar object to keep them in position if you pass out. Wrap a garment around yourself if you can to help keep yourself warm. This position helps ensure that as much blood as possible will remain available to your vital organs.

If you don't have a specialty agent such as QuikClot available, one of the most street-proven trauma dressings is a sanitary napkin or a box of Kleenex, something that ought to be in your first aid kit in addition to regular gauze pads and bandages. Key first aid methods for stopping heavy bleeding include:

- Covering the wound with a sterile dressing such as a gauze pad. If the dressing becomes soaked with blood, apply additional layers over the top of it without removing the original dressing.

- Applying direct pressure to the wound. If bleeding does not stop through a combination of dressings and pressure, remove the dressings, pack the wound with QuikClot (or a similar hemostatic agent), and reapply new sterile dressings. Use a pressure bandage to hold everything in place if available. If you do not have access to specialty agents, you may have to apply direct pressure to a nearby artery to slow the flow of blood. On the arm, the best point is along the inside of the upper arm between the shoulder and elbow. On the leg, the best point is at the crease at the front of the hip in the groin area.

- Elevating the wound above the level of the heart if possible. If you suspect head, neck, or back injuries or broken bones, however, or it may be prudent to remain in place. Moving may increase severity of the damage.

- Never removing imbedded objects before you get to the hospital. Doing so may increase hemorrhaging and severely reduce your chances of survival. Bulky dressings should be placed around the object and bandaged in place to support it so that it won't move around and cause further damage.

- Wrapping severed body parts, if any, in a sterile dressing, placed in a plastic bag, and covered with ice or cold water sufficient to keep the part cool without freezing. Limbs preserved in this manner can frequently be reattached at the hospital. On the other hand, freezing the severed part will cause irreversible damage.

> If you and/or your loved ones have been wounded in a fight, you may have to tend to the injuries yourself until professional help can arrive. Check the incident scene to make sure that it is safe, call 9-1-1 or your local emergency number for help, and then begin to care for the victims. Once you have taken care of your own life-threatening injuries you will also want to treat your opponent. If your adversary is disabled and no longer a threat, it is both prudent and humane to try to keep him from dying from his wounds too.

Head, Neck, and Back Injuries. Head, neck, and back injuries are serious. Do not move the victim unless absolutely necessary. If you do need to move the person, be careful to support the injured area, avoiding any twisting, bending, or other contortions that could cause additional damage. If the person becomes unconscious, you will need to maintain a clear airway and possibly perform rescue breathing or cardio-pulmonary resuscitation.

Concussions. The brain is extraordinarily delicate yet it is protected by a rigid skull and cushioned with cerebrospinal fluid. Trauma to the head, however, can cause the brain to bounce against the skull. This force may damage the brain's function.

There is very little extra room within this cavity, so any resulting swelling or bleeding can quickly become life threatening. In general, a blow to the front of the head is less dangerous than one on the side or back of the head.

Symptoms of a concussion can include severe headache, dizziness, nausea, vomiting, ringing in the ears, mismatched pupil size (left vs. right), seizures, or slurred speech. The person may also seem restless, agitated, or irritable. Often, the victim may experience temporary memory loss. These symptoms may last from hours to weeks, depending on the seriousness of the injury.

Any loss of consciousness or memory resulting from a head injury should be promptly evaluated by a medical professional. As the brain tissue swells, the person may feel increasingly drowsy or confused. If the victim has difficulty staying awake, experiences persistent vomiting, develops seizures, or loses consciousness, medical attention should be sought immediately. These could be signs of a severe injury.

Concussions can run from mild to severe. While only medical professionals can tell for sure, one can surmise what type of concussion has been sustained based upon the observable symptoms. Grade 1 or mild concussions occur when the victim remains conscious after a blow but seems dazed or mildly confused. Grade 2 or moderate concussions occur when the victim remains conscious but continues to be confused for a period of time and does not recall the traumatic event. Grade 3 or severe concussions occur when the victim loses consciousness for a period of time and has no memory of the traumatic event. If you suspect that someone has suffered a Grade 2 or Grade 3 concussion, evaluation from a medical professional should be performed as soon as possible.

Watch the person closely for any changes in level of consciousness until medical help arrives. The victim may need to stay in the hospital for close observation. The standard test to assess post-concussion damage is a computerized tomography (CT) scan. Surgery is not frequently required but may become necessary if swelling persists. Recovery from a traumatic brain injury can be very slow. Sometimes several days can go by without seeing any major visible change. Post-concussion syndrome may also occur in some people. This syndrome generally consists of a persistent headache, dizziness, irritability, emotional instability, memory changes, depression, or vision changes. Symptoms may begin weeks or even months after the initial injury.

Although the symptoms tend to go away over time, some victims will need a rehabilitation specialist to oversee a program for their recovery. People who have had a severe concussion also double their risk of developing epilepsy within the first five years after the injury. There is evidence that people who have had multiple concussions over the course of their lives suffer cumulative neurological damage. A link between concussions and the eventual development of Alzheimer's disease also has been suggested.

Rest is generally the best recovery technique since healing a concussion takes time. For headaches, acetaminophen (Tylenol) or ibuprofen (Motrin) can usually be used, but it is best to avoid aspirin as it can increase the risk of internal bleeding. Check with a doctor before administering medications. Bumps and contusions can be treated with ice packs. Wrap ice in a damp cloth rather than placing it directly against the skin.

Eye Injuries. Do not attempt to treat severe blunt trauma or penetrating injuries to the eye yourself; medical assistance is required in such instances. Tape a paper or Styrofoam cup over the injured area to protect it until proper care can be obtained. As always, if there is an imbedded object, do not attempt to remove it.

In the case of a blow to the eye such as a finger rake, jab, or gouge, do not automatically assume that the injury is minor even if you can see properly afterward. An ophthalmologist should examine the eye thoroughly because vision-threatening damage such as a detached retina could be hidden. Immediately apply an ice compress or bag of frozen vegetables (for example, peas, corn) to the eye to reduce pain and swelling. If you experience pain, blurred vision, floaters (black spots that move around), starbursts (firework-like bursts of color or light), or any possibility of eye damage, see your ophthalmologist or emergency room physician immediately.

The most common type of eye injury is a chemical burn. This is typically from an accident rather than from having something thrown into your face during a fight, but that does happen too on occasion as well since fire extinguishers, hot coffee, and the like make good impromptu weapons on the street. Alkaline materials (such as lye, plasters, cements, and ammonia), solvents, acids, and detergents can be very harmful to your eyes. If you are exposed to these types of chemicals, the eyes should be flushed liberally with water immediately. If sterile solutions are readily available, use them to flush the affected eye. If not, go to the nearest sink, shower or hose and begin washing the eye with large amounts of water. If the eye has been exposed to an alkaline agent, it is important to flush the eye for ten minutes or more. Make sure water is getting under both the upper and lower eyelids.

Chest Wounds. Large chest wounds can cause a lung to collapse, a dangerous situation. Cover the wound with a sterile dressing or clean cloth and bandage it in place. If bubbles begin forming around a wound of significant size (open area that is greater than about an inch in diameter), cover that area with plastic or similar material that does not allow air to pass through. Tape the dressing in place, leaving one corner open to allow air to escape with exhalation.

Most normal stab and bullet injuries will not cause a sucking chest wound because the hole from the wound is smaller than the opening in the trachea. Consequently, it will not cause negative pressure, which inhibits breathing. If you seal a wound that does not need it, you run the risk of tension pneumothorax, which can cause a complete cardio respiratory arrest and subsequent death. If advanced medical care is readily available it is generally more important to transport the victim to the hospital quickly than it is to seal off the wound with anything more than a breathable sterile dressing.

Abdominal Injuries. For abdominal injuries, try to keep the victim lying down with his or her knees bent if possible. If organs are exposed, do not apply pressure to the organs or push them back inside. Remove any clothing from around the wound. Apply moist, sterile dressings or clean cloth loosely over the wound. Keep the dressing moist with clean, warm water. Place a cloth over the dressing to keep the organs warm.

Broken Bones. Broken bones should usually be splinted to keep the injured part from moving and increasing the damage. There is a variety of ways to create an effective splint. The method you choose will be based in part on what materials you have available, the position you find the injury, its location on the body, and a variety of other factors. The most important thing is to pad and immobilize the injury to the extent possible. A basic rule of splinting is that the joint above and below the broken bone should be immobilized to protect the fracture site. For example, if the lower leg is broken, the splint should immobilize both the ankle and the knee.

Anatomic splints affix the injured body part to a convenient uninjured one such as tying one leg to the other. A soft splint can be made from a towel, blanket, jacket, or similar material. A rigid splint can be made from boards, tightly rolled magazines, and similar materials.

Shock. Shock can occur whenever there is severe injury to the body or the nervous system. Because shock can cause inadequate blood flow to the tissues and organs, all bodily processes can be affected. Vital functions slow down to dangerous levels. In the early stages, the body compensates for a decreased blood flow to the tissues by constricting blood vessels in the skin, soft tissues, and muscles. This causes the victim to have cold, clammy, or pale skin; weakness and nausea; rapid, labored breathing; increased pulse rate; and decreased blood pressure. As shock progresses, the victim will become apathetic, relatively unresponsive, and eventually lapse into unconsciousness.

One quick and dirty way to identify shock is by observing a delayed capillary refill response at the fingertips. Press downward on the tip of the fingernail until the skin underneath begins to turn white and then release the pressure. A normal pink appearance should return within two to three seconds. If it takes four to six seconds or longer for normal color to return, the victim is experiencing low blood pressure at the extremities, a clear sign of shock.

You should have already treated any major injuries such as bleeding or broken bones before treating for shock. This care will help ameliorate the source of the shock, but there is more that you can do. Keep the victim lying down, elevate his legs about a foot or so above his chest, and cover him with a blanket or coat to prevent loss of body heat. If the femur (thighbone) has been broken from a gunshot or blunt traumatic injury, however, do not elevate the injured leg as bone fragments may shift around and cause serious internal bleeding. Check the victim's airway, breathing, and circulation on a regular basis until medical help arrives. It is not advisable to give liquids to shock victims.

Infection. If you have been injured by a weapon that breaks the skin, infection is a possibility even after medical treatment. If the wound area becomes red or swollen, throbs with pain, discharges pus, or develops red streaks, contact medical personnel immediately.

If you begin to develop a fever, it may also be a sign of infection. Seek direction from your physician as to how to bandage your injury, how frequently to change the dressing, and how best to clean the wound to minimize the chances of infection.

It's smart to learn first aid. Even if you never have to use it to care for yourself, odds are good that you will find opportunities to help others. If you study martial arts and learn how to hurt other people, it's even more important to understand how to help them as well.

Handling Blows to Your Self Esteem

Prohibit the taking of omens, and do away with superstitious doubts.
— *Sun Tzu*

If you attain and adhere to the wisdom of my strategy, you need never doubt that you will win.
— *Miyamoto Musashi*

Physical blows are oftentimes easier to endure than mental ones. For example, Wilder knows an aikido instructor who was in the wrong part of town at the right time and got into a nasty brawl. He not only lost, but also lost badly, taking a severe beat down. While it's tough to lose a fight, it's especially tough for a martial arts instructor. In this case, it shook the very foundation of his *dojo*, with students questioning the validity of their training and their instructors' expertise. In fact, it took great effort to prevent their organization from flying apart.

Knowing this instructor's method of practice and ideas regarding fighting, Wilder believes that he sought perfection in the situation when it called instead for whatever it took to get the job done. While you normally can't do that and expect to prevail, the reason the guy took a beating is less important than how he handled it afterward. There were physical injuries to deal with, of course, but the blow to the man's self-esteem was particularly severe.

What happens if you lose a fight? How much it affects you depends a lot on your worldview. If you're an average guy or faced weapons or multiple opponents, you might consider yourself lucky to have gotten through it in one piece, shrug things off, and go on about your life. Perhaps you'll be a bit more careful about where you go and/or whom you hang out with, but it likely won't be a world-changing experience for you. At the very least, you will take self-defense a bit more seriously and will make a better effort to avoid fighting in the future by working on such things as your situational awareness and verbal de-escalation skills.

Losing a fight can be very scary. It can leave physical as well as emotional scars. Oftentimes you will be motivated to study martial arts or pick up a knife or a gun so that you will have the ability to fight back. If you decide to go that route, examine your motivation carefully.

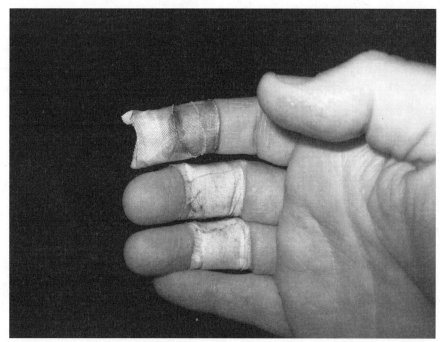

Self-defense is really about not being there, using awareness, avoidance, and de-escalation to eliminate the need to fight. Fighting is what you do when you've totally screwed up your self-defense.

While it's great to be able to defend yourself, it's easy to slip into vigilante mode, subconsciously looking for opportunities to get payback for your loss or otherwise prove your manhood in another fight as Bernard Getz may have done. Don't start doing dangerous things like cutting through alleys or hanging out in the wrong bars in order to provoke another attack where you might get a chance to redeem your honor.

Guns, knives, and martial arts skills do not ward off danger. They help you deal with it more effectively, and only in select circumstances. Never forget that self-defense is really about not being there, using awareness, avoidance, and de-escalation to eliminate the need to fight. Fighting is what you do when you've totally screwed up your self-defense. If you train yourself to fight or decide to carry a weapon, you are working on the two to five percent of the time that those skills will come in handy. Don't get us wrong; those skills are great, oftentimes lifesaving. Just don't go looking for opportunities to try them out unnecessarily.

If you ultimately decide to carry a weapon, be sure to do your homework first, researching the applicable laws in the jurisdictions where you live, work, and frequently travel. Be sure to obtain the appropriate licenses or permits where applicable too. Use of a contraband weapon can turn what should have been a legitimate case of self-defense into a long prison term or possibly even a death sentence. While all fights can have repercussions, odds of serious consequences dramatically increase when weapons are involved.

If you think of yourself as a "fighter" and then wind up getting beat down, things may be much worse for you mentally. If you are a big time martial artist like the aforementioned aikido instructor, if that is the center of your whole world, losing a street fight can be extraordinarily traumatic. It's a major blow to your self-esteem, much more so than a regular, everyday person would typically suffer. You will probably begin to have thoughts like:

- I can't believe that (technique) didn't work!
- What did I do wrong?
- What will the other guys at the *dojo* think?
- I'm such an idiot!
- What I know has no street value; I've been wasting my time all these years!
- What the hell is wrong with me?

If you were badly hurt or otherwise failed to protect yourself or someone you care about, it can be pretty rough. It's important to put things into perspective. Use the loss as a learning opportunity. After all, anything you live through can be a good thing so long as you learn something from it.

> Losing a fight can affect people in different ways. If you're an average guy or found yourself hopelessly outmatched, you may be less traumatized than if you considered yourself a real "fighter" yet got beat down regardless. Anything you live through can be a good thing so long as you learn something from it. Wallowing in misery does you no good. Wait a few days to regain your emotional equilibrium, dispassionately evaluate your objectives, and then figure out what, if anything, you should do differently in the future.

Begin by taking a hard look at yourself and your actions before the fight. Did you do everything you could to calm things down or were you raring to go, looking for an opportunity to prove how tough you are? Think about things like why you got into the fight in the first place. Did you do everything you could to de-escalate the situation? If it was unavoidable and you were simply outmatched, that's a different story than if you set yourself up for the fall. Past behavior predicts future behavior unless you make a concerted effort to change it. If you find that you need to make a change, commit yourself to doing so.

Let's say that you did everything right, all you could do to avoid fighting but found yourself in an altercation anyway. And you got beat down hard. Now what?

There are many bad martial artists out there, but few truly bad martial arts. If you think your art let you down in a fight, it is most likely the other way around. You probably haven't learned it correctly. For example, if you don't truly understand the strategy and architecture in which your tactics and techniques can be most effective, you have not yet mastered your art. You can do what looks like the right thing but totally miss the mark. In such cases, it's important to refocus your training to understand not only the techniques but also the nuances that make them work. In addition to working with your instructor, the book *Becoming a Complete Martial Artist: Error Detection in Self-Defense and the Martial Arts* by Marc MacYoung and Tristan Sutrisno is an excellent resource to help you with that.

You may have a different problem though. As we've stated previously, there's a big difference between sport, fighting, and combat. It's easy to be good at fighting or good at sport, but really tough to be good at both simultaneously. If you've been approaching martial arts from a sports perspective there's nothing wrong with that. It's great exercise and provides positive feedback, trophies, and other rewards for strong performance. The challenge is that it's not necessarily going to be your best bet for self-defense on the street if things get violent.

Wait a few days to regain your emotional equilibrium, and then try to evaluate your objectives dispassionately. If you really want to learn street defense but realize that you are practicing a sport, perhaps you're in the wrong *dojo* or maybe even studying the wrong art. If concepts like awareness, avoidance, and de-escalation are not part of the curriculum, then you're really not studying self-defense. If scenario training is not available or if the legal aspects of countervailing force are not taught along with the techniques, your education is incomplete insofar as practical street defense goes. Sparring and competition are great, but may not really be what you are looking for.

By sorting out your objectives and figuring out what you might do in the future, you are taking proactive steps to get over the loss. That's all for the good. Hand wringing, second-guessing, and beating yourself up are dysfunctional pursuits. The faster you regain your equilibrium after a traumatic event, the less likely you are to have long-lasting negative effects. Consequently, wallowing in misery doesn't help. Setting a course of action does. Debriefing, counseling, psychotherapy, or other forms of mental health treatment may be necessary as well. We will address these issues a bit in the next section.

Dealing with Psychological Trauma

Post Traumatic Stress Disorder (PTSD), critical incident amnesia, and similar forms of psychological trauma were not understood nor addressed by Sun Tzu or Miyamoto Musashi in their writings. Every warrior society has developed some sort of purification ritual to help returning warriors deal with their guilt, however. Throughout time, these rituals helped reassure them that whatever they did in combat was good and proper, necessary for the safety and security of their tribe, tangentially addressing these psychological issues.

It is perfectly normal to experience grief and anguish after traumatic events. You'll tend to replay the incident over and over again in your mind, second-guessing your actions and wondering what you could have done differently. This tends to dissipate naturally over time, however. If you have been involved in a violent altercation and experience recurring emotional effects for more than a week or two, it is a good idea to consider professional counseling to facilitate a healthy recovery. The faster you regain your equilibrium the better.

Unfortunately, many guys don't get the help they need. One theory is that while society seems to presume that women will experience emotional issues after a violent experience such as a rape, men are often expected to take horrendous violence in stride and not let it affect them psychologically. That's just silly. While you may feel embarrassed or unmanly for seeking help to deal with emotional issues after a fight, it's important to get it if you need it. Even Special Forces soldiers, the world's elite fighting corps, seek psychological counseling after their missions as the situation warrants. There are things that ordinary, well-adjusted people simply aren't meant to experience. Dealing with that sort of stuff often takes help.

For most people, the emotional effects of violent incidents tend to subside after a few weeks. If symptoms last longer than a month or two, you may need a professional diagnosis to see if you have developed a psychiatric disorder such as Post Traumatic Stress Disorder (PTSD). PTSD is a psychological condition caused by exposure to or confrontation with highly stressful experiences, typically involving participation in or witnessing of death or serious physical injury. This stressful experience, when combined with feelings of intense fear, helplessness, or horror may lead to PTSD, particularly when the experience is caused by another person such as in a violent confrontation.

These problems can occur whether you win, lose, or merely witness the violent encounter. They can appear after you have taken direct action to harm another person as well as when you have chosen not to get involved.

Symptoms can include re-experiencing phenomena via nightmares and flashbacks, emotional detachment (or hyper control), sleep abnormalities, irritability, excessive startle (hyper vigilance), and uncontrolled rage, among other indicators. Experiences likely to induce this condition include most any form of combat or violent physical attack, rape, emotional abuse, or even catastrophic natural disasters (for example, hurricanes, earthquakes). PTSD often becomes a chronic condition but can usually improve with treatment or, rarely, even spontaneously. There is also the possibility of other psychiatric disorders that may be experienced simultaneously.

Despite the seriousness of these symptoms, most people who experience traumatic events will not develop PTSD. It is possible, however, to have a delayed onset of PTSD years or even decades later. Delayed triggers usually come in the form of life-changing events such as the death of a relative or close friend or diagnosis of a serious medical condition.

The good news is that PTSD and other psychological trauma associated with violence have been thoroughly studied. There are varieties of clinical techniques that mental health professionals and clergy members can use to help victims make a full recovery. With

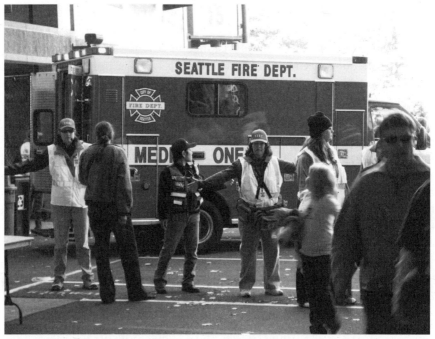

For most people, the emotional effects of violent incidents tend to subside after a few weeks. If symptoms last longer than a month or two, you may need a professional diagnosis to see if you have developed a psychiatric disorder such as Post Traumatic Stress Disorder.

counseling, survivors of traumatic events are able to confront their memories and emotions while working to de-link them from any kind of physiological response.

Autogenic training techniques and structured debriefing sessions are helpful in this process. Similar to biofeedback techniques, autogenic training teaches your body to respond to your verbal commands in order to achieve deep relaxation and reduced stress. These commands help you control your breathing, blood pressure, heartbeat, and body temperature when you want to. Structured debriefing is a psychiatric intervention that follows a trauma episode to promote recovery and minimizing disruption.

The important thing is to get help if you need it. Don't worry about what others might think. Do what's necessary for your continued health and well-being.

Understanding Critical Incident Amnesia

Critical incident amnesia was not addressed by Sun Tzu or Miyamoto Musashi in their writings.

Traumatic situations are frequently associated with memory impairment, a condition commonly described as "critical incident amnesia." The greater the stress, the greater the potential of memory problems as victims have difficulty in transferring information from short-term memory to long-term memory. There are several root causes for this phenomenon, including sensory overload, tunnel vision, and adrenal stress.

Combatants frequently encounter post-incident amnesia immediately after a traumatic experience, failing to remember the majority of the information they observed during the encounter. After a healthy night's sleep, there is usually a significant memory recovery, resulting in an ability to remember a majority of what occurred. You will have the most reliable memories of what occurred at this period. Alcohol interferes with REM sleep; you may sleep more, even easier, but it won't be as deep or as effective, so stay away from alcohol right after the incident. Sleeping pills and other medications affecting the quality of your sleep should be avoided as well, unless prescribed by your doctor.

> It is perfectly normal to experience grief and anguish after traumatic events. Exposure to highly stressful experiences when combined with feelings of intense fear, helplessness, or horror may lead to serious psychological trauma. Symptoms can occur whether you win, lose, or even witness a violent encounter. If you have been involved in an altercation and experience recurring emotional effects for more than a few weeks it is a good idea to consider professional counseling to facilitate a healthy recovery.

The most complete memory recovery will happen within about 72 hours, but it will inevitably include at least partially reconstructed (and therefore somewhat contaminated) information. Inevitably, an individual who has experienced some level of memory loss will discuss the event with others and seek retrieval clues from external sources such as media reports.

Human memory is a fallible process. It includes active construction in which prior experiences, knowledge, beliefs, prejudices, and expectations are constantly shaping, filling in the gaps, and potentially distorting our perception of what actually occurred; a reason that eyewitness testimony is not always reliable. Since memory is a product of perception, it can become distorted whenever our perception becomes distorted or disrupted.

Vision is a huge contributor to memory because it is the primary mechanism by which we observe the world around us. Hearing, touch, taste, and smell play a role too, of course, but not to as great a degree in most people. Under extreme stress, visual exclusion or tunnel vision narrows our field of view by as much as 70 percent. Similarly, stress-induced pupil dilation can disrupt our ability to focus (especially on close objects), degrading our depth perception. Since the visual field is disrupted or narrowed, the amount of information we collect from it will be incomplete.

We are constantly bombarded by stimuli from the world around us, much of which is disregarded as unimportant and not transferred from short term to long term memory. Even in individuals with so-called "photographic memories," focused attention is required to ensure that transfer. Focused attention to certain stimuli can preclude attention to others, resulting in a flashbulb-like effect where only certain aspects of an event are actually remembered (for example, something new or unusual).

Immediately after a traumatic incident, much of what occurred is still in the brain, but it has not been processed in such a manner that it can be retrieved. One of the key factors in being able to access such information is sleep. The brain focuses on problem solving and the resolution of emotional concerns during sleep, particularly during REM sleep (which is when most dreaming occurs). This sleep cycle helps the brain consolidate unusual information that requires a good deal of adaptation in order for it to be absorbed. In fact, REM sleep cycles happen more frequently and last longer for individuals who are placed in circumstances in which they must process great quantities of new information. Although you may not remember much about a traumatic incident right after it occurs, you should experience significant memory recovery after a good night's sleep.

> Traumatic situations are frequently associated with critical incident amnesia. The greater the stress, the greater your potential of experiencing memory problems. Although you may not remember much about a traumatic incident right after it occurs, you should experience significant memory recovery after a good night's sleep. Do everything you can to safeguard your first night's sleep after any violent encounter.

If your initial night's sleep is disturbed, however, memory recovery may be disrupted. Further, if you are rendered unconscious or injured to the extent that you require an operation involving general anesthesia, there is a good possibility that normal memory recovery will be greatly disrupted. Your ability to remember crucial details about a violent incident and subsequently to defend yourself in court is greatly influenced by the memory recovery process. Do everything you can to safeguard your first night's sleep after any violent encounter.

Expect to be debriefed by law enforcement professionals shortly after a fight. If your memory about what occurred is fuzzy, take extra caution to avoid guessing to fill in the blanks. Anything you guess about may be held against you in a court of law. Better still; wait until your attorney is present before making any statements.

Don't Exaggerate, Don't Threaten

Hence the saying: if you know the enemy and know yourself, your victory will not stand in doubt; if you know Heaven and know Earth, you may make your victory complete.

– Sun Tzu

When you opponent is hurrying recklessly, you must act contrarily, and keep calm. You must not be influenced by the opponent. Train diligently to attain this spirit.

– Miyamoto Musashi

"They have never hung a mute. Anything you say can and will be used against you in court of law." That is what an attorney told Wilder some fifteen years ago. He was right then and he is right now. Don't exaggerate; it will be interpreted in the worst light when it is read in court. And don't threaten because there is no question, no doubt without exception, that it is going to be used against you in court. Celebrities, politicians, and other powerful individuals often attempt to throw their weight around when dealing with the police, thinking that their name, reputation, or wealth will buy them special treatment. Despite some notorious and highly publicized exceptions, it usually ends badly for them, and almost certainly will for you, too, if you try to go that route.

When the police arrive, they will talk to everybody and write down everything they hear. What is written is neither screened nor reviewed. It is put into the report and the report goes into the official record. Any half-truths, lies, or whatever you utter will get written down and it will be read into court as fact. Don't hang yourself with your own words.

Officers are there to ascertain the truth, gathering unbiased facts and evidence about what transpired. They are not there to hand you a medal for heroism under adversity even if you really did act heroically. If, in their best judgment, there is probable cause that you should be locked up because you committed a crime, then that's exactly what will happen. Not exactly fair, but common enough nevertheless, especially if you used a weapon and there is no compelling evidence (for example, witnesses, closed circuit video tape) that you used it in self-defense. The way you interact with police officers when they arrive is critical to your continued well-being. No matter how upset, injured, angry, insulted, or unsettled you are, never forget that your words and demeanor can significantly affect the tone of the entire encounter and the eventual outcome.

Whether or not you are arrested hinges on a concept known as "probable cause." Probable cause means that the responding officer has a reasonable belief that a crime has been committed and that you are the perpetrator. This belief can be based upon several factors, including direct observation, professional expertise, circumstantial evidence, or factual information. Officers will make a decision based upon what, if anything, they saw during the incident, what they can infer about the incident based upon professional experience, physical evidence or other factors at the scene, statements from witnesses, victims, or suspects, available video surveillance, and other relevant data.

Approach the responding officer(s) positively. Police are people too. They likely have the same emotional makeup that you do. Officers arriving on the scene will be encountering an unknown, potentially hostile environment, where one or more combatants may have been, and possibly still are, armed. Like any sane person, they will be concerned, cautious, and likely at least a little bit scared. Since they do not know exactly what transpired, they also do not know who the good guy is and who the bad guy is yet.

A confrontational attitude will do you no good and may well guarantee that you will be arrested or possibly even shot. Even undercover officers have been killed on occasion by their uniformed counterparts when they failed to follow directions immediately and/ or did not identify themselves properly. For example, on January 12, 2001 undercover police officer William Alberto Wilkins was shot and killed by fellow officers in Oakland California. Detective Wilkins, a seven-year veteran with the Oakland PD, was working a narcotics stakeout when he spotted a stolen car pass by. He pursued and caught the car thief near San Leandro and was holding the suspect at gunpoint in a driveway when the two uniformed officers arrived. Misunderstanding the scene, at least one of the responding officers opened fire, striking Wilkins several times in the upper torso. Eleven shell casings were found at the scene. Wilkins died at Highland Hospital a few hours later. He was survived by his wife and ten-month-old son.

If you are training a weapon on a subdued attacker, be sure to follow responding officer's instructions immediately without any hesitation. While the officer does not know whether you are the good guy, he knows with absolute certainty that you are armed and dangerous. You don't want to survive a violent confrontation only to be killed afterward due to a preventable misunderstanding.

Be respectful, courteous, obedient, and kind but remember that the officer(s) is not your friend—not your enemy either, but still not your friend. The officer's job is to secure the environment, provide for aid, gather facts, and enforce the law. Consequently, he or she will not necessarily be on your side no matter how prudently you acted, at least not until all the facts are known.

You may not be arrested, but if you are, do not resist for any reason. Similarly, do not interfere with an attempt to arrest anyone who is with you at the time. Attempting to flee, evade, or elude responding officers is almost certainly going to make you look guilty and result in a chase and subsequent detention.

Control your emotions to the extent possible. Carefully and calmly, explain what happened so that the responding officer(s) will know that you are the good guy. Retain your composure and conduct yourself in a mature manner at all times, avoiding any words or actions that may appear threatening or volatile. Never forget that police are trained interrogators. They will note your body language, speech patterns, and eye movements to help ascertain your probable guilt or innocence when deciding whether to make an arrest. Worse yet, officers will err on the side of caution, so even a suspicion of guilt may be enough to earn you a night in jail.

Remember the section on critical incident amnesia? Your memory will probably not be firing on all cylinders. Say as little as possible. Here is an example of something you might say that is perfectly honest and should be relatively well received:

> *"This was very traumatic experience. I think I'm in shock. I don't think I should say anything until I'm calmer. Can I please call [your attorney or contact person]?"*

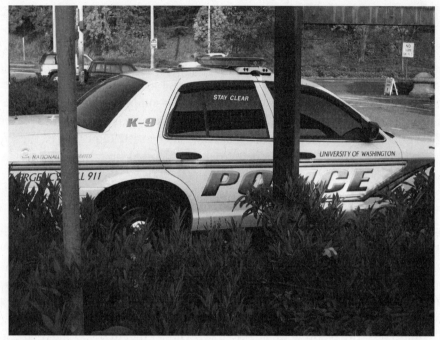

Approach the responding officer(s) positively. A confrontational attitude will do you no good and may well guarantee that you will be arrested or possibly even shot if they perceive a significant enough threat.

Do not, under any circumstances, make any incriminating statements that may be used against you at a later time. Do not confess to any crime, even if you think you exercised poor judgment or are actually guilty. Having said that, however, do not withhold any information that can affect the responding officer's safety either. Bad guys may still be roaming; armed friends may have melted into the crowd.

Officers usually distinguish between a debrief/interview conducted at the police station where legal representation is appropriate and a tactical debrief which takes place at the scene to make sure the situation is really resolved and that you are really safe. If you withhold information that endangers officers, you will not make friends and could get someone seriously hurt, but information you give could (rarely but theoretically) incriminate you. It could also break down your resistance to talking and get you blabbing, which is generally unwise.

While there may be a fine balance between implying guilt through silence and being overly talkative, err on the side of caution. You really do not have to say anything at all without an attorney present though it is generally prudent to identify yourself, state that the other person attacked you, and that you were in imminent and unavoidable danger, fearing for your life. You may even wish to explain why you could not simply run away.

If you used a weapon and have a concealed weapons permit, it is generally a good idea to let the officers know that as well.

The Fourth Amendment generally prohibits seizure of persons without a warrant. However, in some instances a warrant may not required. These instances can include felonies, misdemeanors, danger to the public, and violent crimes. A fight probably qualifies for warrantless arrest under any of these conditions. If you are arrested and taken into custody, be sure to understand why.

You should always carry the phone number of an attorney you trust (see "Find a Good Attorney" later on in this section for more information) and of a person who can contact an attorney for you if your lawyer is not immediately available. Ask permission to telephone your attorney or contact person immediately after being booked into jail.

Be polite and respectful to the jail guards. They can deny you phone access and generally make your life even more miserable if you act inappropriately. In most jurisdictions, you must be taken before an officer of the court (for example, judge, magistrate) within 24 hours of your arrest, except on weekends. You should always secure counsel and have legal representation before this initial court appearance. If you cannot afford an attorney, you can be represented by a public defender though that is generally not preferable.

> Officers arriving on the scene will be encountering an unknown, potentially hostile environment, where one or more combatants may have been, and possibly still are, armed. Like any sane person, they will be concerned, cautious, and likely at least a little bit scared. Since they do not know exactly what transpired, they also do not know who the good guy is and who the bad guy is yet. Retain your composure and conduct yourself in a mature manner at all times. A confrontational attitude will do you no good and may well get you arrested or possibly even shot. Don't exaggerate; it will be interpreted in the worst possible light when it is read in court. Don't threaten; there is no question that it will be used against you if you do.

When responding officers arrive, don't exaggerate, and don't threaten. Be calm, polite, honest, and non-confrontational, saying as little as possible until you have an opportunity to consult with your attorney.

Police Officers Don't Like Fighting, So They Don't Like You

Supreme excellence consists in breaking the enemy's resistance without fighting.
— Sun Tzu

The spirit of fire is fierce, whether the fire be small or big; and so it is with battles.
— Miyamoto Musashi

The fight is over, the police have arrived, and somebody is going to jail. Responding officers really don't care a whole lot about how it started or what you were fighting about. A couple of questions to make an assessment, a professional assessment based on their experience, and more often than not, somebody gets arrested. Officers will err on the side of caution, prudently letting a judge determine guilt or innocence. They just want to eliminate the immediate threat and control the danger that you and/or your adversary caused to the public welfare.

You might think that what you are involved in is the most important thing in the world at that moment. You might be fighting over the love of your life, defending your honor, trying to get paid for a bet or a loan, or collecting sports memorabilia that was stolen from you. It might be very important to you, yet these officers have just left a scene just like yours to deal with you. And the odds are good that they'll get another half a dozen calls just like yours before the night is over.

> Law enforcement officers have to have a shell; without it, they can't function. They are not bad people, but they simply see, hear, and feel too much to allow an emotional attachment for every person and every problem. You with your petty problems don't have a chance at cracking that shell. Police officers don't like fighting, so if you get into a fight they almost certainly are not going to be all that thrilled with you.

From the jaded perspective of a veteran officer, you're really not that special. You're barely a name, let alone a face. Your story, your issues, they mean absolutely nothing to these guys. The officers cannot afford to get emotionally involved; they have a job to do. Now don't take that as an anti-cop comment because it is not. They have a dirty, unglamorous, rotten job to do that few are willing to take. We should all be damned thankful that there are people willing to step up and do it. The challenge is that in order to survive on the mean streets of most any city, a certain level of emotional detachment has to come with the territory.

To illustrate this point, Wilder was standing in the control center of a jail with a police officer friend of his when an internal call came in. A young woman was going through drug withdrawal and had started having seizures. The ambulance was called and the mobilization process was underway to get her to the hospital.

Holding the chart in his hand, Wilder's officer friend read the file. "May I see it too?" Wilder asked. The officer closed it and handed it to him as he turned to the issues at hand. Wilder looked at the file and after scanning it said, "Wow, twenty-seven, pretty, and strung out, what the hell?"

"Yup, you can't afford to get involved," his friend said as he reached for the file.

"No," Wilder replied, "You can't, but I can."

His friend gave a small smile and nodded. Simply put, law enforcement officers have to have a shell; without it, they can't function. They are not bad people, they just see, hear, and feel too much to allow an emotional attachment for every person and every problem. You with your petty problems don't have a chance at cracking that shell.

Find a Good Attorney

Attorneys and legal counselors were not addressed by Sun Tzu or Miyamoto Musashi in their writings. Feudal warlords developed judicial codes that were administered by the sword without complicating factors or intricacies of modern laws. A disgraced samurai, for example, was expected to salvage his honor by committing seppuku, ritual suicide.

If you've been in a fight, there is a very good chance that you'll be charged with a crime. When that happens, you need a professional on your side to help you navigate the complex legal system and give you the best odds of prevailing. As the old saying goes, "Lawyers who represent themselves in court have idiots for clients." Seriously, the average person is woefully unprepared to defend himself in court. That's like a weekend golfer trying to compete with Tiger Woods. You could get in a lucky shot and win a hole or two, but your odds of victory over an 18-hole course are miniscule at best.

You need the best attorney (or team of attorneys) you can afford to help you out. The legal fight is just as dangerous if not more so than the physical fight you just survived. Lose this one and you may very well lose your freedom, your job, your house, your relationships, and your money. Relying on an underpaid, overworked public defender appointed by the court is the last thing you should do unless you absolutely have no other choice. You want someone fully committed to win your case.

It is very useful to have an attorney in mind before you actually need one. It's

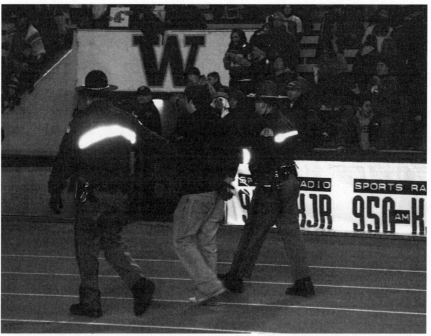

Officers tend to err on the side of caution, prudently letting a judge determine guilt or innocence. They want to eliminate the immediate threat and control the danger that you and/or your adversary have caused to the public welfare.

downright imperative if you have a concealed weapon permit and carry a firearm or work in a violence-prone vocation (for example, bouncer, bounty hunter, security guard). The challenge is that surfing the net or browsing the yellow pages is a time-consuming, haphazard way to find one. A good place to find a solid reference is through a friend or relative. Even if they have only used someone for civil matters such as creating a will, their attorney will likely know someone who specializes in criminal defense law. If you are enrolled in college, you can check with the law school there. They will often have an excellent referral service. You can also contact the Bar Association where you live or work to find solid referrals.

It's important to find a lawyer who has a long track record in the applicable field of law, someone who has successfully worked on cases like yours in the recent past. For example, a DUI* attorney might be the top player in his field, a real expert at defending accused drunk drivers, yet totally incompetent to handle a murder case. Further, since many violent crime cases like murder or aggravated assault are settled with a plea bargain instead of going to trial, you will want someone who has experience adjudicating a case like yours through the whole process. If you truly are innocent, pleading guilty to a lesser offense would be highly inadvisable in most instances. Take your attorney's advice on that though, not ours.

In firms with multiple attorneys, different lawyers may represent different cases or different aspects of the same case. Be sure to meet the person who will actually be representing your case. If a team is likely to be involved, be sure to meet with each specialist before agreeing to anything. This reasonable request should be readily accommodated. After all, you are the paying customer. It is your welfare on the line.

Understand what and how you will be charged for the case. You will undoubtedly want to hire the best attorney you can possibly afford, but you should always understand the pricing structure before signing any contract. For example, research work may include activities performed by clerks, investigators, or analysts in addition to the attorney who heads up your case. Expert witnesses may be retained as well. Understand how the fees for each aspect of the case will be handled and what options, if any, there are. Some attorneys quote flat fees while others charge by the hour. Some accept payment schedules while others require payment prior to performance of the service.

Ascertain how reliable, available, and responsive your prospective lawyer is likely to be. Most attorneys keep a running backlog of cases, managing multiple clients at the same time. Regardless, it is important that you be able to contact your attorney whenever you need assistance throughout the legal process as well as whenever any new information about your case may arise. Understand your prospective attorney's schedule and availability, asking questions such as how often you will be able to meet with him or her. You may be relying on this person not only to defend you in a criminal court but also in any

---

* Driving Under the Influence (DUI) or Driving While Intoxicated (DWI) in some jurisdictions, is a crime committed by a person who operates a motor vehicle while impaired by alcohol or drugs.

follow-on civil procedure as well, so you don't want someone who's too busy to give you his or her best work.

Once you have selected someone to defend you, you will need to be patient and cooperate. Never forget that your attorney is literally your lifeline, protecting your freedom and reputation. While you are bound to be anxious and generally afraid, the justice system moves rather slowly at times.

Ask about the costs, benefits, and risks of pursuing any particular legal strategy. Cooperate with your defense attorney to help expedite the process by promptly providing information. Be willing to do some of your own legwork, gathering documents and information as requested. Keep a log of any questions you might have so that you can discuss them during regular consultations rather than contacting your attorney every time something pops into your head.

As your case progresses, your attorney will work with you to develop a plan for securing your freedom and restoring your reputation. Criminal defense strategies can include alibis, justifications, procedural defenses, and excuses. While the particulars of each case will be different, alibis and justifications are fairly common and are generally effective defense strategies. Procedural and excuse defenses can be challenging to prove in a court of law. There are a few other innovative defenses as well, but they are unorthodox, fairly rare, and not generally effective.

- An alibi is based upon a premise that you are completely innocent, attempting to prove that you were in another place when the alleged act was committed and could therefore not possibly be guilty.

- A justification is where you admit that you committed the act but should not be held liable for your actions because of certain special or extenuating circumstances. A justification for murder, for example, is a legitimate claim of self-defense (which makes it not a murder in the eyes of the court).

- A procedural defense attempts to prove that while you broke the law, you cannot be held criminally liable because the state violated a procedural rule. Examples include entrapment, prosecutorial misconduct, double jeopardy, or denial of a speedy trial. In these instances, you may have done something wrong but cannot be found guilty.

> The average person is woefully unprepared to defend himself in court. That's like a weekend golfer trying to compete with Tiger Woods. You could get in a lucky shot and win a hole or two, but your odds of victory over an 18-hole course are miniscule. You need the best attorney you can afford to help you out. Relying on an underpaid, overworked public defender appointed by the court is the last thing you should do unless you absolutely have no other choice. You want someone fully committed to win your case. This legal fight is just as dangerous if not more so than the physical fight you just survived. You may be facing both criminal and civil litigation with your freedom, your job, your house, your relationships, and your money on the line.

- An excuse is an argument that you were not liable for your actions at the time a law was broken. Examples include diminished capacity, duress, or insanity. While you may not be criminally liable in such instances, you may still be civilly committed to professional counseling in order to assure that you recover from the illness that let you off the hook.

- Other so-called "innovative defenses" can include allegations of long-term abuse, premenstrual syndrome, battered women's syndrome, urban survival syndrome, and other creative things that lawyers occasionally use to try to convince a jury to acquit a defendant. These things rarely work, however, and are generally not something a prudent attorney would try. Be cautious if your attorney suggests pursuing this line of defense.

If you face a legal fight in the courtroom, it can be just as dangerous if not more so than the physical fight you survived on the street. You may be facing both criminal and civil litigation with your freedom, your job, your house, your relationships, and your money on the line. Find the best attorney you can afford, someone with the knowledge, skills, and experience necessary to help you win.

Realize That Courts Are About Resolution, Not Justice

The art of war, then, is governed by five constant factors, to be taken into account in one's deliberations, when seeking to determine the conditions obtaining in the field. These are: (1) The Moral Law; (2) Heaven; (3) Earth; (4) The Commander; (5) Method and discipline.

— *Sun Tzu*

Until you realize the true Way, whether in Buddhism or in common sense, you may think that things are correct and in order. However, if we look at things objectively, from the viewpoint of laws of the world, we see various doctrines departing from the true Way.

— *Miyamoto Musashi*

If you are looking for justice from the courts, you are playing a fool's game. Courts are not interested in justice, they are interested in resolution. While judges are honorable, hardworking individuals, the courts are jam-packed with cases, notoriously understaffed, and in some cases, truly overwhelmed. Your case is a minor blip to the average judge. You may think that your case is different, special, or unique, but it is not. Your case means nothing; these judges have seen thousands of people just like you. They don't have the emotional investment in your case that you do. They are not bad people by any means, yet like police officers, they simply cannot get that emotionally involved with every person they come across while performing their official duties. Frankly, the three cases that came on the docket before yours are probably the same. It all becomes a blur after enough time.

Look at the lists of people with rap sheets five feet long who are still out on the streets—these guys became professional criminals a long time ago. If there were justice, they wouldn't be out preying on the weak, vulnerable, aged, and defenseless of our society. Jail to these professional criminals means three free meals a day, long showers, plenty of sleep, and a great opportunity to study up on what they did wrong and refine their technique. It is a nice respite to help them get ready for their next go in the world of violence and crime.

Facing a shortage of bed space, severe overcrowding, and a lack of taxpayer willingness or political wherewithal to build additional facilities, prisons throughout the country are forced to make tough decisions. They use a variety of processes to identify low-risk offenders, such as prison matrixing, to routinely releasing prisoners early. Unfortunately, there is rarely such a thing as "low risk" when it comes to criminal offenders.

According to the Bureau of Justice Statistics, recidivism rates are very high. About three percent of the adult population has spent time in prison. That's not jail, mind you, but prison, the place where you are sent for serious crimes with convictions that result in long-term sentences. Jail, on the other hand, is where inmates are locked up for a relatively short time, such as awaiting trial or serving a short-term sentence. Almost three quarters of parolees are re-arrested for felonies or serious misdemeanor crimes within three years of release. About half of those are re-convicted for a new crime.

You, most likely, are not a professional criminal. That means that you are just the kind of person that the justice system likes. You are inclined to make bail (that costs you money). You are likely to show up in court with an attorney (that costs too). You are looking to earn some sort of parole (that takes time, and time equals money). Depending on what you have been accused of, you might well be assigned a psychiatric examination (that costs money) and a violence education program (that takes a lot time, the cost for which you have the privilege of paying too).

In short, as a regular, generally law-abiding citizen, you are also an easy mark for the courts. You will bear the full brunt of the legal system. You can pad their conviction statistics by pleading guilty to a lesser crime in order to avoid the risk of an extended prison stay. In most cases, you probably shouldn't cop a plea, but you certainly may be tempted to. After all, you value your life and your lifestyle. The professional criminal, on the other hand, couldn't care less what the judge says. All he hears is, "Quack, quack, woof, woof, ninety days, yadda yadda..." The threat of a jail stay or prison term is not an earth-shattering, life-changing event as it would be to the rest of us. It is, rather, a minor inconvenience.

Courts are designed to process people and come to resolution. Justice is an expensive commodity. The police do their job and the courts do theirs. Unfortunately, if you

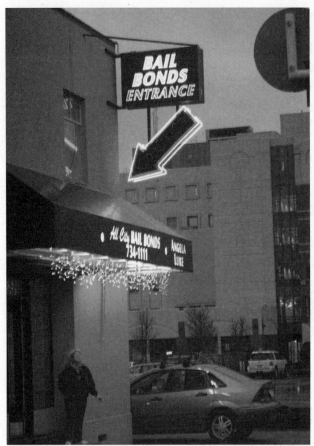

For the professional criminal, a jail stay or prison term is a minor in-convenience. Recidivism rates are high; roughly 75 percent of felons are re-arrested within three years of release and about half of those re-arrested are re-convicted of a new crime.

engage in violence you will get pinched in the middle.

If you still think that courts are about justice, go ask Nicole Simpson or Ronald Goldman what justice is all about. Oops, you can't... because they are dead. Their murderer, O.J. Simpson, has been living in Florida, playing golf as a free man. Well, legally he wasn't the murderer now was he? He was acquitted in criminal court. Even though Simpson lost the subsequent civil trial, the victims' families have not been compensated for their losses. A Florida bankruptcy court awarded the rights to Simpson's book *If I Did It: Confessions of the Killer* to the Goldmans in August 2007 to satisfy partially the unpaid wrongful death judgment, which had risen, with interest, to over $38 million.

To further illustrate the point that the courts are about resolution rather than justice, here are a few more examples. These situations involved law enforcement professionals, the very people who go out there and protect the rest of us every day. The system failed them too. All three of these events took place in Seattle, Washington, over a four-month period in 2006.

- On August 13th, Seattle Officer Joselito Barber, 26, was killed when her car was hit by the vehicle that Mary Jane Rivas was driving. Rivas, who had just been released from prison, was accused of being high on cocaine at the time of the incident and was subsequently charged with vehicular homicide. She pled guilty in King County Superior Court on September 21, 2007.

- On November 13th, Seattle Police Officer Beth Nowak was killed on her way to work when a convicted felon, Neal Kelley, with an outstanding warrant for his arrest, crashed a stolen Honda into Nowak's vehicle. Kelley died at the scene as well.

• On December 2nd, Sheriff's Deputy Steve Cox responded to reports of shots being fired in the White Center neighborhood and was interviewing several people at a house party when one of them ambushed and killed him. Deputy Cox was shot in the head twice by one of the witnesses, Raymond Porter, a convicted felon who was on active supervision by the state Department of Corrections. After fatally wounding Cox, Porter shot and killed himself as well.

It works the same way in civil court too. For example, administrative law judge Roy L. Pearson, Jr. filed a 54 million dollar lawsuit against a drycleaners that lost his pants. While Pearson ultimately lost his infamous case, the defendant, Soo Chung, was run through the emotional wringer and had to pay out thousands of dollars in legal fees to defend himself. The case was filed in June of 2005, cycled through two judges, three settlement offers, dozens of exhibits, and hundreds of pages of court filings before culminating in an emotional two-day trial. During the proceedings, both the plaintiff and the defendant burst into tears. The case was finally wrapped up in June of 2007. Tired of the whole ordeal, the Chungs sold their business and closed up shop three months later. According to news reports, Pearson is expected to appeal so it may not be over yet. If a mundane matter like a lost pair of pants can bring about this much heartache, imagine what a wrongful death lawsuit might be like.

> Courts are not interested in justice, they are interested in resolution. For the professional criminal, a jail stay or prison term is a minor inconvenience. Recidivism rates are high; roughly 75 percent of felons are re-arrested within three years of release and about half of those re-arrested are re-convicted of a new crime. Justice is an expensive commodity. The police do their job and the courts do theirs. Unfortunately, if you engage in violence you will get pinched in the middle.

We've all seen examples in the news where celebrities who can afford handlers, fixers, and small armies of attorneys can get away with things that the average citizen cannot. Despite the tabloids and the headlines, however, the justice system really does work pretty well much of the time. Even the rich and famous can wind up doing hard time when they get caught. Imagine how much worse it might be for you, the not so rich, and mostly anonymous. Your best bet is keeping your nose clean, of course, but if you ever do find yourself caught up in the legal system, it is paramount that you find yourself an excellent attorney to help you navigate the process.

Courts are interested in resolution, not justice. If you find yourself caught up in the legal system it will cost you. The police do their job and the courts do theirs. If you engage in violence, you are bound to get caught in the middle. It's expensive, time-consuming, and fraught with peril. Think about that the next time you're in the mood to hit someone.

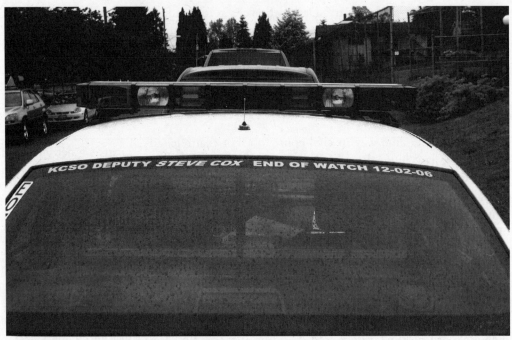

A tribute to slain Sheriff's Deputy Steve Cox. Deputy Cox was gunned down on December 2nd, 2006, by a convicted felon who was on active supervision by the state Department of Corrections at the time of the shooting.

Be Wary of the Press

In the times of Sun Tzu and Miyamoto Musashi, the ruling aristocracy controlled the media. Warlords and kings commissioned songs and plays to honor their names and legacies. An independent press was unheard of; hence, reporters were never discussed in their works.

Dealing with the press is dangerous. You may be excited to do an interview or get in front of the cameras, but it is very important to look before you leap into headlines. Never forget that your fifteen minutes of fame could easily be used against you in a court of law. Much as you'd like to have a moment in the spotlight, it is critical that you check with your attorney before accepting any interviews. Be prepared to have him or her either coach you or handle questions in your stead.

Hardly anyone is truly fair and balanced. Almost all humans have biases, even reporters. In fact, there is an ongoing debate in the United States about the liberal/conservative bias of the media. Whatever side of the line you fall on, if you get cross-wise with a member of the press you may not be treated fairly. This is important because any interviews you may provide to the press could be taken out of context in a manner that can adversely affect your case.

For example, a Rabbi we know accidentally struck and killed a pedestrian while driving his daughter to school. Since he was talking on a cell phone at the time, he was charged with a crime and eventually tasked to perform community service, a light sentence that caused a lot of anger and even some anti-Semitic incidents. The local news media focused on this man's poor driving record; he'd been in fender-benders before, but the media did not fully explain the circumstances surrounding the accident that took place that morning. The person he hit was wearing dark clothing, listening to an iPod, and stepped out into the crosswalk directly in front of him without looking. Even though he was traveling just under the speed limit, neither the Rabbi nor anyone in his vehicle (or even the car behind him for that matter) saw the victim in the early morning darkness. All these facts came out in the trial where he was acquitted of 15 of the 16 charges against him.

While what was reported was not factually incorrect, it was not the whole story either. This man and his family were devastated not only because he accidentally killed someone but also because the incomplete reporting turned the community against him. His life will never be the same.

It is prudent to consider that if you speak with a reporter about a violent incident you were involved with, you may well be dealing with a hostile audience. We all know that reporters should be completely objective, of course, but that does not necessarily mean that they always are. It is important to understand what angle a story is likely to take. If the reporter is evasive, tread lightly. It may be useful to pull up copies of other stories the person has written or produced to get a feel for how you might be treated.

It is generally considered taboo for a reporter to send you a copy of a story to review or approve, so do not expect to be able to do that regardless of how much you may want the opportunity to do so. Always get the reporter's contact information and find out when and where the piece will appear so that you can view the end result however.

> You may be excited to do an interview or get in front of the cameras, but it is very important to look before you leap into headlines. Never forget that your fifteen minutes of fame could easily be used against you in a court of law. Avoid talking to reporters unless specifically advised by your attorney that it will help your case to do so.

On- and off-camera interviews should be handled a bit differently. Here's some advice:

- For on-camera interviews, ask for some warm-up questions so that you can compose yourself before you speak. If you can get a hold of the questions you will be asked ahead of time, you will have some time to think of answers that are meaningful and hard to be misinterpreted or taken out of context.
- If it is an off-camera interview, take your time to answer, and then say what you feel. Be sure to check in with the reporter and understand whether he or she understood your message. If the person repeats back your quotes and paraphrases his understanding, you will have a chance to clear up any confusion.

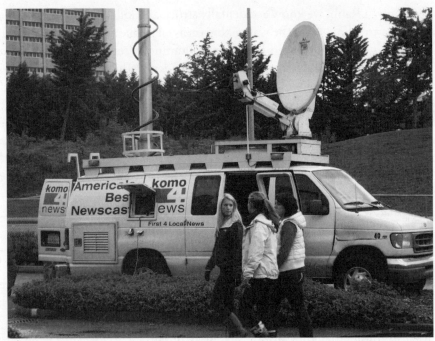

Dealing with the press is dangerous. You may be excited to do an interview or get in front of the cameras, but never forget that your fifteen minutes of fame could easily be used against you in a court of law later on.

Once the interview is published or the story is aired, you can call or e-mail the writer or editor and request a correction if you were misquoted or there is an egregious error. Better still, avoid talking to reporters altogether, unless specifically advised by your attorney that it will help your case to do so. Be wary of the press.

Beware the "Friday Night Special"

At first, then, exhibit the coyness of a maiden, until the enemy gives you an opening; afterwards emulate the rapidity of a running hare, and it will be too late for the enemy to oppose you.

– Sun Tzu

Or, in single combat, start by making a show of being slow, then suddenly attack strongly. Without allowing him space for breath to recover from the fluctuation of spirit, you must grasp the opportunity to win. Get the feel of this.

– Miyamoto Musashi

Dispute the presumption of innocence in most jurisprudence, as a man you are almost always assumed guilty when it comes to domestic violence. Domestic violence can be very serious so courts tend to err on the side of caution. Consequently, when the police arrive for a domestic violence call, someone has to be arrested and taken to jail. If you are it, as guys almost always are, you will have the expensive proposition of proving that you are innocent.

Various states and municipalities have different laws governing how domestic violence is governed, yet the following is a general overview of what you can expect. This scenario is what some attorneys call the "Friday Night Special."

Let's pretend for a moment that you and your spouse (or girlfriend) have been having some troubles lately. Not too unrealistic a starting point, right? After all what relationship doesn't have a few rough spots? So you come home on a Friday night after a long day at work or school, have a beer, and get into a spat with your significant other. She dials 9-1-1 and reports you for domestic violence.*

Maybe something happened and maybe it did not. Maybe you were the one who got shoved or hit or perhaps you initiated the confrontation. Sadly, it makes absolutely no difference to the arriving police; they are going to arrest you because that is the law. A report of domestic violence means that somebody goes to jail. If she made the call, you are the one who's going.

The beer on your breath isn't helping either. After being handcuffed and arrested, probably right in front of your child if you have one, you get processed into the jail. This could take hours. You get a statutory phone call, but reaching an attorney on a Friday night is simply not going to happen. The attorneys will be back in the office on Monday, so unless you've got his home phone number and a solid relationship, you're stuck until then. Regardless, in most jurisdictions you must be held for 24 hours before you are eligible for release.

Saturday morning rolls around and you share a phone with several other men in the cell while trying to reach some relative or an attorney to bail you out. Here's where it often gets really ugly: While you are on the phone trying to make bail, your significant other has gone to the bank and removed all of the money from your joint account.

Sunday rolls around and you still are not out of jail yet, but you discover that there is a twenty day Temporary Restraining Order (TRO) against you that she has imposed by simply asking for it. In most cases, no proof is needed for a TRO, only an accusation. Since the law errs on the side of caution when it comes to accusations of domestic violence and spousal abuse, it is pretty easy for her to get a TRO. Hearings to evaluate the merits of the TRO will follow but that does you no good right now.

---

* Domestic violence typically means: (a) Physical harm, bodily injury, assault, or the infliction of fear of imminent physical harm, bodily injury or assault, between family or household members; (b) sexual assault of one family or household member by another; or (c) stalking of one family or household member by another family or household member. This definition is from the Revised Code of Washington 26.50.010. That "infliction of fear of..." part gives responding officers and prosecutors a lot of leeway.

On Monday afternoon, you finally get bailed out. You ask your friend who has secured your release to take you back to your place to get a new set of clothes. Before you get there, you suddenly realize that you can't get any of your possessions from your house or apartment because of the temporary restraining order. The TRO states that if you come within sixty feet of her, you will be in violation of the order and immediately go back to jail where you will be held until your trial date.

Since going home is not an option, you go to the bank to get some money for a set of new clothes and some food instead. Unfortunately, the teller tells you that you don't have an account with this bank anymore; your significant other withdrew all the money and closed it. Now, you're broke! Oh, and don't forget that you still need to call your boss and tell him or her why you didn't make it to the office on Monday.

Finally you talk one of your friends into lending you some couch space and a set of clothes. A day or two later, you're back at work, but it's still not over yet. While you have been setting your life back in order, she is preparing a yard sale for your stuff, assuming it hasn't already been placed on the curb with a "Free" sign on it.

Want to do something and get your possessions back? Sadly, you can't because it is only hearsay as to what is hers and what is yours. The police are not going to stop a yard sale and you'd better not break the restraining order by showing up, and even asking that your stuff not be sold or you go back to jail.

A week later, the landlord calls your cell phone because the rent is late. You explain the situation and he says, "It's your name in the lease. You gotta pay up!"

Suddenly you recognize that your credit is at risk too. You open you eyes wide and grasp the fact that you have a joint credit card. Frantically you make that fateful call to the credit card company only to discover that your worst fear has been realized—your card is maxed out too! Hanging up the phone, you realize that

- You have been arrested for domestic violence.
- Your job was placed at risk.
- You have lost all your possessions in a yard sale.
- Your credit is ruined.
- You are in debt, deep.
- You owe an attorney.
- You have to take time off from work to go to court.
- ...but wait, it is not over yet...

Last weekend she left the apartment, took your kid(s), and moved in with her mother in a state that has no reciprocity agreement. This means that the state she has left for does not recognize your state's laws. You didn't file for divorce or separation because you didn't think about it and, frankly, you didn't have the money even if you had wanted to. And you couldn't take the time off of work to meet with an attorney and file papers, so now you have no standing in the eyes of the court.

What does this mean? It means you may never get to see your child(ren) again. Let's hope she doesn't accuse you of molesting the kid too. That's a common enough tactic and will almost certainly bar you from ever seeing your child again.

Oh and don't forget the truck she took was registered in your name and the payments are late. *Ka-ching...* again.

Done? Nope, not yet... You get to pay child support for a child you will likely never see. Refuse to pay and suddenly you're a "deadbeat dad." If you become one, you are going to get reported; guess by whom? Now the state will garnish your wages to get the money you owe her.

Now jump ahead a couple of years. You could not afford an attorney so either you've had an incompetent public defender who let you get convicted, you actually were guilty, or you simply pled to a lesser charge to get things over with. Your life is somewhat back in order, you've got a little money, so now you go and try to rent a nice place to live. Unfortunately, you've still got bad credit.

But wait, it gets worse still. When you get to the checkbox on the application that asks, "Have you ever been convicted of a crime; if yes please explain," what are you going to do? That is just what the landlord wants in his or her place, a dangerous domestic violence offender. Oh, and you will find that checkbox on your next job application too.

Never lie about the domestic violence conviction. Tell the truth by checking the little box and you get rejected for that great job that would have almost doubled your annual income. However, lie about the case to get the job and you will always have that Sword of Damocles hanging over your head. And rest assured it will be found out sooner or later. No matter how good you are at the job, you are out the door looking for a new job as soon as someone uncovers the truth.

What do you think about this little scenario? An exaggeration you think? Sure, we presented the worst-case scenario, but we know a couple of real live individuals that a number of these things have happened to. So, do this little drill: Go ahead and cut half of the events out of the story. Still looks pretty grim doesn't it? Now cut the story in half once again. Not a whole lot of improvement, is there?

What can you do about it? First off, to state the obvious, choose wisely when entering into a long-term relationship with anyone. Whoever you let move in with you will have an unprecedented level of access to you and your stuff. While it might seem a bit paranoid to conduct a background check on your prospective partner, it can be a good (and relatively inexpensive) way to protect yourself. Since everyone puts on their best face forward while they are dating, you may not discover a history of mental illness, deviant behaviors, sexually transmittable diseases, financial difficulties, or legal problems until it's too late. Consider hiring a private investigator or using a resource like www.netdetective. com, www.ussearch.com, www.crimcheck.com, or www.sentrylink.com before taking a major step such as moving in together. Regardless of whether you do a background check or not, pay attention to any mental alarm bells that go off while you are together (see "Listen to the Subtle Warnings You Get" in Section One for a refresher on the signs of an abusive relationship).

If you have a solid partnership, domestic violence, and accusations thereof should never become an issue. Relationships are a two-way street, however, so you'll need to hold up your end of the bargain. Work on your active listening and communication skills to ensure that little problems don't fester to become big ones. If you sense signs of trouble brewing and cannot resolve them on your own, consider professional counseling or, potentially, ending the relationship before things can get ugly. If you do get into an argument, watch your temper. No matter how mad you get, never be the aggressor, at least not physically. Do your best to respond rather than react so that you cannot be goaded into starting something that you will regret.

According to many experts, serious relationship problems are often rooted in two areas: sex and money. Infidelity and financial difficulties are two of the leading causes of divorce. Until you are married, it is relatively easy to deal with the sex thing by either staying committed or breaking things off if you're tempted to stray. If you plan on getting married, be faithful to your wife. A few moments of pleasure is never worth the consequences of getting caught cheating, particularly when your soon-to-be ex-wife can use the legal system to make your life a living hell in retribution. False accusations of domestic abuse often stem from resentment. Hell hath no fury, and all that…

The money issue can be a bit more of a challenge, but nothing insurmountable. Never commingle your assets by conjoining your bank accounts, sharing credit cards, buying a house, or making investments together without the legal protections of marriage. Strongly consider a pre-nuptial agreement as well. Many couples find that they can eliminate much of the stress by maintaining separate bank accounts while collaborating on large purchases after they are married too. This type of arrangement also makes it much harder for your partner to pilfer your bank account without your knowledge.

There is no excuse for beating a woman. Unfortunately, even the accusation of abusing your significant other can land you in serious trouble. While both men and women can instigate violence, men are statistically more likely to be the perpetrator. Consequently, the laws of domestic violence are written and enforced to err on the side of caution. This means that they are stacked against you as a man. Act accordingly.

A Fight Can Take Place Over Time; It's Called a Feud, and It Is Bad

In war, then, let your great object be victory, not lengthy campaigns.
– Sun Tzu

The essence of strategy is to fall upon the enemy in large numbers and to bring about his speedy downfall.
– Miyamoto Musashi

A fight can take place over a long period of time. It's called a feud, and it's bad. For example, in 1878 a hog was stolen in the Appalachian Mountains. Twelve years later, in 1891, the result of the feud was

- One deserted pregnant woman (the guy left her for her cousin).
- One kidnapping.
- More than a dozen men dead, one stabbed 26 times and subsequently shot.
- About twelve bounty hunters presumed dead as they never returned and were never found.
- The call up of the West Virginia National Guard.
- Intervention by The U.S. Supreme Court.
- Seven life imprisonments.
- And, one hanging.

Want to get even with someone? Want to bump up against the law for your brand of justice? Just remember the Hatfields and McCoys because over a hundred years ago they got into a feud not too different from the one you might be thinking about. Nothing good will come of it. Don't start a feud. Oh, and in case you are wondering, nobody is really sure what happened to the hog.

Could something like this happen to you? Could you start something that you can't stop? Absolutely! Perhaps you have a girlfriend that wants to go out with some guy from the other fraternity so you decide to have a blanket party* and beat him senseless. His fraternity brothers subsequently get together and come gunning for you. Guess what? You've just started a feud.

Is this sort of thing real? You bet. Though he was not involved in the violence, something just like this happened in 1986 while Kane was in college. The instigator supposedly told his buddies that the other guy had raped his girlfriend, a claim she vehemently

---

* A "blanket party" is when a group of guys tackles their victim, wraps him up in a blanket, and beats on him with baseball bats or similar bludgeons until he stops squirming and making noises. It's positively brutal.

denied. No one died but there was at least one hospitalization, a very long recovery for the victim, several visits from the police, and more than one arrest.

Fistfights, acts of vandalism, and serious hard feelings between these two fraternities lasted for years, long after the guys involved in the incident had graduated and moved away. On one occasion, about a year after the original incident, Kane had to band together with a group of his fraternity brothers to prevent another guy, Ron, from bringing his gun to one of the subsequent brawls. Had they not intervened, someone would undoubtedly have been killed in that street fight.

> A fight can take place over a long period of time. It's called a feud and it's bad. Feuds tend to begin because one party correctly or incorrectly perceives itself to have been insulted, wronged, or attacked by another. A long-running cycle of retaliation then ensues. Feuds can last for generations, even in modern times where certain cultures practice revenge killings today. Often the original cause is forgotten, yet the cycle of violence continues simply because it is perceived that there has always been a feud. Consider this before you do something stupid.

Violence is bad. Long-running violence is particularly so. Feuds tend to begin because one party correctly or incorrectly perceives itself to have been insulted, wronged, or physically attacked by another. Like the Hatfields and McCoys, a long-running cycle of retaliation, often involving the original parties' family members and/or associates, then ensues. Feuds can last for generations, even in modern times where certain cultures practice revenge killings today.

For example, American hip-hop and rap stars are famous for taking verbal potshots at each other. This war of words occasionally turns into physical violence, sometimes even murder. Perhaps the most infamous incident of this type was the dispute between Tupac Shakur and Christopher Wallace, known to his fans as The Notorious BIG. These two principles may or may not have been directly involved with the violence, yet it nevertheless escalated out of control. There were several attacks on both of these rap stars as well as on their friends and associates, including several shootings. The feud ended after Shakur was gunned down on September 13, 1996 in a drive-by shooting and Wallace was subsequently assassinated on March 9, 1997.

A fight can take place over a long period of time; it's called a feud and it's bad. Consider this before you do something stupid. Just because you think it's over doesn't mean that the other guy agrees. Once the ball gets rolling, it may not stop until someone is dead. And maybe not even then.

Summary

The following is a brief recap of the content you have read in this section.

- The fight itself is only the beginning. Win or lose, there's always a cost to violence. Once you survive a violent conflict, there are a host of other consequences to address, including triage, legal issues, managing witnesses, dealing with the press, interacting with law enforcement, and dealing with psychological trauma.

- If you have been wounded in a fight you may have to tend the injuries yourself until professional help can arrive. Check the incident scene to make sure that it is safe, call 9-1-1 or your local emergency number for help, and then begin to care for the victims. Once you have taken care of your own life-threatening injuries you will also want to treat your opponent too.

- If you're an average guy or found yourself hopelessly outmatched you may be less traumatized than if you considered yourself a real "fighter" yet got beat down regardless. Anything you live through can be a good thing so long as you learn something from it. Wait a few days to regain your emotional equilibrium, dispassionately evaluate your objectives, and then figure out what, if anything, you should do differently in the future.

- It is perfectly normal to experience grief and anguish after traumatic events. Exposure to highly stressful experiences may lead to serious psychological trauma. Symptoms can occur whether you win, lose, or even witness a violent encounter. If you have been involved in an altercation and experience recurring emotional effects for more than a few days, it is a good idea to consider professional counseling to facilitate a healthy recovery.

- Traumatic situations are frequently associated with critical incident amnesia. The greater the stress, the greater your potential of experiencing memory problems. Although you may not remember much about a traumatic incident right after it occurs, you should experience significant memory recovery after a good night's sleep.

- Retain your composure and conduct yourself in a mature manner at all times when interacting with law enforcement personnel at the scene. A confrontational attitude will do you no good. Don't exaggerate; it will be interpreted in the worst possible light when it is read in court. Don't threaten; there is no question that it will be used against you if you do.

- Law enforcement officers have to have a shell; without it, they can't function. They are not bad people, but they simply see, hear, and feel too much to allow an emotional attachment for every person and every problem. Police officers don't like fighting, so if you get into a fight they almost certainly are not going to be all that thrilled with you.

- The average person is woefully unprepared to defend himself in court. You want someone fully committed to win your case. This legal fight is just as dangerous if not more so than the physical fight you just survived. You may be facing both criminal and civil litigation with your freedom, your job, your house, your relationships, and your money on the line.

- Courts are not interested in justice; they are interested in resolution. While the thought of jail might be abhorrent to you, to the professional criminal a jail stay or prison term is a minor inconvenience. Recidivism rates are very high. If you engage in violence, you can expect lengthy and expensive criminal and/or civil litigation proceedings.

- You may be excited to do an interview or get in front of the cameras, but it is very important to look before you leap into headlines. Never forget that your fifteen minutes of fame could easily be used against you in a court of law. Avoid talking to reporters unless specifically advised by your attorney that it will help your case to do so.

- There is no excuse for beating a woman. Unfortunately, even the accusation of abuse can land you in serious trouble. The laws of domestic violence are written and enforced to err on the side of caution. Consequently, they are stacked against you as a man. Know this and act accordingly.

- A fight can take place over a long period of time. It's called a feud and it's bad. Feuds can last for generations, even in modern times where certain cultures practice revenge killings today. Consider this before you do something stupid.

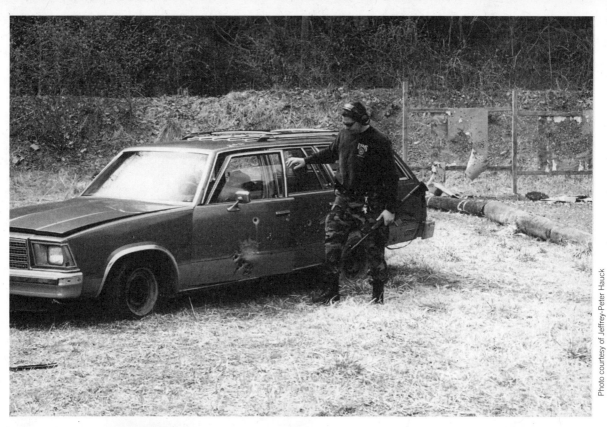

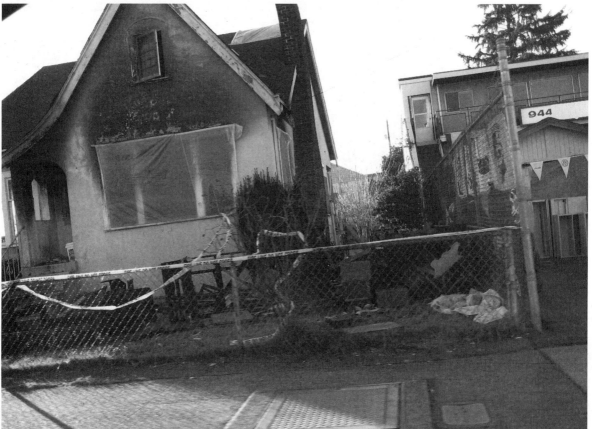

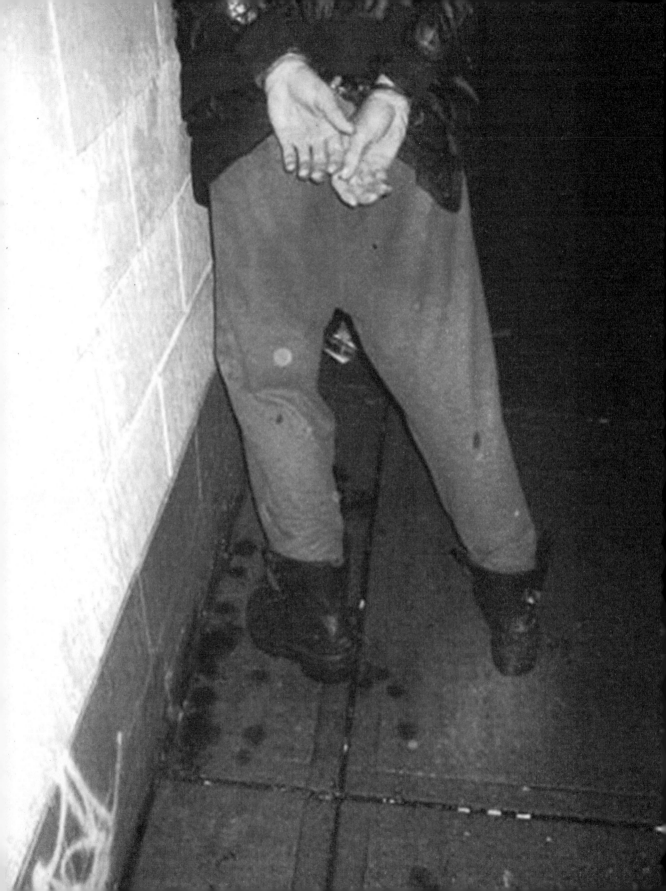

Conclusion

I cleansed the mirror
of my heart – now it reflects
the moon.
                    – Renseki (1701–1789) [9]

Violence is a complex and disturbing subject, one that requires careful study and first-hand experience to truly understand. In this book, we have presented what we hope is a clear, thorough, realistic, and thought-provoking analysis of violence. You have read real-life examples of violent people, examined their brutal behavior, and have a good understanding of the harsh realities of the aftermath of violence.

You have probably noticed by now that the "before" section is much longer than the "during" or "after" sections of this book. That was done intentionally because, let's face it, you have a lot more control about what happens to you before a confrontation gets physical than you do during the fighting or after the smoke has cleared. Once you get violent, much of what follows places your fate in the hands of others.

Now that you have finished the book, you should be able to recognize behaviors, both in others as well as in yourself, that may lead to a fight. Understanding these situations can help you make the right choices for success in conflict resolution. Sometimes you really do need to fight yet most of the time it's the wrong thing to do.

To summarize what you've read we would like to leave you with these four simple rules of self-defense:

- Rule Number One: "Don't get hit." That's primarily about using awareness, avoidance, and de-escalation to eliminate the need to fight in the first place. Where a physical confrontation is unavoidable, it's also about warding off the other guy's blows so that you can counterattack successfully.

- Rule Number Two: "Stop him from continuing to attack you." A purely defensive response is insufficient in a street fight as it can only keep you safe for a very short period of time. You must stop the assault that is in progress so that you can escape to safety or otherwise remain safe until help arrives. Your goal is to be safe, not to kill your attacker or teach him a lesson.

- Rule Number Three: "Always have a Plan B." No matter how good a fighter you are, whatever you try is not necessarily going to work. The other guy will be doing his damnedest to pound your face in, pulling out every dirty trick he can think of in an effort to mess you up. It is prudent, therefore, to have a Plan B, some alternative you can move to without missing a beat when things go awry.

- Rule Number Four: "Don't go to jail." This is about judicious use of force, both knowing when it is appropriate to take action as well as knowing how much force to apply. The AOJP principle can hold you in good stead during conflict situations.

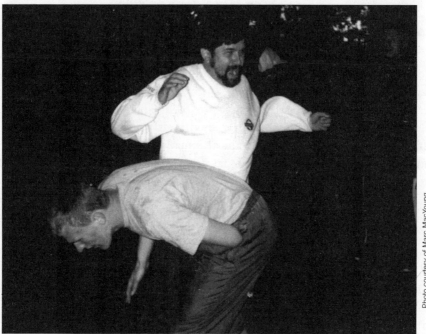

Photo courtesy of Marc MacYoung

Now is the right time to put some heavy thought into what you have learned. Flip back to the checklist in Appendix A. See if what you have read changes any of your original answers.

Be smart, use your head, and stay safe.

Afterword (by Lt. Colonel John R. Finch)

I have seen convicted murderers suddenly awake screaming from a sound sleep and try to run from what they later, I believe, honestly describe as the hands of their victims reaching for them through the walls of their room. As we staff intercepted these scared criminal patients, we realized that despite their crimes, there was more to their punishment than that meted out by the legal system.

Lawrence Kane was kind enough to ask me to write a few words about what I have described as "the cost of it" as related to the area interpersonal violence. I have written previously that the phrase is derived from my work in the U.S. Army where I researched many areas for classes presented at the U.S. Army Command and General Staff College (CGSC). During these efforts, I once again came across a painting by the famed combat

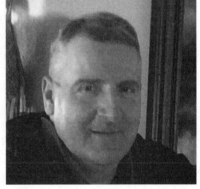

artist Tom Lea, titled "The Price," depicting a terribly wounded U.S. combatant as he struggled forward during the fighting at Peleieu during WWII in the Pacific (www.pbs.org/theydrewfire/gallery/large/019.html).

In my various experiences, mostly as a soldier, I have come to the conclusion that for most of us, lethal force confrontations ultimately extract a cost, potentially for the rest of our lives. When forced to fight, and perhaps even to kill another human being, there are the well-known possible court-related consequences and costs, even when you are found legally justified. Not so widely acknowledged are the likely long-term effects on the survivor of interpersonal violence, be it in conflicts like those in Iraq or Afghanistan in the war against terror, or on the mean streets here at home as a law enforcement officer, security guard, or private citizen.

The authors have included in Appendix A, a checklist they have titled "How Far Am I Willing to Go?" They ask that you complete it before reading their book. I second their recommendation as I feel that your answers, if honestly given, may serve you well if you ever encounter the need to engage in potentially deadly conflict.

What do I mean by the phrase "the cost of it?" Most of us easily recognize that in lethal force situations, the primary objective is to win, hopefully without loss of life or resulting injury. I contend that there are also psychological costs even when you prevail, that may have, over an extended period, serious life influencing consequences.

As an example, I spent nearly 34 years periodically suffering what I viewed as survivor guilt concerning what I believed was the eventual death of a teammate from burn wounds suffered in Vietnam when his helicopter was shot down near Kontum and the wreckage caught fire. My friend was evacuated with serious burns and I lost touch with his wife after he arrived at Brooke Army Hospital for treatment. Years later, not finding his name on the "Wall" in Washington, D.C. at the Vietnam War memorial, I concluded that maybe he was alive, or that a mistake had been made. I made some initial inquiries based upon a faded old document with his name and Social Security Number on it but they were fruitless. Occupied with my own life and family, I relegated his status to a fading memory, but I never forgot.

Then in 2006, additional information from a Kontum related Web site led to some Internet searches, use of private investigators, and contacting surviving MACV Team 33 survivors in an effort to gain closure. The faded war document that had provided that Social Security number, ultimately proved to have a reversed digit due to a wartime typographic error. Despite this setback, additional efforts by team survivors eventually recovered the correct SSN and an ironic form of closure was gained.

Ironic? Yes, the "dead" comrade was actually alive. He had "died" on the operating table at Brooke, but had, through a variety of what might be called medical miracles, survived, though badly scarred by his trial by fire. We eventually reunited, and it was an emotional and at times psychologically painful occasion. My survivor guilt had been lifted, 34 years after the event… I had remembered his last conversation before that flight, when he showed me a rocket fragment lodged in his flak jacket and said, "Well Jack, they've had their chance. I'm gonna make it."

He later took that fatal flight, I thought at the time to fill in for me to look for NVA tanks, as I had just finished an all-night shift. You can imagine how I felt when I learned of the shoot-down, the loss of the pilot, who was also a good acquaintance, and my friend's burn wounds. During the reunion, he told me that no, his flight was to distribute new communication security codebooks and was not as a replacement for me. Thirty-four years of thinking I was partly responsible for his death… There is a cost to violence… As the authors ask… how far are you willing to go?

Thankfully, I've only shot and killed one enemy soldier that I know died from my bullet only, my pulling the trigger, a teenaged NVA sapper at Kontum in late May 1972. I have written of the story elsewhere over the years, but the bottom line is that it was unexpected, a snap decision (the infamous but accurate 1 to 3 seconds rule of gun fighting), him or me, his ChiCom stick grenade versus my M-16A1. My rifle was held only in my right hand, my left held a baseball grenade, and so the shot was attempted at his chest but as some do in crisis, instead of squeezing the trigger, I jerked too quickly as my hand brought the rifle to bear, and the round instead stuck him fatally in the head. The resulting wound was reminiscent of the JFK head shot in Dallas in November 1963.

It remains etched in my aging mind and memory even to this day. From time to time, I see the old photograph taken by a news photographer who was there that day, and I ponder the irony of its eventual publication in the *Stars and Stripes* and *New York Times*, as I still wonder… Who was the sapper I killed? Did he have a family? What did they think when he did not return? Did they ever learn where and how he died? What might have he become? Thirty plus years later and I still see his face frozen in time as the bullet struck home and ended his life. So what, you say? Forget it… I can't. And I think, that in the dark of night, during fitful sleep, those who are not sociopaths or psychopaths may also recall such violent events from their lives or careers.

Also during the Kontum fighting, there was an engagement at a water tower where an enemy heavy machine gun had already shot down a Vietnamese Air Force A1-E and damaged a U.S. Marine Corps F-4 Phantom. I lost six out of ten Vietnamese soldiers in helping destroy that tower. Here's the hard part to that Silver Star I was awarded. The award was presented by B.G. "Iron Mike" Healy and then Colonel "Barbwire Bob" Kingston. I'd never met either of them, but as the medal was awarded, I remember seeing the faces of those six dead soldiers and thinking of B.G. Healy's dead predecessor, the controversial and legendary John Paul Vann who died flying to Kontum at night in early June 1972. There is a cost to so-called "glory"…

With that thought in mind, for those readers who know they will never be in uniform, be it military or in law enforcement or related service, ponder this. As I now work with psychiatric forensic maximum security patients, you might think that murderers have no such feelings. And in some cases, I would agree. But I have seen convicted murderers suddenly awake screaming from a sound sleep and try to run from what they had done, I believe, honestly describe as the hands of their victims reaching for them through the walls of their room. As we staff intercepted these scared criminal patients, we realized that despite their crimes, there was more to their punishment than that meted out by the legal system. Some of them suffered a continuing cost also.

As you currently scan your various news media, I'm confident that you have been made aware of the increasing numbers of U.S. combatants now diagnosed with various forms of Post Traumatic Stress Disorder (PTSD) related problems following combat operations in various parts of the world. Searches via the Internet will reveal other related problems for law enforcement, emergency responders, and emergency department personnel as they deal with the results of interpersonal violence. Experts like Lt. Col. Dave Grossman (U.S. Army, Retired) have written about the costs of interpersonal violence in books like *On Killing* and with Loren Christensen in *On Combat*. I recommend them to you as excellent sources for attempting to gain a greater awareness of the full meaning of such violence, even for the survivors.

I now live in a state where a citizen can, after meeting certain conditions, legally carry a concealed firearm. I am one of those citizens who do carry such a firearm. My wife and I live in a fairly remote area, and so when strangers come to call we tend to meet them at our outer gate carrying concealed. Sheriff's deputy response time is likely thirty minutes or more to our location, so we are on our own so to speak. With that said, if you are ever "on your own" and have to make that 1 to 3 second lethal force decision, please also remember this old legal adage: If the fired bullet came from your gun, then it's your lawsuit if anything goes wrong, like hitting an innocent bystander.

So, even though I'm now sixty, I follow Massad Ayoob's expert advice and still regularly practice with our weapons—dryfire, presentation, concealed carry options etc.—while always remembering in the back of my mind "the cost of it" that looms if "on that day" I again meet a lethal force threat. Remember... "your bullet, your lawsuit" so try not to miss. When I served as a reserve police officer, that thought was always there during our patrols, especially when responding to calls for assistance. It may serve you well also if you carry a firearm.

I leave you with this thought and image. At the conclusion of Operation Desert Storm in 1991, hundreds of U.S. and allied troops were purposefully brought to the carnage at the so-called "Highway of Death" north of Kuwait City where allied airpower had devastated retreating Iraqi formations. I was already there with a British unit and can still see some un-blooded American troops cheering and laughing as they investigated the destroyed columns and spray painting "US #1" and related sayings on the destroyed hulks still reeking from the heat bloated bodies within. I think the commanders who ordered these tours were trying to ensure that their troops were able to see the battlefield power of the American military.

I'm not so sure they fully contemplated the psychological trauma they may also have inflicted on their units. How many, who may have never slain an enemy combatant are still haunted by those images and smells as they now visit VA hospitals for psychiatric treatment? I do not know, but I ask you to ponder the "cost of it" effect before you voluntarily enter that arena of interpersonal violence.

Be safe,

John R. Finch

Lt. Colonel John R. Finch (U.S. Army, Retired) served twenty-two years as an intelligence officer, seeing combat at Kontum, South Vietnam during the 1972 Eastertide Offensive, in Panama during 1989's Operation Just Cause and finally during participation in the final stages of Operation Desert Storm in 1991. He was awarded the Silver Star for gallantry during the fighting at Kontum in May, 1972. He also served for approximately one year before and after the 9/11 attack as a reserve police officer in Kansas. While stationed at Ft. Leavenworth, KS, he was an instructor with the Combat Studies Institute at the U.S. Army Command and General Staff College. He is a graduate of Massad Ayoob's Lethal Force Institute LFI 1–4 and instructor courses and currently works as a psychiatric RN dealing with forensic maximum-security patients. He holds an MA in History from the University of Kansas.

Notes

1. Ouchi Yoshitaka (1507–1551) was a *samurai* lord, ruler of most of the island of Kyushu, Japan. In 1551, one of his generals rebelled and overpowered his army. He composed this death poem just before committing *seppuku* (ritual suicide). The last two lines of his poem come from the *Kongo-gyo* (Diamond sutra), a Buddhist scripture that teaches that the essence of all is void. Translation from the original Japanese reads:

Both the victor	*Utsu hito mo*
and the vanquished are	*utaruru hito mo*
but drops of dew,	*morotomo ni*
but bolts of lightening	*nyo ro yaku nyo den*
thus should we view the world	*sa ni ze kan*

2. Sunao (1887–1926) was a *haiku* poet who died at the age of thirty-nine. *Haiku* is a traditional epigrammatic Japanese poem based on 17 syllables that are arranged 5 – 7 – 5. Translation from the original Japanese reads:

Spitting blood	*chi o hakeba*
clears up reality	*utsutsu mo yume mo*
and dream alike	*saekaeru*

3. Togyu (1705–1749) was a *haiku* poet. He died on August 15, 1749 at the age of forty-four. Translation from the original Japanese reads:

When autumn winds blow	*Nan no mama*
not one leaf remains	*nokoru ha mo nashi*
the way it was	*aki no kaze*

4. The 1984 movie *Ghostbusters* featured Bill Murray, Dan Aykroyd, Sigourney Weaver, and Harold Ramis at their comedic best. The "don't cross the streams" reference, in case you haven't seen or don't remember it, goes like this:

Dr. Egon Spengler (Ramis):	*"There's something very important I forgot to tell you."*
Dr. Peter Venkman (Murray):	*"What?"*
Spengler:	*"Don't cross the streams."*
Venkman:	*"Why?"*
Spengler:	*"It would be bad."*
Venkman:	*"I'm fuzzy on the whole good/bad thing. What do you mean, bad?"*
Spengler:	*"Try to imagine all life as you know it stopping instantaneously and every molecule in your body exploding at the speed of light."*
Venkman:	*"Right. That's bad. Okay. All right. Important safety tip. Thanks, Egon..."*

5. Sosen (1694–1776) was a *haiku* poet. He died on June 28, 1776 at the age of eighty-two. Translation from the original Japanese reads:

Lotus seeds jump every which-way as they wish	*Hasu no mi no* *tobitokoro ari* *shinjizai*

6. David R. Organ is a retired soldier, peacekeeper, and unarmed combat instructor with the Canadian Armed Forces. After leaving the military, he drifted between a variety of jobs including security guard, private investigator, dishwasher, and bodyguard. He began working as a printer, eventually rising to become technical supervisor of his department. Laid off due to 'restructuring,' he took on the job of manager of a local U-Haul, a job that included tossing drunks, pacifying hostile 'customers,' repossessing stolen vehicles and collecting debts. He now works as the manager of the Creekside Restaurant and Lounge in Westerose, Alberta. Over the past 25 years, Dave has studied a variety of martial arts including karate, judo, and aikido, and now teaches aikido at his *dojo*, Great Wave Aikido, in Westerose, Alberta.

7. Ryushi (1684–1764) was a *haiku* poet. He died on September 6, 1764 at the age of seventy. Translation from the original Japanese reads:

Man is Buddha the day and I grow dark as one	*Mi wa hotoke* *ware to iu hi wa* *kurenikeri*

8. *Miranda v. Arizona*, 384 U.S. 436. Ernesto Miranda was arrested for robbery, kidnapping, and rape in 1963. He was subsequently interrogated by police and confessed to his crimes. Prosecutors offered only his confession as evidence during his trial where he was convicted. The Supreme Court later ruled in 1966 that Miranda was intimidated by the interrogation. Neither understanding his right to not incriminate himself nor his right to have counsel present during the interrogation. On the basis of that finding, the court overturned his conviction. He was later convicted in a new trial where witnesses testified against him and other evidence was presented, serving 11 years for his crimes. This Supreme Court ruling forms the basis of the "Miranda Rights" that all suspects must be read prior to interrogation by law enforcement.
The actual wording states,

"The person in custody must, prior to interrogation, be clearly informed that he has the right to remain silent, and that anything he says will be used against him in court; he must be clearly informed that he has the right to consult with an attorney and to have that attorney present during interrogation, and that, if he is indigent, an attorney will be provided at no cost to represent him"

Police are only required to Mirandize an individual whom they intend to subject to custodial interrogation. While arrests can occur without questioning and without the Miranda warning, the warning must be given prior to any formal interrogation.

9. Renseki (1701–1789) was a *haiku* poet. He died on July 5, 1789 at the age of eighty-eight. Translation from the original Japanese reads:

I cleansed the mirror of my heart—now it reflects the moon	*Harai aria* *kokoro no tsuki no* *kagami kana*

Glossary

Romaji (Romanization) note—we have primarily used the *Hebon-Shiki* (Hepburn) method of translating Japanese writing into the English alphabet and determining how best to spell the words (though accent marks have been excluded), as it is generally considered the most useful insofar as pronunciation is concerned. We have italicized foreign terms such that they can be readily differentiated from their English counterparts (for example, *dan* meaning black belt rank versus Dan, the male familiar name for Daniel). As the Japanese and Chinese languages do not use capitalization, we have only capitalized those words that would be used as proper nouns in English.

Japanese is a challenging language for many English speakers to pronounce correctly. A few hints—for the most part, short vowels sound just like their English counterparts (for example, a as in father, e as in pen). Long vowels are essentially double-length (for example, o as in oil, in the word *oyo*). The u is nearly silent, except where it is an initial syllable (for example, *uke*). Vowel combination e + i sounds like day (for example, *bugeisha*); a + i sounds like alive (for example, *bunkai*); o + u sounds like float (for example, *tou*); and a + e sounds like lie (*kamae*). The consonant r is pronounced with the tip of the tongue, midway between l and r (for example, *daruma*). Consonant combination ts is pronounced like cats, almost a z (for example, *tsuki*).

Although there are a few words here from other languages, the majority of words listed in this glossary comes from Japanese.

Foreign Terms	English Definition
arnis	A Filipino martial art that uses weapons from the very beginning of training. *Arnis* incorporates striking, locking, and throwing techniques performed with short rattan staves, knives, short swords, and empty hand. "Modern Arnis," a widely popular style, was founded by Remy Presas.
dan	black belt rank
dojo	training hall, literally the "place to learn the way"
escalato	The cycle of one-upmanship that almost inevitably leads to physical violence unless one party backs down and breaks off the game.
fa jing	explosive or vibrating power
fudoshin	indomitable spirit
go no sen	late initiative
Goju Ryu	An Okinawan form of karate developed by Chojun Miyagi.
gyaku hishigi	opposite or reverse crushing strangulation technique (guillotine choke)

gyaku juji jime	reverse cross lock choke
hadaka jime	rear naked choke
haiku	a traditional epigrammatic Japanese poem based on 17 syllables which are arranged 5 – 7 – 5
Hapkido	A Korean martial art that uses punches, kicks, throws, and joint locks.
hiki uke	pulling/grasping open-hand block
humerus	upper arm bone
Hyōhō Niten Ichi-Ryu	The two-sword school of swordsmanship founded by Miyamoto Musashi. Roughly translates as "two heavens as one."
ibuki	breath control
ikken hissatsu	one blow one kill, a Japanese phrase
judo	A Japanese martial art and now international and Olympic sport that consists of throwing, grappling, choking, and arm locks founded by Jigoro Kano; literally "the gentle way."
judoka	judo practitioners
jujitsu	A Japanese unarmed combat art that focuses primarily on throwing, grappling, choking, and joint locking techniques.
kamikaze	Literally "divine wind," usually refers to the suicide attacks by Imperial Japanese aviators who smashed their planes into Allied ships attempting to sink them during the closing stages of the Pacific campaign of World War II.
kancho	director, head of an organization (honorific title for the leader of a martial arts organization or martial style)
karate ni sente nashi	"There is no first strike in karate," a saying made famous by Gichin Funakoshi, the founder of *Shotokan* karate.
karate	A (primarily) Japanese or Okinawan martial art that emphasizes weaponless or empty-hand striking techniques (for example, punching/kicking).
karateka	karate practitioners
kata	a logical series of offensive and defensive movements performed in a particular order during solo training, literally "formal exercise"
kiai	a very loud yell, literally "spirit shout"
kongo-gyo	"Diamond sutra," a Buddhist scripture which teaches that the essence of all is void
koshi guruma	hip wheel throw (from judo)

kosoto gake	minor outside hook throw (from judo)
kobudo	A Japanese or Okinawan martial art that specializes in using farm implements and everyday objects from feudal society as weapons.
Kodokan	Judo's world headquarters in Japan. Roughly translated it means "a place for the study or promote the way." It was established by Jigoro Kano, the founder of judo, in 1882.
Krav Maga	A form of self-defense and hand-to-hand combat created in Israel. Israeli security forces. Special Forces use *Krav Maga* because it is fast to learn, effective and swift. *Krav Maga* might not be considered a "martial art" in the classical sense, but more of a self-defense structure. Since its inception, it has been modified for civilians, becoming popular throughout the world.
kubaton	Invented by Takayuki Kubota, the *kubaton* is a hard plastic or metal cylinder about 5 inches to 6 inches long that can be used for striking, pressure point manipulations, and control techniques. It is frequently sold with an attacked key ring as a "self-defense key chain."
kubi hishigi	neck joint crush strangulation technique.
kyu	a colored belt (non-black belt) rank in martial arts.
mokuroku	"teaching certificate," literally a catalog of techniques that a martial arts student has mastered in order to achieve their rank
muay Thai	Thai kickboxing; an art that focuses on knees, elbows, shins, and feet for most fighting techniques
Mixed Martial Arts (MMA)	Mixed Martial Arts is a sport that uses many martial arts disciplines to create a freestyle form of fighting that adheres to the few rules that govern the sport. Popular in Japan, Brazil and the United States, some forms of events are called PRIDE Fighting Championships and UFC (Ultimate Fighting Championship).
nami juji jime	front cross lock choke
nidan	second degree black belt
osoto gari	major outer reaping throw (from judo)
sambo	an abbreviation of the Russian words *Samozashchita Baez Oruzhiya,* literally "self-defense without a weapon"
samurai	the military class in feudal Japan, literally "to serve"
sasae tsurikomi ashi	lifting/pulling ankle block throw (from judo)
sen no sen	simultaneous initiative
sensei	a martial arts instructor, literally "one who has come before"

sen-sen no sen	preemptory initiative
seppuku	ritual suicide by disembowelment, literally "belly cutting"
shihan	Expert instructor, generally a 4th degree black belt or higher who has a specialized certification beyond his or her rank in martial arts alone
Shorei-Shobukan	a style of karate founded by *Kancho* John Roseberry.
Shorinji Ryu	Japanese martial art that incorporates Buddhism, adding a distinctly spiritual emphasis.
shuai-jan	Chinese wrestling
sifu	a martial arts instructor, literally "master"
Sosuishitsu-ryu jujitsu	An ancient unarmed combat art that uses throwing, grappling, choking, and joint locks. It was developed for the Japanese *samurai* to use on the battlefield should they lose their weapon(s). The classic grips and attacks reflect the opponent wearing battlefield armor.
taekwondo	a Korean martial art and Olympic sport, literally "the way of the foot and the hand"
uke	to receive (or block) an attack

How Far Am I Willing to Go?

You need to seriously think about what you're willing to do, what you are not willing to do, and what you are willing to have done to you far before violence occurs. Such decisions cannot rationally be made during a tense, dangerous encounter. The following table lists a variety of scenarios that you might encounter. Spend some time thinking about each one and determine where your values lie. You can undoubtedly add to this list on your own as well (there are spaces at the bottom where you can do so).

There is always a cost in terms of physical and/or emotional well-being to both taking action as well as to not taking action. There is no right or wrong answer. The important thing is to evaluate realistically where you stand.

At minimum, this questionnaire should be completed before *and* after you read this book. Use a pencil or make a photocopy so that you can do it twice. It is a good idea to reevaluate periodically where you stand as time progresses too.

Check the appropriate boxes in each column.

I am willing to...

- ❑ Admit when I am wrong and sincerely apologize
- ❑ Allow myself to be blindfolded
- ❑ Allow myself to be captured by a criminal and moved to a secondary crime scene
- ❑ Allow myself to be tied up to live a little longer
- ❑ Allow others to call me names without responding
- ❑ Avoid a place (for example, neighborhood, pool hall, nightclub, public park, eatery) where a specific race or ethnic group congregates
- ❑ Avoid a place (for example, street corner, housing complex, store, area in a mall, fast food restaurant, tavern) where there might be trouble
- ❑ Ban someone from my home and/or place of business
- ❑ Be raped
- ❑ Be stolen from
- ❑ Be threatened by a loved one
- ❑ Be threatened by a stranger

I am not willing to...

- ❑ Admit when I am wrong and sincerely apologize
- ❑ Allow myself to be blindfolded
- ❑ Allow myself to be captured by a criminal and moved to a secondary crime scene
- ❑ Allow myself to be tied up to live a little longer
- ❑ Allow others to call me names without responding
- ❑ Avoid a place (for example, neighborhood, pool hall, nightclub, public park, eatery) where a specific race or ethnic group congregates
- ❑ Avoid a place (for example, street corner, housing complex, store, area in a mall, fast food restaurant, tavern) where there might be trouble
- ❑ Ban someone from my home and/or place of business
- ❑ Be raped
- ❑ Be stolen from
- ❑ Be threatened by a loved one
- ❑ Be threatened by a stranger

294   The Little Black Book of Violence

I am willing to...

- ☐ Call 9-1-1 (or local emergency number) to report a crime in progress
- ☐ Carry a knife or a firearm on a daily basis
- ☐ Chase a thief or other criminal in my car
- ☐ Chase a thief or other criminal on foot
- ☐ Cooperate with the police
- ☐ Defend a weaker friend
- ☐ Defend a weaker stranger
- ☐ Defend my honor
- ☐ Eliminate contact with a friend, relative, or acquaintance who is a known trouble-maker
- ☐ Fight a group by myself
- ☐ Fight one-on-one
- ☐ Fight over an insult to my favorite sports team
- ☐ Fight when I drink or use drugs
- ☐ Gouge out someone's eye in self-defense
- ☐ Hand over my hard-earned money to a mugger
- ☐ Interfere in another person's argument
- ☐ Join a gang
- ☐ Just walk away from a potential problem no matter how much others might criticize me for it
- ☐ Kick someone when he's down
- ☐ Kill in self-defense
- ☐ Kill a close friend or relative in self-defense
- ☐ Let my car be broken into or defaced
- ☐ Let my personal items be broken or defaced
- ☐ Listen attentively, even when I am angry
- ☐ Lose face in private, in front of a close friend, relative, or significant other
- ☐ Lose face in public amongst friends or acquaintances
- ☐ Lose face in public amongst strangers
- ☐ Maim, permanently disable, or kill another person in self-defense
- ☐ Own a weapon

I am not willing to...

- ☐ Call 9-1-1 (or local emergency number) to report a crime in progress
- ☐ Carry a knife or a firearm on a daily basis
- ☐ Chase a thief or other criminal in my car
- ☐ Chase a thief or other criminal on foot
- ☐ Cooperate with the police
- ☐ Defend a weaker friend
- ☐ Defend a weaker stranger
- ☐ Defend my honor
- ☐ Eliminate contact with a friend, relative, or acquaintance who is a known trouble-maker
- ☐ Fight a group by myself
- ☐ Fight one-on-one
- ☐ Fight over an insult to my favorite sports team
- ☐ Fight when I drink or use drugs
- ☐ Gouge out someone's eye in self-defense
- ☐ Hand over my hard-earned money to a mugger
- ☐ Interfere in another person's argument
- ☐ Join a gang
- ☐ Just walk away from a potential problem no matter how much others might criticize me for it
- ☐ Kick someone when he's down
- ☐ Kill in self-defense
- ☐ Kill a close friend or relative in self-defense
- ☐ Let my car be broken into or defaced
- ☐ Let my personal items be broken or defaced
- ☐ Listen attentively, even when I am angry
- ☐ Lose face in private, in front of a close friend, relative, or significant other
- ☐ Lose face in public amongst friends or acquaintances
- ☐ Lose face in public amongst strangers
- ☐ Maim, permanently disable, or kill another person in self-defense
- ☐ Own a weapon

I am willing to...

- ❏ Participate in a mob
- ❏ Physically intervene in a fight
- ❏ Report another student or coworker who is carrying a weapon on the premises
- ❏ Report another student or coworker who is making threats to harm others
- ❏ See another person's position
- ❏ Sell drugs
- ❏ Shoot a person in self-defense, knowing that he might die or be crippled for life
- ❏ Show respect
- ❏ Stab a person in self-defense, knowing that he might die or be crippled for life
- ❏ Strike first if I feel that violence is imminent
- ❏ Take risks such as cutting off other drivers, tailgating, or traveling through undesirable neighborhoods in order to save time on my commute
- ❏ Testify in court against a violent offender whose crimes I have witnessed even if he threatens retribution
- ❏ Threaten another person to get what I want
- ❏ Train in a martial art like karate, taekwondo, or boxing
- ❏ Turn my back to an armed individual when ordered to do so
- ❏ Use a weapon to injure or kill another person
- ❏ Use anything as a weapon (for example, hot coffee, hedge shears, power saw, vehicle, baseball bat, iron skillet, fire extinguisher, or beer bottle) to protect my life or another's life
- ❏ Use whatever force is necessary to neutralize an adult who is threatening me with a weapon
- ❏ Use whatever force is necessary to neutralize a child who is threatening me with a weapon
- ❏ Visit a location (for example, street corner, housing complex, store, nightclub, restaurant, or tavern) where violence has recently occurred

I am not willing to...

- ❏ Participate in a mob
- ❏ Physically intervene in a fight
- ❏ Report another student or coworker who is carrying a weapon on the premises
- ❏ Report another student or coworker who is making threats to harm others
- ❏ See another person's position
- ❏ Sell drugs
- ❏ Shoot a person in self-defense, knowing that he might die or be crippled for life
- ❏ Show respect
- ❏ Stab a person in self-defense, knowing that he might die or be crippled for life
- ❏ Strike first if I feel that violence is imminent
- ❏ Take risks such as cutting off other drivers, tailgating, or traveling through undesirable neighborhoods in order to save time on my commute
- ❏ Testify in court against a violent offender whose crimes I have witnessed even if he threatens retribution
- ❏ Threaten another person to get what I want
- ❏ Train in a martial art like karate, taekwondo, or boxing
- ❏ Turn my back to an armed individual when ordered to do so
- ❏ Use a weapon to injure or kill another person
- ❏ Use anything as a weapon (for example, hot coffee, hedge shears, power saw, vehicle, baseball bat, iron skillet, fire extinguisher, or beer bottle) to protect my life or another's life
- ❏ Use whatever force is necessary to neutralize an adult who is threatening me with a weapon
- ❏ Use whatever force is necessary to neutralize a child who is threatening me with a weapon
- ❏ Visit a location (for example, street corner, housing complex, store, nightclub, restaurant, or tavern) where violence has recently occurred

I am willing to...

- ☐ Visit a location (for example, street corner, housing complex, store, nightclub, restaurant, or tavern) where violence has recently occurred
- ☐ Visit a location (for example, street corner, housing complex, store, nightclub, restaurant, or tavern) where violence is common
- ☐ Watch a loved one be beaten down without intervening
- ☐ Watch a loved one be kidnapped or taken hostage without intervening
- ☐ Watch a loved one be murdered without physically intervening
- ☐ Watch a loved one be raped without intervening
- ☐ Watch a stranger be beaten down without intervening
- ☐ Watch a stranger be kidnapped or taken hostage without intervening
- ☐ Watch a stranger be murdered without intervening
- ☐ Watch a stranger be raped without intervening
- ☐ _____
- ☐ _____
- ☐ _____
- ☐ _____
- ☐ _____
- ☐ _____
- ☐ _____
- ☐ _____
- ☐ _____
- ☐ _____
- ☐ _____
- ☐ _____
- ☐ _____

I am not willing to...

- ☐ Visit a location (for example, street corner, housing complex, store, nightclub, restaurant, or tavern) where violence has recently occurred
- ☐ Visit a location (for example, street corner, housing complex, store, nightclub, restaurant, or tavern) where violence is common
- ☐ Watch a loved one be beaten down without intervening
- ☐ Watch a loved one be kidnapped or taken hostage without intervening
- ☐ Watch a loved one be murdered without physically intervening
- ☐ Watch a loved one be raped without intervening
- ☐ Watch a stranger be beaten down without intervening
- ☐ Watch a stranger be kidnapped or taken hostage without intervening
- ☐ Watch a stranger be murdered without intervening
- ☐ Watch a stranger be raped without intervening
- ☐ _____
- ☐ _____
- ☐ _____
- ☐ _____
- ☐ _____
- ☐ _____
- ☐ _____
- ☐ _____
- ☐ _____
- ☐ _____
- ☐ _____
- ☐ _____
- ☐ _____

APPENDIX B

Words You Can Use

Anyone who stumbles across a fight in progress won't know who's who unless you make it clear. Consequently, it's good to shout something that points out who the bad guy is while you counterattack. It's easy to yell but extraordinarily hard to articulate under extreme stress in combat, so it's important to practice. Select a few phrases that are natural and easy for you to use in a variety of situations and incorporate them into your training regimen. You can come up with something on your own, or if you're having problems thinking of something good, choose from the following list.

- ☐ Back off now!
- ☐ Back up, you're too close to me!
- ☐ Calm down and step back!
- ☐ Don't come any closer!
- ☐ Don't crowd me!
- ☐ Don't hurt me!
- ☐ Don't make me hurt you!
- ☐ Don't touch me!
- ☐ Drop the weapon!
- ☐ Five feet!
- ☐ Get away from me!
- ☐ Get off me!
- ☐ Get the hell away from me!
- ☐ Give me five feet now!
- ☐ Give me five feet!
- ☐ Go on your way!
- ☐ He's got a gun!
- ☐ He's got a knife!
- ☐ Help, he's got a knife!
- ☐ Help, he's trying to kill me!
- ☐ Hold it right there!
- ☐ I don't have any money, go away!

- ☐ I don't want any trouble!
- ☐ I don't want to fight with you!
- ☐ I don't want to talk to you!
- ☐ I don't want you any closer to me!
- ☐ I said stand back!
- ☐ I want to leave now!
- ☐ I want you to back up!
- ☐ Leave me alone!
- ☐ Let me out now!
- ☐ Move on your way!
- ☐ Oh my god, don't cut me with that knife!
- ☐ Put down the weapon!
- ☐ Stand back!
- ☐ Stay away from me!
- ☐ Stay back; leave me alone!
- ☐ Step back!
- ☐ Stop fighting me!
- ☐ Stop right there!
- ☐ That is far enough!
- ☐ Turn around and go away!
- ☐ You're getting too close to me!
- ☐ You're standing too close to me!

APPENDIX C

The Will to Kill

by Marc "Animal" MacYoung

Murder is easy. Dealing with someone who's coming at you just as hard, ain't.

When discussing the subject of self-defense, there is one subject that always comes up sooner or later: the "will" to kill. While most of the talk is rather poetic (if not posturing, posing, and woofing), the will to kill isn't as simple as many people make it out to be. In fact, most are leaving out a critical component:

You gotta be willing to die.

More importantly, you gotta be willing to risk being permanently maimed. Dying would be easy in comparison to living a crippled lifestyle. And while we are on the subject, you gotta be willing to do that and still fail.

Desmond Morris says in his book *Manwatching: A Field Guide to Human Behavior*, as the opening of the "Fighting Behavior" chapter (page 156), the following:

> *Fighting represents the failure of threat display. If intimidation signals cannot settle a dispute, then extreme measures may be called for, and conflict may develop into full-scale bodily assault. This is extremely rare in human societies, which are remarkably non-violent, despite popular statements to the contrary, and there is a sound biological reason for this. Every time one individual launches a physical attack on the body of another, there is a risk that both may suffer injury. No matter how dominant the attacker may be, he has no guarantee of escaping unscathed. His opponent, even if weaker, may be driven into a desperate frenzy of wild defensive actions, any one of which could inflict lasting damage.*

For the record, this is why most bullying is psychological. It is the looming and constant threat of violence, rather than actual act of violence, that makes up an overwhelming majority of the bully's behavior. If you actually look at the time spent intimidating and posing (and include the amount of obsession the victim pours into the threat), you will see that actual violence is microscopic. So way more time is spent threatening violence than actually doing it. Still, I've seen timid people reach a snapping point and eat the bullies' lunches. And this is almost as entertaining as watching bullies decide to fuss with the wrong person. (The guy was in the marching band! Who knew drummers were so strong?)

I often say, "Murder is easy. Dealing with someone who's coming at you just as hard, ain't." Recognize that there is a distinct difference between killing and murder.

Manslaughter is usually the taking a life during the moment. For example, in the heat of an argument someone pulls a gun and *ka-pow*. (This is also critical as to why one must understand the importance of threat displays, predatorial vs. territorial violence and the dangers of escalato, because, face it, the stupidest last words ever spoken while looking down the barrel of a gun are, "You don't have the guts," (especially when said in Spanish). This also can include someone falling down and cracking his skull during a fight or drunken driving. While killing someone was not the intent, both are conditions that could have been avoided.

Generally speaking, murder is the taking the life of someone incapable or unlikely to defend oneself or in a situation where the person doesn't have a chance. And putting in a legal definition, it is thought out and, if not evil overlord's worth, to some degree planned. Generally, if there is an altercation, the heat of the moment has passed, and now it has festered into something else. Another legal definition of murder is a killing that occurs during the commission of a crime. In both cases, there are intentional and willful steps towards the commission of this killing (for example, running home, getting a gun, and coming back to shoot someone or robbing a place using the threat of force).

While murder tends to be much rarer, manslaughter is the more common charge. Most of the time, you will see people so wrapped up in their game of escalato that violence isn't combat per se, it is in fact another stage of threat display. No lie, the intent to kill wasn't there, the waving a weapon around was just another ante into the pot trying to get the other guy to fold. This is especially true in light of the "Oh sh*t, I killed him!" so commonly seen after the heat of moment has passed.

Homicide just means the killing of a human by another (*Homo sapiens*, ergo homicide). Homicide can occur for many different reasons, including self-defense. I tend to use the term 'killing' for 'homicide,' because people understand it better. I bring these distinctions up because they are important to understand how death can occur with risks and without risks to the individual. For example, a drunken driver can hit a pedestrian with very little danger to himself. This also is true in the case of a murder. The person committing the murder is doing so with minimum risk to self.

On the other hand, two guys 'fighting' are taking a risk of injury. The degree of resulting damage may be far greater than either intended. This brings us to combat, which—as I define it—is when two or more combatants ARE intent on killing each other and actively engaged in the act. In these circumstances, the risks of death and injury to everyone involved are very great. This is why fighting is rare—and combat even more so—it's too damned dangerous.

Many moons past a group of questions were asked of gang bangers. Basically, the questions were: "Is _____ worth killing over?" The answers were unanimously, "YES!" If someone did this to them, they'd cap his ass. These kids were willing to kill over these subjects. Then the questions were rephrased as: "Is _____ worth dying over?"

"WHOA! Wait a minute! Nobody said anything about US dying now! It's okay for him to die over this, but I ain't volunteering!"

Now gosh golly gee, isn't it an interesting point, that most of their strategies and tactics reflect this same attitude? Take a look at a drive-by shooting. They're willing to kill, but they don't want to risk their own precious hides.

Here you run into some things that were mentioned in the clip of Steve Pinker speaking at the Technology Entertainment Design (TED) conference. He mentions Payne James Payne's views about places where "life is cheap" the hesitation to use violence is less. It is interesting because while I have not read Payne's works, I agree wholeheartedly with that sentiment... with a very distinct clarification. Pinker ascribes to Payne, "When pain and early death are every day features in one's own life, one feels fewer compunctions about inflicting them on others." It would be easy to think, "Okay, you live in a violent world, therefore violence is no big thing" which is true. However, I personally think it goes a little deeper than that.

Look at Pinker's/Payne's next line: "As technology and economic efficiency lengthen and improve our lives, we place a higher value on life in general." It is here that we realize it ain't just about violence; we're also talking about living a hard scrabble existence chock full of 'death professions,' disease, starvation and being 'expendable.' I'm talking this is the danger you face every day WITHOUT the threat of violence. "Oh yeah, violence, that can kill me too... get in line."

It is here that we have to take a look at Maslow's *Hierarchy of Needs* and realize that someone who is living on the lower rungs has a totally different mindset than these gang bangers. Ever seen what a life of death professions can do to a man? Torn and twisted bodies and 45-year-old men moving like they're 80. Manual labor, if it doesn't kill you outright, will kill you sooner than later. (As an aside, this is where gender feminism got it wrong; they were speaking from a postindustrial perspective and totally ignored the fatality rate among the men doing this kind of work). Under these hardscrabble conditions then, yes, life is very cheap. I mean who's afraid of violence when your job is guaranteed to kill you? And yet death professions are taken by these men because they are the only way to support one's family.

And that is where the real difference between these gang bangers and—for example—suicide bombers can be seen. The gansta's aren't really in a hardscrabble existence. They aren't always a hair's breadth away from starvation, disease, or death (a.k.a. real poverty). Their biggest threat to life and limb is violence brought about by their lifestyle choices. Contrast this, however, to a poor suicide bomber—whose death will ensure the financial comfort of his family. (That's another factor, but we'll get to that in a minute).

Pinker/Payne is correct that the better the life conditions one has the more value one puts on life—especially one's own. This brings us back to the issue of if you engage in violence you risk injury/death.

Often youths claim that they aren't afraid of dying. In fact, often death is looked at as an escape route from a f%&ked up and emotionally painful existence. However, let me add something that a friend's grandfather used to tell him, "Don't worry about the man who isn't afraid of dying. Worry about the man who doesn't mind."

People who aren't afraid to die can usually be easily accommodated (a.k.a., they're most often sloppy). Whereas someone who is willing to kill you, but isn't willing to die himself in the process, is also usually pretty easy to handle. All you gotta do is shoot back. Usually their desire to whack you evaporates in light of the realization that their butts are on the line, too. It's the guy who is intent on achieving a goal and who calmly accepts that he might have to go down in the process who is going to require some overtime on your part.

People who talk about the "will to kill" almost all forget that part of you also has to have the willingness to die. "No, no, no!," I hear them squeak. "You have to be willing to kill so you can survive Ragnarök!'" Yeah, right ... and that's how come they so often choke when it comes down to it. Despite all their posing and grandstanding, they freeze up in the actual face of "there ain't no such thing as guaranteed survival."

While we're at it, there ain't no such thing as guaranteed success either ... which is another 'hold the phone' issue when it comes to dying. I'm not just talking about you didn't achieve your goal of whacking someone. That's, "Oh well, I missed. Golly gee. Guess I'll go home and watch *The Simpsons*." Nor am I talking about a grand and glorious last stand where you die while heroically protecting others or achieving a great and grand end.

I'm talking about you both dying AND failing. I'm talking about a *kamikaze* pilot who gets shot down and flames out in the ocean. I'm talking about the suicide bomber who gets isolated and is left standing there alone with nobody else to kill. I know of only one guy who blew himself up in those conditions, and it's questionable if he or his handlers did it. I'm talking about the assassin who flubs the hit and gets taken down without killing his target. I'm talking about a valiant effort that gets you killed, as well as the person you are trying to save.

In more affluent lifestyles, we like to think that our lives mean something. And by extension, we hope that our early deaths would, too. That's part of the reason why stone killers scare people. It's nothing personal. We at least want our deaths to have some significance. We just hate to think that our deaths would go something like this:

> *"Do you remember that guy you killed last week?"*
> *"Which one?"*
> *"On Thursday."*
> *"Which one?"*
> *"Thursday morning."*
> *"Early or later?"*
> *"Early."*
> *"Sorta ... why?"*

---

* In Norse mythology, Ragnarök is the battle at the end of the world.

Wow, what a bummer! Not to be remembered. And dying for no good reason because you failed to achieve your goal. This is frickin' scary!

We often use the word *kamikaze* or suicide bomber, but those aren't true suicides... they are homicidal acts aimed at an external goal. Granted they are acts that one isn't going to survive, but that external goal gives them value. True suicide doesn't have an external goal.

ALL of this has to be factored into the subject of the WILL. Yes, there are many people who are willing to murder another person. But that is done with absolutely the most minimum danger to the murderer.

This is why self-defense is such a tricky subject. People think that it's a matter of survival when, in fact, you might not survive. And you need to know that going in. You could fail and end up being Thursday's statistic. What's more is that a half-baked attempt at defense actually increases the odds of you getting killed.

Even harder is being the one who goes into a dangerous situation to save someone else or for some "greater goal." Not only is there a good chance of dying, but there ain't no guarantees you're going to succeed. You hope for the best, but that ain't how it always works out.

Stop and think about your reactions to these concepts. You can see them in manifest in many movies. In fact, the original *Die Hard* movie was a great example of all of these motives. The deputy police chief, ignoring McClane's (Bruce Willis') warnings about the entrenched positions of the terrorists, sends in SWAT and an assault vehicle (useless deaths). The rage and blind hatred of Karl seeking to avenge his brother's death (murder and in the end failure). Han's (Alan Rickman's) losing and attempting to take Holly McClane (Bonnie Belinda) with him into death and failing. (And this brings out a cheer from the audience when he died AND failed). We want to see the "bad guy" not only die, but also fail to achieve his goal.

Contrast this with the shoot out at the end of *Open Range*. Where after listening to his partner (Kevin Costner) line out the tactics they will be facing, Robert Duval says, "Sounds like you got things pretty well figured out." Costner replies, "Yeah, except how we're going to survive." And yet, despite this, they go out and engage with the cattle baron and his men.

So I'm kind of the opinion that the issue of "will" is a whole lot more complex than do you "have it" or not. Because basically, a big-assed factor is how much are you willing to pay? And it is a crapshoot that you might fail in the process.

Vital Area Targets

If you have to hurt someone in a fight, you will need to target a vital area of his body, someplace that can be damaged relatively easily. Punching someone in the stomach, for example, may only piss him off while striking him in the temple may render him unconscious. When executed correctly, vital area attacks are extremely dangerous stuff. **Do not abuse this knowledge**. Such areas should only be forcefully struck or manipulated in true life-or-death, self-defense situations from which you can only escape through violence.

Not every vital area blow will have consequences such as we list here. It depends on how hard and accurately you strike as well as what you hit with. Most people can deliver a pretty strong blow using their fists or unshod feet, while a severe blow requires help from some sort of solid object such as a baseball bat or steel-toed boot to increase the effectiveness of their strike. Highly skilled martial artists can often do extraordinary damage unaided. It is important to note, however, that individuals who are stimulated by adrenaline, fear, drugs, alcohol, or even sheer willpower may not be incapacitated from any blow that is not immediately physiologically disabling, even if mortally wounded.

While you read this chart, it helps to have a good anatomy book on hand.

Vital Area	Description
Crown of the head	A strong blow to the crown of the head at the coronal suture can dislocate the frontal bone, causing severe damage to the motor regions of the brain resulting in paralysis or death.
Fontanelle	Located between the crown of the head and the forehead. A strong blow to this location can cause fatal damage to the brain and cranial nerves.
Temple	The temple is the weakest structural area of the skull where it flattens at the sides, about two-finger widths back from each eye. The weakness exists because curves are architecturally much stronger than flat surfaces. Shock transmits through the skull most easily at these points. A strong blow to the temple can cause massive hemorrhaging of the meningeal artery, coma, and eventually death.
Ears	A concussive slap to the ears can cause pain, disorientation, and severe trauma to the eardrum, particularly if the hand is slightly cupped.
Summit of the nose	A strong blow to the summit of the nose at the center of the forehead can shock the frontal lobes causing unconsciousness, while a severe blow can cause death.

Circumorbital region	Located above and below the eyes. Hard strikes to this area can transmit shock to the frontal lobes of the brain resulting in unconsciousness.
Eyeballs	Eye strikes can cause anything from watering to blindness depending on severity. When the adversary is standing, the eyes are usually attacked with a raking motion. When he is on the ground such that his head can be immobilized, gauges or displacements may be used. This is frequently done by pressing the thumb or a finger into the side of the socket, which displaces and potentially ejects the eyeball. Excruciating pain and psychological trauma from this type of application usually render the victim unconscious. Permanent eye injuries may be sustained.
Intermaxillary suture	Located just under the nose at the philtrum. The nerves are very close to the surface in this area such that even a light blow can cause pain, watery eyes, and disruption in most people. This sensitive area can also be used for control techniques when leveraged from behind (pushing in and up to manipulate the head/neck and control the spine). Strong blows can transmit shock through the upper jawbones into the braincase, thereby causing unconsciousness or death.
Center of the lower jaw	A blow here transmits shock through the jaw into the inner ear, shaking the brain. Injuries can include broken teeth, dislocation of the jaw, whiplash, dizziness, or unconsciousness. Really severe blows such as those from mass weapons (for example, baseball bat, sledgehammer) can dislocate the skull from the top of the spinal column resulting in instant death.
Mastoid process	Located behind the ears at the sides of the neck. Blows to this area can affect the facial nerve, causing pain and rapid disorientation. Neck "cranks" are often performed in this area as well.
Nape of the neck	Located at the third intervertebral space, the nape of the neck is the weakest point of the spinal column. A strong blow here can cause disorientation, unconsciousness, paralysis, or death depending on severity.
Carotid sinus	Located at the side of the neck in front of the sternocleidomastoid muscle, a blow to this area can disrupt the baroreceptors, which regulate blood pressure flowing through the carotid artery into the brain. This can cause the heart rate to instantly, though temporarily, drop leading to disorientation or unconsciousness. This point is also used for strangulation techniques where applying pressure can cut off the blood flow leading to unconsciousness or death. It has also been used by emergency room technicians and paramedics to temporarily stave off dangerously high blood pressure until medication can be administered.
Base of the throat	The windpipe is very vulnerable just above the suprasternal notch. A blow or strangulation technique here can crush the cartilage of the trachea leading to suffocation and death. A finger jab or push can elicit severe pain.

Summit of the breast-bone	Located where the manubrium and sternum meet. A strong blow here can cause trauma to the heart, bronchus, lungs, thoracic nerves, and/or pulmonary arteries leading to unconsciousness or death.
Xiphoid process	Striking this point, particularly with a rising blow, can bruise the heart, liver, and/or stomach leading to unconsciousness or possibly even death.
Solar plexus	Located just below the xiphoid process. A blow to this area can shock the diaphragm rendering the recipient temporarily incapable of breathing. A powerful blow in this area can cause internal bleeding in the stomach and/or liver leading to severe pain, unconsciousness, and even death.
Subaxillary region	Located below the armpits, approximately between the fifth and sixth ribs. A strong blow here, especially when performed with a single knuckle, can cause trauma to the lungs disrupting breathing. This area can also be raked with a knuckle causing considerable pain in many, but not all, people.
Hypochondriac region	Located between the seventh and eighth ribs, approximately one hand width below the solar plexus. A blow to the right side can severely damage the liver causing internal bleeding. A blow to the left side can damage the stomach and/or spleen, once again causing internal bleeding. Either blow can have fatal consequences.
Kidneys	A strong blow to this region can cause internal bleeding, shock, and death. This area is frequently targeted using kicking techniques.
Floating ribs	The eleventh and twelfth ribs are only attached at one end making them more vulnerable than other ribs to breakage. A blow to the right side can damage the liver, while a blow to the left can damage the stomach and/or spleen.
Lower stomach	Located approximately one inch below the navel. A strong downward blow to this area can damage the bladder and large intestine causing extreme pain and loss of bladder control.
Shoulder	This joint can be dislocated or hyper extended, rendering the arm unusable for combat.
Back of the upper arm	A strike to this area can affect the radial nerve, causing pain and weakness. A forceful rub in this area can affect the triple warmer (plexus of the radial, ulnar, and medial nerves), causing pain in many individuals and an involuntary rotation of the arm. This facilitates controlling techniques such as an arm bar.
Elbow joint	A strike to the area about an inch above the elbow can affect the ulnar nerve (this area is sometimes referred to as the funny bone), causing pain and weakness. The joint can be dislocated or hyper extended, rendering the arm unusable for combat.

Wrist	The joint can be dislocated or hyper extended resulting in temporary or permanent loss of use of the hand. The wrist is much harder to damage using joint manipulation techniques than the elbow or shoulder.
Inside of the wrist	Located where the pulse can be felt. A blow here can affect the median nerve eliciting pain and weakness. Arteries are very close to the surface in this area making them vulnerable to damage, especially from edged weapons.
Back of the wrist	A blow to the back of the wrist can affect the median nerve eliciting pain and weakening the grip.
Back of the hand	The radial nerve is exposed between the thumb and index finger, and the radial and ulnar nerves meet between the knuckles of the middle and ring fingers. A sharp blow to these areas will cause additional pain and weakness, though a powerful strike to anywhere along the back of the hand can damage delicate bones. Digging the knuckles into the back of an opponent's hand can break his grip. The fingers may be attacked or manipulated too.
Groin	Severe blows to this region can elicit pain, shock, nausea, vomiting, unconsciousness, or even death in male victims. A firm grab to this area can also be incapacitating. Upward blows to the pelvic girdle of a female opponent can elicit similar results, though it takes a bit more force and accuracy.
Coccyx	Located at the base of the spine. Because the major nerves feeding the lower limbs originate in this sacral plexus region at the tailbone, a blow to this area can elicit severe pain. The coccyx is fairly easy to break with an upward strike severely hampering an opponent's ability to move.
Inguinal region	Located at the inside the upper thigh where it joins with the torso. A strike to this area can affect the femoral artery as well as the femoral nerve, weakening the whole leg. A severe blow can cause temporary paralysis. Any cut that damages the femoral artery can cause the victim to exsanguinate (bleed to death) very quickly.
Gluteal fold	Located just below the buttocks. The sciatic nerve, the largest in the body, is located here. A solid blow can cause cramping, loss of control of the leg, and pain throughout the hips and abdomen.
Lateral part of the lower thigh	Lateral part of the lower thigh, about halfway down on the outside of the vastus lateralis (the large muscle). A blow here can cause pain and temporary paralysis of the thigh.
Knee joint	One of the weakest areas of the human body when struck from the proper angle, this joint can be hyperextended or dislocated to disrupt balance and effectively take an opponent out of a fight.

Peroneal nerve	Located at the center point of the tibia (shin bone) and fibula (splint bone on the outside of the leg). A blow delivered about two-thirds of the way down the shin can hit the peroneal nerve, eliciting pain and weakening the leg.
Base of the calf	Blows to the inside of the lower leg at the base of the calf can cause pain and temporary paralysis of the leg muscles.
Ankle joint	This joint may be hyperextended, dislocated, or crushed by a solid blow, causing severe pain, disabling an opponent's balance, and reducing his ability to move and fight.
Instep	A blow to the upper surface of the instep can damage the plantar and peroneal nerves causing pain throughout the leg, hip, and abdomen, weakening the leg.
Top of the foot	Like the hand, small bones in the foot are easily crushed, disabling an opponent's balance and reducing the ability to move and fight.

The vital areas listed above describe targets that are vulnerable to blunt force trauma, the type of damage typically meted out by the fist or foot, though occasionally by instruments such as baseball bats, batons, bricks, boots, and other solid objects. When it comes to bullets, ballistic performance (for example, penetration, expansion, energy transfer) and wound trauma (for example, level of physiological disruption) both affect stopping power, though shot placement is paramount. The only truly incapacitating targets are the brain and upper spinal cord, though the wounds to the heart, major arteries, and lungs may prove severely disabling if not fatal in rather short order. Damage to the head or neck that does not disrupt the central nervous system, as well as hits to the arms, legs, stomach, and groin, may prove sufficiently painful to stop an attacker, though they are generally not immediately disabling and can be shrugged off by a committed adversary.

Common targets that have proven lethal or severely disabling with blade weapons include the heart, subclavian artery (behind the collarbone), stomach, brachial artery, radial artery, carotid artery, femoral artery, axiliary artery, groin, and kidneys. Knife thrusts are generally more damaging than slashes yet they also require you to move deeper into your opponent's target zone where he can easily reach you with his weapon if he is similarly armed. Consequently, other frequent targets include the hands, wrists, and elbows, which may be cut at somewhat less risk of riposte. Such damage, while not immediately disabling, may convince an attacker to break off and retreat though you certainly cannot count on that happening in every situation.

APPENDIX E

Reading List

The topic of violence is far greater than anyone can cover in a single book. The following is a list of authors whose texts we highly recommend for further study. The authors are arranged alphabetically.

Massad Ayoob

Massad Ayoob is director of the Lethal Force Institute, an organization that trains 800 to 1,200 personnel per year in the judicious use of deadly force, armed and unarmed combat, threat management for police, and advanced officer survival in four countries. A retired police lieutenant, firearm, weapon, and unarmed combat expert, his books, articles, and classes teach law enforcement professionals and civilians realistic, street-worthy self-defense techniques. He appears selectively as a court-accepted expert witness in the areas of dynamics of violent encounters, weapons, self-defense, police training, and survival/threat management tactics and principles.

- Ayoob, Massad. *Gun-Proof Your Children*. Concord NH: Police Bookshelf, 1986.

When Kane was eight years old, he spent the night at his friend Craig's house for a sleepover birthday party. One of the boys discovered a loaded .38 caliber revolver hidden in a dresser drawer, pulled it out to show the rest of the kids, and began passing it around. Remembering what his father had taught him about safety, Kane checked the cylinder, discovered that the gun was loaded, and removed the ammunition before handing it to one of the other kids to play with, undoubtedly saving someone's life, quite possibly his own. If you own firearms and have children or have relatives who have children who may visit you, this book is a must read. Even if you hate firearms, it is good to know a bit about gun safety. This book is fairly short, yet well written, with practical advice that can keep your children safe.

- Ayoob, Massad. *In the Gravest Extreme: The Role of the Firearm in Personal Protection*. Concord NH: Police Bookshelf, 1980.

This book was required reading for a defensive handgun course that Kane took over 20 years ago and still remains relevant today. Among other things, it answers the all important question, "when can I pull the trigger and stay out of jail." This book is well written, easy to read, and offers truly sound advice. It covers several important subjects such as common sense about carrying guns,

guns in your store, guns in your car, guns in your home, guns on the street, how to choose a defensive firearm, basic gun fighting techniques, what caliber bullet is appropriate for self-defense, and gun safety. The aftermath of violence section is also outstanding. The only drawback is that some technologies have changed a bit since its original release. For example, the Glock handgun, the .40 S&W caliber bullet, and pre-fragmented self-defense ammunition all did not exist at that time. Nevertheless, the vast majority of the information remains relevant and useful today.

- Ayoob, Massad. *Stressfire, Vol. 1: Gunfighting for Police: Advanced Tactics and Techniques.* New York, NY: Bantam Books (Police Bookshelf), 1983.

This is a serious a book on gun fighting, something you will hopefully never have to do, but should you carry a weapon for self-defense, you must be able to understand and anticipate. Having debriefed hundreds of gunfight survivors, the author describes the tactics, techniques, and, most importantly, mindset, that can give you the best odds of survival. It covers important aspects such as stances, sighting, muzzle control, trigger control, and ammunition management in a well written, easy to read and understand, manner.

- Ayoob, Massad. *The Truth About Self-Protection.* New York, NY: Bantam Books (Police Bookshelf), 1983.

Although some of the material is a bit dated, we still consider this one of the finest tomes on the subject matter ever written. It discusses what to do before, during, and after a violent encounter—morally, legally, and ethically identifying the appropriate to use countervailing force. It covers everything from walking down the street, to driving your vehicle, to securing your home. All manner of makeshift weapons as well as open hand defensive scenarios are discussed. It also provides a holistic set of criteria and considerations to help civilians decide whether to carry a firearm for self-defense.

Loren W. Christensen

Loren Christensen began his martial arts training in 1965, earning eleven black belts over the years, eight in karate, two in *jujitsu*, and one in *arnis*. He is a retired police officer with 29 years of experience in military and civilian law enforcement, where he specialized in street gangs, defensive tactics, and dignitary protection. A prolific author, he has written more than thirty books and hundreds of articles on the martial arts, self-defense, law enforcement, nutrition, prostitution, gangs, and post-traumatic stress disorder. He has also produced several DVDs.

- Christensen, Loren and Dr. Alexis Artwohl. *Deadly Force Encounters: What Cops Need To Know To Mentally And Physically Prepare For And Survive A Gunfight.* Boulder, CO: Paladin Enterprises, Inc., 1997.

While written for law enforcement officers, this important book can be very meaningful for civilians as well. It focuses not on tactics, but rather on the mental aspects of combat, especially the aftermath of violent encounters. The goal is to teach readers how to survive physically, mentally, and legally. It analyzes the nature of violence, provides a thorough explanation of fear and its effects on a person in combat, and portrays dozens of real-life survival stories to drive the important points home in a meaningful way. The insight on Post Traumatic Stress Disorder is particularly valuable for anyone who observes or participates in a violent incident.

- Christensen, Loren. *Far Beyond Defensive Tactics: Advanced Concepts, Techniques, Drills, and Tricks for Cops on the Street.* Boulder, CO: Paladin Enterprises, Inc., 1998.

While it is primarily aimed at police officers, martial artists and those interested in practical self-defense can really benefit from these materials as well. The author's experience, sense of humor, and real-life adventures make it a quick, interesting read. Readers learn how to stay safe patrolling (or simply walking) the streets, protect their weapon, deal with multiple attackers, handle stronger, larger opponents, and otherwise deal with deadly threats. It is especially good for folks who do not have a martial arts background. It is a bit more strategic than tactical yet hits just the right blend. There is an introduction to the "right demeanor" (which is reminiscent of *Verbal Judo* by George Thompson), a large section on control techniques, principles and concepts, and important insights into the nature of fighting. The various scenarios in the training section are truly excellent. The chapter on how to create a witness is really outstanding and particularly useful.

- Christensen, Loren. *Gangbangers: Understanding the Deadly Minds of America's Street Gangs.* Boulder, CO: Paladin Enterprises, Inc., 1999.

Gangs are not only ubiquitous but also growing, becoming more pervasive and deadlier despite society's best efforts to stamp them out. The author interviews current and former gang members, law enforcement officers, school officials, lawyers, social workers, and other experts to provide chilling insight into the minds of those who join street gangs. A quick and easy read, this provocative book provides terrific insight into gang culture and etiquette. Respect, reputation, and revenge are integral to gang life. For example, the so-called "commandments of the 'hood" include thou shalt handle thy business, get girls, get respect, get thy money on, carry a gat (gun), and be down for thy homeboy right or wrong, and thou shalt not snitch. This book is a fascinating and worthwhile read.

• Grossman, Dave and Loren Christensen. *On Combat: The Psychology and Physiology of Deadly Conflict in War and Peace.* Belleville, IL: PPCT Research Publications, 2004.

If you are a soldier, a police officer, a martial artist, the holder of a concealed weapons permit, or just live in a bad neighborhood, you really ought to read this book. Christensen has engaged in deadly conflict, been forced to kill, and learned to survive the experience yet continue to conduct himself as a decent human being. Grossman has studied all aspects of the subject in depth and is considered one of the world's foremost experts on the psychology and physiology of combat. Not only do the authors know what they are talking about, but also they are introspective enough to understand a larger picture of what they have endured and are clearly articulate this hard won wisdom. Their thought provoking, insightful work definitively examines every aspect of the psychology and physiology of deadly conflict. Along with Grossman's book *On Killing*, this text is required reading at West Point, the U.S. War College, and the FBI Academy, among other units and academies (for example, USMC).

The book begins by describing what happens to a person anatomically during a battle then covers the perceptual distortions that take place in combat. The second half of the book covers why people put themselves in harms way and what happens to them after the smoke clears. It talks about Post Traumatic Stress Disorder, survivor's guilt, and a host of related subjects. The research is great. The various vignettes and quotes are quite interesting. Even if you are never involved in a deadly encounter, the book really helps you understand and have a new appreciation for those who are.

• Christensen, Loren. *Surviving Workplace Violence: What to Do Before a Violent Incident, What to Do When the Violence Explodes.* Boulder, CO: Paladin Enterprises, Inc., 2005.

The author does a great job of making readers aware of the threat and presents solid strategies for keeping us safe. It is pretty short, a mere 105 pages, yet extremely valuable nevertheless. Its pithiness positions it as an excellent reference manual that just about anyone can read and understand in a few short hours. The vignettes in this book are startling and very informative. For example, it describes a situation where a 70-year-old salesman attacked and killed his former boss with a mason's hammer several months after she fired him for spitting on another employee. This clearly points out that just about anyone can be a potential hazard.

Christensen describes warning signs (employee behaviors) that may indicate a higher likelihood of threat. The book covers essential survival strategies for the employer (for example, company policies/committees), as well as for the employee. The latter include awareness, stages of alertness, hiding places, escape routes, incident response, combat breathing, mental imagery, and fighting back. He offers specific techniques that can be used against common weapons (for example, knife, handgun, or rifle) as well as descriptions of how to use everyday implements (for example, stapler, pen, or coffee cup) to help you fight back should you be forced to do so.

Peter Consterdine

Consterdine is acknowledged as one of the world's leading authorities on personal security and unarmed combat. He has written numerous books and produced many DVDs on the subject, giving seminars on security awareness and defensive tactics throughout the world. An 8th *dan* black belt in karate, he has over forty continuous years of martial arts training behind him. Along with Geoff Thompson, Consterdine is joint Chief Instructor of The British Combat Association, Europe's leading association for the promotion of self-defense and practical combat.

- Consterdine, Peter. *Fit to Fight: The Manual of Intense Training for Combat.* Chichester, UK: Summersdale Publishers, 1998.

  This book prepares you mentally and physically for a violent confrontation. It covers human physiology, biology, aerobic and anaerobic training, strength training, stress work, aggression drills, hill work, and motivation. The proper use of equipment, partner, and solo drills are described as well. The author offers practical, street-worthy advice to get you into shape for combat.

- Consterdine, Peter. *Streetwise: A Complete Manual of Security and Self Defense.* Chichester, UK: Summersdale Publishers, 1998.

  A no-nonsense book about personal safety, the author addresses principles of personal security, the threat pyramid, security on the street, fear and adrenal responses, personal threat analysis, legal aspects of self-defense, ranges, tools, handling multiple attackers, situational awareness, psychology of conflict, conflict resolution, and a whole lot more. Home, mobile and office security are covered as well. It is holistic, well written, and imminently practical.

- Consterdine, Peter. *Travelsafe: A Travel Security Guide for the Tourist and Business Traveler.* Leeds, UK: Protection Publications, 2001.

  One of the few books of its kind specifically written for travelers, this is an outstanding reference. It covers everything from risk analysis to travel and health, surviving hotel fires, hotspots of the world, hostage survival and anti-kidnap procedures, crisis planning and evacuation, and a whole lot more. Personal, hotel, airport, expatriate, and road travel security are described in a clear and concise manner. A wonderful resource!

Gavin DeBecker

Gavin DeBecker is acknowledged by many as the world's greatest expert on the prediction and prevention of violence and the management of fear. He wrote an international bestselling book on the subject, *The Gift of Fear*. His consulting firm advises media figures, public figures, police departments, transnational corporations, government agencies, universities, and at-risk individuals on the assessment and management of situations that might escalate to violence.

• DeBecker, Gavin. *The Gift of Fear: Survival Signals That Protect Us From Violence.* New York, NY: Dell Publishing, 1998

Several years ago Kane's friend Carol tried to break up with her boyfriend. He couldn't handle the rejection, threatened to kill her, and tried a couple of times, yet the Temporary Restraining Order was ineffective. After the first couple of weeks, the police were not much help either. Kane remembers trying to fall asleep on her couch while holding a shotgun, wondering why she hadn't seen this train wreck coming a whole lot sooner. Long story short, ex-boyfriend is in jail; she's fine. She did not go on another date for more than two years afterward, however, until Kane bought her this book. It is illuminating and empowering—the best, most holistic treatise on the subject available.

It seems like every time there is a tragedy in the news where someone goes on a rampage, some reporter interviews the shocked neighbors who thought the guy or gal was perfectly normal until one day they snapped. Gavin DeBecker puts this nonsense to rest. There is always an indication ahead of time if you are trained to see it. This book is a step-by-step guide on how to identify these cues and avoid danger. The same thing works on a national scale too. When the President or Homeland Security asks us to be vigilant, what the heck does that mean? DeBecker sums it up quite well, "Before the courageous FBI raid, before the arrest, long before the news conference, there is a regular American citizen who sees something that seems suspicious, listens to intuition, and has the character to risk being wrong or seeming foolish when making the call to authorities." This is an outstanding book. Though it was written a bit more for women than men, it is invaluable for everyone. Buy it. Read it. Keep yourself safe!

Marc "Animal" MacYoung

Growing up on gang-infested streets not only gave Marc MacYoung his street name "Animal," but also extensive firsthand experience about what does and does not work for self-defense. Over the years, he has held a number of dangerous occupations including director of a correctional institute, bodyguard, and bouncer. He was first shot at when he was 15 years old and has since survived multiple attempts on his life, including professional contracts. He has studied a variety of martial arts since childhood, teaching experience-based self-defense to police, military, civilians, and martial artists around the world. His has written dozens of books and produced many DVDs covering all aspects of this field.

- MacYoung, Marc. *A Professional's Guide to Ending Violence Quickly.* Boulder, CO: Paladin Enterprises, Inc., 1993.

  This is the definitive book about how to handle a violent situation without resorting to extreme force. The author does an excellent job of explaining the different kinds of social violence you might have to deal with and how to handle it effectively. Kane has successfully applied many of MacYoung's techniques to escort drunken football fans out of a stadium without being hurt, sued, fired, or otherwise getting into trouble!

  For those with reasonably advanced martial arts training, you may be better off following whatever system you study while keeping MacYoung's ideas in mind so that they can't be pulled on you. If you are not a black belt or don't care to be, what he writes about is extremely effective with a bit of practice. More than just the techniques, however, his insight into violence, escalato, and mind games is well worth the price of admission. The writing style is cynical, in your face, and very entertaining. The language is, however, a bit crude at times.

- MacYoung, Marc. *Cheap Shots, Ambushes, and Other Lessons: A Down And Dirty Book On Streetfighting & Survival.* Boulder, CO: Paladin Enterprises, Inc., 1989.

  This is a real no-nonsense book on the reality of street fighting from a guy who's been there, done that, and lived to tell the tale. It's rude, crude, and very eye opening. Important subjects such as the difference between fighting and combat, set-ups blows, anger, bullies, berserkers, sucker punches, low blows, dirty tricks, and weapons are all covered in detail. The stories and personal insights are entertaining and enlightening as well.

- MacYoung, Marc. *Fists, Wits, and a Wicked Right: Surviving On the Wild Side of the Street.* Boulder, CO: Paladin Enterprises, Inc., 1991.

More or less an extension of *Cheap Shots…*, this book is more tactical than strategic. If you are not a trained martial artist, the various techniques, targets, and combat insight can truly enhance your ability to survive a street fight. Once again, the language is by no means politically correct, but still highly entertaining.

- MacYoung, Marc. *Floor Fighting: Stompings, Maimings, and Other Things to Avoid When A Fight Goes To The Ground.* Boulder, CO: Paladin Enterprises, Inc., 1993.

It is imperative to understand and appreciate the differences between a wrestling match and a real-life struggle for survival on the ground. This book is a no-holds barred look at the reality of ground fighting. We hope that we've already managed to convince you that despite what many grapplers think, the ground is a really bad place to be in a fight. This book gives you practical advice to help you avoid going there. It also teaches you how not to get hurt when/if you do. Topics covered include breakfall techniques, offensive and defensive ranges, what happens when you hit the floor, counters, floor-fighting positions, triangle defense, defending against stomps, and striking from the floor, and keeping the other guy down.

- MacYoung, Marc. *Knives, Knife Fighting, And Related Hassles: How To Survive A Real Knife Fight.* Boulder, CO: Paladin Enterprises, Inc., 1990.

You already know by now that there is no such thing as a knife "fight"; it is really more of a knife ambush, an assassination attempt. Unless you are fortunate enough to run into a dominance display rather than a wholehearted attack, are extraordinarily lucky, or are very highly trained, you will never see it coming should someone attempt to stab you with a knife. That's why you need to develop superb situational awareness. This means that you need a comprehensive understanding of where, how, and why street thugs conceal their knives to pull off an effective assassination, all topics covered in this excellent book. The information is illuminating and very possibly life saving as well. You'll learn a bit about how to use a blade offensively too.

- MacYoung, Marc. *Pool Cues, Beer Bottles, & Baseball Bats: Animal's Guide to Improvised Weapons for Self-Defense and Survival.* Boulder, CO: Paladin Enterprises, Inc., 1990.

A comprehensive look at improvised weapons you might encounter on the street such as beer bottles, pool cues, baseball bats, brass knuckles, fighting rings, saps, chains, shovels, bricks, and the like. Even hairbrushes and orange juice, two of the more unusual things the author has actually been assaulted with, are covered along with solid principles of how to spot, utilize, and defend yourself from these potentially deadly objects. Importantly, the book also delves into awareness, covering in depth some of the subtle and not-so-subtle cues that people tend to give when preparing to attack as well as patterns of trouble, diversions, distractions, and other things to look out for.

- MacYoung, Marc. *Street E & E: Evading, Escaping, and Other Ways to Save Your Ass When Things Get Ugly.* Boulder, CO: Paladin Enterprises, Inc., 1993.

Let's face it, unless you are a law-enforcement professional there are very few legitimate reasons to get into a fight. Rule number one for survival, as we've already stated, is "don't get hit." The best way to do that is not being there. Before things get ugly, leave. On occasion, however, you can't just strap on those Nikes, make like brave Sir Robin, and beat a hasty retreat. The bad guys have a nasty habit of getting in the way.

MacYoung shows you how to survive when you're outnumbered or outgunned. Real life isn't like a kung fu movie. Rather than wading in with fists and feet flying, you need to learn to apply hit-and-run tactics, use the environment to your advantage, and use your attacker's weaknesses against them. This book is chocked full of street survival lessons from a guy who knows. His writing style is engaging, entertaining, and sarcastically witty. The knowledge he imparts is realistic, practical, and very important.

- MacYoung, Marc. *Taking It to the Street: Making Your Martial Art Street Effective.* Boulder, CO: Paladin Enterprises, Inc., 1999.

Real fights have no rules. They tend to be short, fast, and brutal. While the average criminal does not hit nearly as hard as the average martial artist does, they frequently hit harder, faster, and more aggressively than the average martial artist, boxer, or sports fighter has ever felt. Consequently, it is important to understand how to bridge the gap between the structured safety of drills in the *dojo* and the mayhem of a full-on, back-alley brawl. Contents include the realities of street violence, centerlines, blocking, dealing with kicks, footwork, and dirty tricks, among other important elements. The author not only teaches practitioners how to identify and resolve gaps in their training to make it more effective for real-life encounters, but also provides important tips on what to do after you have survived an attack, dealing with witnesses, legal issues, revenge seekers, and one's own mental welfare in the aftermath.

- MacYoung, Marc. *Violence, Blunders, and Fractured Jaws: Advanced Awareness Techniques and Street Etiquette.* Boulder, CO: Paladin Enterprises, Inc., 1992.

This book truly helps readers refine and strengthen their situational awareness for survival on the street. It can help you instantly and easily identify the fighters, hustlers, workers, spectators and troublemakers using the same tricks that bouncers, law enforcement officers, prison guards, drug dealers, bikers, and street people utilize so effectively. It goes in-depth into subjects like family group operating systems, personal operating systems, utilizing and refining your personal radar, turf, territory, personal space, rural versus urban reactions, gambling, tacking, scarring, piercing, tattoos, etiquette, eye contact, and other issues that are commonly known only to a very small segment of society. Reading this book is a very eye-opening, mind-expanding experience.

Sergeant Rory Miller

Sergeant Miller has studied martial arts since 1981. He has received college varsities in judo and fencing and holds *mokuroku* (teaching certificate) in *Sosuishitsu-ryu jujutsu*. He is a corrections officer and tactical team leader who teaches and designs courses in defensive tactics, close quarters combat and Use of Force policy and application for law enforcement and corrections officers. A veteran of hundreds of violent confrontations he lectures on realism and training for martial artists and writers. Both Wilder and Kane have trained with him and know first-hand that Miller truly knows what he is talking about.

- Miller, Rory A. *Meditations on Violence: A Comparison of Martial Arts Training and Real World Violence.* Wolfeboro, NH: YMAA Publication Center, 2008.

  Violence is the soul of chaos. Martial arts are clean and structured, even simple in a way, yet somehow one arose from the other. Maybe it is the human need for structure that somehow converted a bloody, smelly, terrifying experience of combat into the beauty and structure of *kata*. Experienced martial artist and veteran correction officer Sergeant Rory Miller distills what he has learned from jailhouse brawls, tactical operations and ambushes to explore the differences between martial arts and the subject martial arts were designed to deal with—violence.

  This book is a refreshingly frank, honest, and in-depth assessment of the subject. Readers will learn how to think critically about violence, how to evaluate sources of knowledge, and how to identify strategies and select tactics to deal with it effectively. One of the most important aspects of the book is Miller's insights on how to make self-defense work. He examines how to look at defense in a broader context as well as how to overcome some of your own subconscious resistance to meeting violence with violence. It's truly outstanding stuff!

Peyton Quinn

Peyton Quinn is considered by many the "dean" of barroom brawling. He began his training in formal martial arts systems in 1964, eventually achieving black belts in karate, judo, and aikido. While he continues to respect and explore Asian martial arts systems, his real-world experience has shown him that for most people, training in martial arts alone is not enough for real fighting. He has written numerous books and created several DVDs on the subject.

- Quinn, Peyton. *Bouncer's Guide to Barroom Brawling: Dealing with the Sucker Puncher, Streetfighter, and Ambusher.* Boulder, CO: Paladin Enterprises, Inc., 1990.

  Quinn's writing style is very similar to Marc MacYoung's, right down to the expletives. Similarly, his no-nonsense advice is hard hitting and right on point. This excellent book begins by pointing out that avoiding violence is an essential technique in and of itself, just as valuable as knowing how to throw a good punch or deliver a strong kick. The fundamental elements of avoidance tactics section is important information. There are also solid sections on the realities of fighting that, as experienced warriors understand, is nothing like what you see in the movies. It is ugly stuff best avoided. Even when you triumph, there are legal (and medical) ramifications that can come back to haunt you. The author's "stay out of prison plan" is excellent. Advanced practitioners should appreciate this information but won't get a lot out of the rest of the book. The principles of defensive and offensive techniques are fairly basic, but well written and comprehensive. He covers striking, grappling, and movement in good detail. Chapter 7, which covers how to select an appropriate martial art for your own personal safety, is an outstanding overview for beginners that can help you find one.

- Quinn, Peyton. *Real Fighting: Adrenaline Stress Conditioning through Scenario-Based Training.* Boulder, CO: Paladin Enterprises, Inc., 1996.

  In a violent encounter, your heart rate can jump from 60 or 70 beats per minute (BPM) to well over 200 BMP in less than half a second. While this adrenal dump gives you a survival edge by making you more resilient during combat, it severely degrades your motor skills, hand-eye coordination, and sense of timing making complicated techniques very challenging, if not impossible, to perform. This stress can even cause you to experience tunnel vision, suffer temporary memory loss, become hyper-vigilant, lose rational thought, or even lose the ability to consciously move or react. If your training does not account for adrenaline, it will be of dubious value on the street. That's what this excellent book is all about. Contents include the fear factor, combat mindset, muscular memory, strategy, training methods, scenario based training, and using weapons.

Bibliography

Books

Ayoob, Massad. *In the Gravest Extreme: The Role of the Firearm in Personal Protection.* Concord NH: Police Bookshelf, 1980.

Ayoob, Massad. *The Truth About Self-Protection.* New York, NY: Bantam Books (Police Bookshelf), 1983.

Christensen, Loren and Dr. Alexis Artwohl. *Deadly Force Encounters: What Cops Need To Know To Mentally And Physically Prepare For And Survive A Gunfight.* Boulder, CO: Paladin Enterprises, Inc., 1997.

Christensen, Loren. *Far Beyond Defensive Tactics: Advanced Concepts, Techniques, Drills, and Tricks for Cops on the Street.* Boulder, CO: Paladin Enterprises, Inc., 1998.

Christensen, Loren. *Gangbangers: Understanding the Deadly Minds of America's Street Gangs.* Boulder, CO: Paladin Enterprises, Inc., 1999.

Christensen, Loren. *Riot: A Behind-the-Barricades Tour of Mobs, Riot Cops, and the Chaos of Crowd Violence.* Boulder, CO: Paladin Enterprises, Inc., 2008.

Christensen, Loren. *Surviving Workplace Violence: What to Do Before a Violent Incident, What to Do When the Violence Explodes.* Boulder, CO: Paladin Enterprises, Inc., 2005.

Consterdine, Peter. *Fit to Fight: The Manual of Intense Training for Combat.* Chichester, UK: Summersdale Publishers, 1998.

Consterdine, Peter. *Streetwise: A Complete Manual of Security and Self Defense.* Chichester, UK: Summersdale Publishers, 1998.

Consterdine, Peter. *Travelsafe: A Travel Security Guide for the Tourist and Business Traveler.* Leeds, UK: Protection Publications, 2001.

Covey, Stephen R. *The 7 Habits of Highly Effective People.* New York, NY: Simon and Schuster, 1989.

DeBecker, Gavin. *The Gift of Fear: Survival Signals That Protect Us From Violence.* New York, NY: Dell Publishing, 1998

Grossman, Dave and Loren Christensen. *On Combat: The Psychology and Physiology of Deadly Conflict in War and Peace.* Belleville, IL: PPCT Research Publications, 2004.

Hoffman, Yoel. *Japanese Death Poems: Written by Zen Monks and Haiku Poets on the Verge of Death.* Rutland. Vermont: Tuttle Publishing, 1986.

Kane, Lawrence A. *Surviving Armed Assaults: A Martial Artists Guide to Weapons, Street Violence, and Countervailing Force.* Boston, MA: YMAA, 2006.

Kane, Lawrence and Kris Wilder. *The Way of Kata: A Comprehensive Guide to Deciphering Martial Applications.* Boston, MA: YMAA Publication Center, 2005.

Kane, Lawrence and Kris Wilder. *The Way to Black Belt: A Comprehensive Guide to Rapid, Rock-Solid Results.* Wolfeboro, NH: YMAA Publication Center, 2007.

(Lichtenfeld) Sde-Or, Imi and Eyal Yanilov. *Krav Maga: How to Defend Yourself against Armed Assault*. Tel Aviv, Israel: Dekel Publishing House, 2001.

Lutrell, Marcus and Patrick Robinson. *Lone Survivor: The Eyewitness Account of Operation Redwing and the Lost Heroes of SEAL Team 10*. New York, NY: Hachette Book Group, 2007.

MacYoung, Marc. *A Professional's Guide to Ending Violence Quickly*. Boulder, CO: Paladin Enterprises, Inc., 1993.

MacYoung, Marc and Tristan Sutrisno. *Becoming a Complete Martial Artist: Error Detection in Self-Defense and the Martial Arts*. Guilford, CT: The Lyons Press, 2005.

MacYoung, Marc. *Cheap Shots, Ambushes, and Other Lessons: A Down And Dirty Book On Streetfighting & Survival*. Boulder, CO: Paladin Enterprises, Inc., 1989.

MacYoung, Marc. *Fists, Wits, and a Wicked Right: Surviving On the Wild Side of The Street*. Boulder, CO: Paladin Enterprises, Inc., 1991.

MacYoung, Marc. *Floor Fighting: Stompings, Maimings, and Other Things to Avoid When A Fight Goes To The Ground*. Boulder, CO: Paladin Enterprises, Inc., 1993.

MacYoung, Marc. *Knives, Knife Fighting, And Related Hassles: How To Survive A Real Knife Fight*. Boulder, CO: Paladin Enterprises, Inc., 1990.

MacYoung, Marc. *Pool Cues, Beer Bottles, & Baseball Bats: Animal's Guide to Improvised Weapons for Self-Defense and Survival*. Boulder, CO: Paladin Enterprises, Inc., 1990.

MacYoung, Marc. *Street E & E: Evading, Escaping, and Other Ways to Save Your Ass When Things Get Ugly*. Boulder, CO: Paladin Enterprises, Inc., 1993.

MacYoung, Marc. *Taking It to the Street: Making Your Martial Art Street Effective*. Boulder, CO: Paladin Enterprises, Inc., 1999.

MacYoung, Marc. *Violence, Blunders, and Fractured Jaws: Advanced Awareness Techniques and Street Etiquette*. Boulder, CO: Paladin Enterprises, Inc., 1992.

Miller, Rory A. *Meditations on Violence: A Comparison of Martial Arts Training and Real World Violence*. Wolfeboro, NH: YMAA Publication Center, 2008.

Morgan, Forrest. *Living The Martial Way*. Fort Lee, NJ: Barricade Books, Inc., 1992.

Musashi, Miyamoto. *A Book of Five Rings: The Classic Guide to Strategy*. Woodstock, NY: The Overlook Press, 1974.

Quinn, Peyton. *Bouncer's Guide to Barroom Brawling: Dealing with the Sucker Puncher, Streetfighter, and Ambusher*. Boulder, CO: Paladin Enterprises, Inc., 1990.

Quinn, Peyton. *Real Fighting: Adrenaline Stress Conditioning through Scenario-Based Training*. Boulder, CO: Paladin Enterprises, Inc., 1996.

Rapaport, Samuel. *Tales and Maxims from the Midrash*. 1907 (http:\\www.sacred-texts.com/jud/tmm/tmm17.htm]).

Tzu, Sun. *The Art of War: Text Only No Commentary*. Translator: Lionel Giles. The Project Gutenberg eBook, December 28, 2005 [eBook #17405]

Articles

Ayoob, Massad. The Ayoob Files – One Gun, No Hands: The Marcus Young Incident. *American Handgunner*, Sept–Oct, 2004.

DVDs and Videos

Barroom Brawling: The Art of Staying Alive in Beer Joints, Biker Bars, and Other Fun Places (with Peyton Quinn and Marc MacYoung), Paladin Press, 1991.

Street Safe: How to Avoid Becoming a Victim (with Marc MacYoung), LOTI group productions, 2007.

Street Smarts: How to Avoid Being a Victim (with Detective J. J. Bittenbinder). Video Publishing House, Inc., 1992.

Web Sites

Bureau of Justice Statistics (www.ojp.usdoj.gov/bjs)

Crime Check (www.crimcheck.com)

Federal Bureau of Investigation Uniform Crime Reports (www.fbi.gov/ucr/ucr.htm)

In The Line of Duty's web site (www.lineofduty.com)

Marc "Animal" MacYoung's web site (www.nononsenseselfdefense.com)

Net Detective (www.netdetective.com)

Seattle Post Intelligencer web site (www.seattlepi.nwsource.com)

Sentry Link (www.sentrylink.com)

The Art of War (www.chinapage.com/sunzi-e.html)

The Book of Five Rings (www.samurai.com/5rings)

The Mayo Clinic (www.mayoclinic.com)

The Seattle Times (www.seattletimes.com)

U.S. Search (www.ussearch.com)

Yahoo news (http://story.news.yahoo.com)

Index

About the Authors

Kris Wilder

Beginning his martial arts training in 1976 in the art of *taekwondo*, Kris Wilder has earned black belt-level ranks in three arts: *taekwondo* (2nd Degree), *Kodokan* judo (1st Degree) and *Goju Ryu* Karate (5th Degree), which he teaches at the West Seattle Karate Academy. He has trained under Kenji Yamada, who as a *judoka* won back-to-back United States grand championships (1954–1955); Shihan John Roseberry, founder of *Shorei-Shobukan* Karate and a direct student of Seikichi Toguchi; and Hiroo Ito, a student of *Shihan* Kori Hisataka (Kudaka in the Okinawan dialect), the founder of *Shorinji-Ryu Kenkokan* Karate.

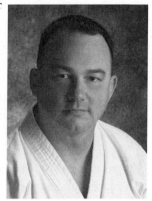

Though now retired from Judo competition, while active in the sport Kris competed on the national and international level. He has traveled to Japan and Okinawa to train in karate. He is the author of *The Way of Sanchin Kata* and *Lessons from the Dojo Floor* and co-author (with Lawrence Kane) of *The Way of Kata* and *The Way to Black Belt*. He has also written guest chapters for other martial arts authors and has had articles published in *Traditional Karate*, a magazine out of the U.K. with international readership. Kris also hosts the annual Martial University, a seminar composed of multidisciplinary martial artists. He also regularly instructs at seminars.

Kris lives in Seattle, Washington with his son Jackson. He can be contacted via e-mail at kwilder@quidnunc.net or through the West Seattle Karate Academy website at www.westseattlekarate.com.

Lawrence Kane

Lawrence Kane is the author of *Surviving Armed Assaults* and *Martial Arts Instruction*, as well as co-author (with Kris Wilder) of *The Way of Kata* and *The Way to Black Belt*. He has also published numerous articles about teaching, martial arts, self-defense, and related topics, contributed to other author's books, and acts as a forum moderator at www.iainabernethy.com, a website devoted to traditional martial arts and self-protection.

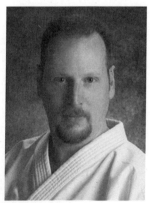

Since 1970, he has participated in a broad range of martial arts, from traditional Asian sports such as judo, *arnis*, *kobudo*, and karate to recreating medieval European combat with real armor and rattan (wood) weapons. He has taught medieval weapons forms since 1994 and *Goju Ryu* karate since 2002. He has also completed seminars in modern gun safety, marksmanship, handgun retention and knife combat techniques, and he has participated in slow-fire pistol and pin shooting competitions.

Since 1985, Lawrence has supervised employees who provide security and oversee fan safety during college and professional football games at a Pac-10 stadium. This part-time job has given him a unique opportunity to appreciate violence in a myriad of forms. Along with his crew, he has witnessed, interceded in, and stopped or prevented hundreds of fights, experiencing all manner of aggressive behaviors as well as the escalation process that invariably precedes them. He has also worked closely with the campus police and state patrol officers who are assigned to the stadium and has had ample opportunities to examine their crowd control tactics and procedures.

To pay the bills he does IT sourcing strategy and benchmarking work for an aerospace company in Seattle where he gets to play with billions of dollars of other people's money and make really important decisions. Lawrence lives in Seattle, Washington with his wife Julie and his son Joey. He can be contacted via e-mail at lakane@ix.netcom.com.

BOOKS FROM YMAA

more products available from...
YMAA Publication Center, Inc. 楊氏東方文化出版中心
1-800-669-8892 • ymaa@aol.com • www.ymaa.com

YMAA
PUBLICATION CENTER

BOOKS FROM YMAA (continued)

VIDEOS FROM YMAA

DVDS FROM YMAA

more products available from...
YMAA Publication Center, Inc. 楊氏東方文化出版中心
1-800-669-8892 • ymaa@aol.com • www.ymaa.com

YMAA
PUBLICATION CENTER